To John Fry

Without whose help and encouragement,
this book would never have been written

COMMON MEDICAL PROBLEMS

A Clinical Guide

Gerald Sandler, MD, FRCP
Consultant Physician
District General Hospital
Barnsley

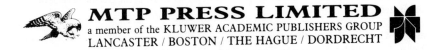

MTP PRESS LIMITED
a member of the KLUWER ACADEMIC PUBLISHERS GROUP
LANCASTER / BOSTON / THE HAGUE / DORDRECHT

Published in the UK and Europe by
MTP Press Limited
Falcon House
Lancaster, England

British Library Cataloguing in Publication Data

Sandler, Gerald
    Common medical problems.
    1. Diagnosis
    I. Title
    616.07′5   RC71

    ISBN 0-85200-715-9

Published in the USA by
MTP Press
A division of Kluwer Boston Inc
190 Old Derby Street
Hingham, MA 02043, USA

Library of Congress Cataloging in Publication Data

Sandler, Gerald, 1928–
    Common medical problems

    Includes index.
    1. Internal medicine–Case studies. I. Title.
[DNLM: 1. Diagnosis, Differential. 2. Internal
medicine. WB 141.5 S217c]
RC66.S26   1984   616   84-3852
ISBN 0-85200-715-9

Typeset by Georgia Origination, Liverpool
Printed and bound by Butler and Tanner Ltd., Frome and London

CONTENTS

'More than the calf yearns to suck
does the cow yearn to suckle'

Rabbi Akiba (ca. 40 AD–135 AD)

Acknowledgements

I am greatly indebted to Garry Swann for all the artwork, except for the illustration of a patient with left ventricular failure which was kindly drawn for me by Steven Hurst. It is a pleasure to acknowledge the help I received from Dr Ronald Grainger and Dr Tom Powell with illustrative X-rays. I would also like to thank Mr D. L. Broatch for his help in organizing the artwork, and Mr Bob Walker for assistance with photographs and X-rays.

I would like to thank Anne Patterson, Managing Editor of Update, for permission to use material from my series of articles on 'The Art of Diagnosis', published 1982/3.

I am very grateful to Dr John Fry for allowing me to use data and illustrations from his book *Common Diseases*, 3rd Edn. (1983, MTP Press Ltd.).

I would like to express my sincere gratitude also to my secretary Ann Youell who so generously undertook the considerable work involved in preparation of the manuscript, in addition to her extensive normal duties.

Last, but by no means least, I would like to acknowledge and thank my wife, Ella, for her great patience and forbearance in putting up with the inevitable neglect resulting from all the time I had to spend in writing the book.

Preface

The Oxford English Dictionary defines diagnosis as: 'Identification of a disease by careful investigation of its symptoms and history'.

Regrettably, the value of the history in the diagnosis of disease often seems to be neglected in both undergraduate and postgraduate medical education.

The considerable advances in medical technology have made it easy to carry out a multiplicity of tests. As a result, there is frequently an unfortunate tendency to rely on the results of tests before decisions are taken on diagnosis and treatment, even though such tests are often of limited value in the management of the patients.

This book is an attempt to redress the balance and place the proper emphasis on the diagnostic value of a well-taken and perspicacious history. The main purpose of the book is to show that most of the clinical problems encountered in daily practice can be dealt with effectively and satisfactorily on the basis of a good clinical history. This should be supplemented by a problem-orientated clinical examination, the primary function of which is either to confirm and amplify the diagnosis provided by the history, or to refute it.

Each chapter deals with an instructive case history exemplifying common medical problems. The importance of the history, and the examination, are made clear in arriving at the diagnosis. The use of investigation in the management of each patient is placed in its proper perspective, which should surely be to provide an answer to a specific clinical question relating to diagnosis or treatment only when there is doubt as to either.

Where the result of a test is unlikely to change either the diagnosis or the management of the patient, there can be little justification for asking for it.

Medicine is an ancient art based on observation, communication, experience and common sense. Hippocrates always stressed the importance of symptoms and signs in diagnosis and treatment of patients. This advice is as valid today as in Hippocrates' time and it is hoped that this book will help to make some small contribution towards showing how soundly-based this advice is in the medical practice of our own day.

1

Chest pain

PRESENT HISTORY

A 46-year-old motor mechanic presented with chest pain which had been present about 2 years, and had been getting worse recently. On more detailed enquiry it appeared that he actually had two different kinds of chest pain, one over the left side of his chest and a more recent pain in the front of his chest, and it was the development of the frontal chest pain which had worried him and made him seek medical advice (Figure 1.1).

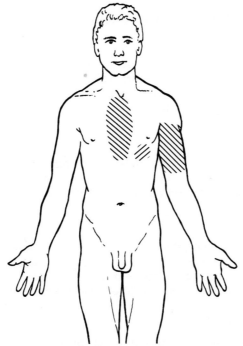

Figure 1.1 The patient's two types of chest pain

1

The chest pains

The left-sided chest pain had been present intermittently and irregularly for the previous 2 years and he felt he could put up with this. He described this pain as sometimes stabbing and sometimes aching and fairly localized in the region of the left breast or below. Although he denied any strict relationship to physical effort, he would tend to get this pain after a heavy day's work, usually in the evening when he was sitting watching television. This ache would last often till he went to bed.

He was more concerned about a different type of pain which affected the front of the chest and had come on only over the previous 2 months or so. He described it as a 'gripping' or 'squeezing' pain which he had noticed especially if he was working on a heavy vehicle. It would usually last about 10 minutes and he would have to ease up on his work or it became more uncomfortable. He did not think that the sternal pain radiated anywhere, though he had some-times noticed a feeling of discomfort in his left arm when he had the pain – he said the arm felt 'heavy' and 'useless' while the pain was on. He thought that his pain was becoming more frequent and he had experienced occasional similar attacks recently when he wasn't undertaking any exertion, and even once in bed, but it still lasted no more than 10 minutes or so. He did not think that either this pain or his left-sided chest pain were related in any way to eating, bending or lying in bed.

Other relevant facts on direct enquiry

Neck pain

The only other symptom which emerged on direct systematic enquiry was that he occasionally had a bit of discomfort in his neck and left shoulder, especially when working in the garage pit on the underside of a vehicle. He denied any undue breathlessness or palpitations.

Dyspepsia

In the past history, he had an operation on his stomach some years previously for what he thought was a 'burst ulcer'. Since then he has had occasional flatulence and heartburn, especially after a heavy meal.

FAMILY HISTORY

His father had died of a heart attack at the age of 67 years, and he thought his mother, aged 69 years, had mild 'blood pressure'. He had a younger brother, aged 41 years, who had some kind of heart trouble for which he was taking tablets, but he didn't know what kind of heart trouble it was.

PERSONAL HABITS

The patient used to smoke 25 cigarettes a day but gave up 2 years ago because of the increasing cost. He drank 5–6 pints (3–3·5 litres) of beer at most weekends.

2

EXAMINATION

General

He was not clinically anaemic or overweight but had distinct xanthelasma affecting both eyes and an arcus senilis (Figure 1.2). He was not breathless. The neck veins were not distended and there was no leg oedema.

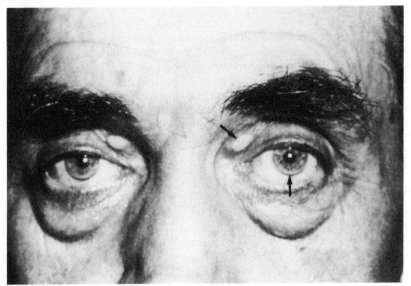

Figure 1.2 Xanthelasma and arcus senilis

Cardiovascular system

His pulse was 96 per minute regular.

The radial artery was not thickened but his brachial artery was easily visible and slightly tortuous.

The blood pressure was 170/105 initially, falling to 155/98 at the end of the examination when the pulse had also fallen to 78/min.

His apex beat was normal in site and character.

The heart sounds were normal with no triple rhythm or murmurs.

The femoral, posterior tibial and dorsalis pedis pulses were all easily felt and considered normal.

Respiratory system

The only abnormal findings were a few scattered fine crepitations at both lung bases but they soon cleared with coughing.

Abdomen

Abdominal examination was normal. The fundal arterioles were slightly irregular and there was early arteriovenous nipping.

3

Cervical spine

There was some limitation of lateral flexion, especially to the left, with some discomfort to the patient.

ANALYSIS OF THE HISTORY

Chest pains

Chest pain is one of the commonest presenting symptoms and may be one of the most difficult to diagnose, especially when the characteristics of the pain are vague or the patient is a poor historian. Additionally, the patient may have more than one kind of chest pain, as in the present case. The most important decision to be made in this case is whether the patient does have angina, since angina remains a notoriously unpredictable condition and a missed diagnosis may be potentially lethal, while the correct diagnosis enables the patient to benefit considerably from the recent advances in management of this condition.

Angina

This patient has two different causes of the chest pain. There is little doubt that his more recent central chest pain is angina. The diagnosis of angina is made primarily on the basis of several important characteristics of the pain (Table 1.1).

Table 1.1 Assessment of anginal pain

```
• site
• radiation
• character
• duration
• precipitating factors
• relieving factors
• associated symptoms
```

The classical *site* of angina is behind the upper sternum, and less commonly either the left side of the chest alone or rarely the right side.

Typical anginal pain *radiates* across the chest and down the left arm: also, typically it may radiate up into the throat or jaw, and for all practical purposes radiation from the chest into the lower jaw is pathognomonic of angina (Figure 1.3). Occasionally, anginal pain will radiate into the left scapular or interscapular area. Very rarely it will reverse its direction of radiation, start in the arm and radiate centrally into the chest. Although this patient denied radiation of his pain from his chest to his arm, the regular association between the chest pain and the discomfort in his left arm is the significant factor.

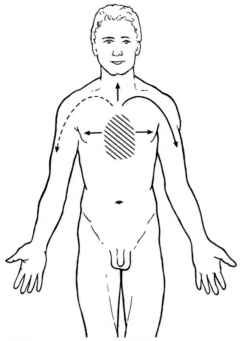

Figure 1.3   Site and radiation of angina

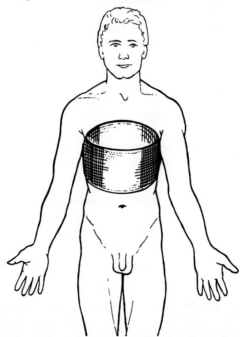

Figure 1.4   Typical character of anginal pain

5

The *character* of the chest pain is important in diagnosing angina, and there are a number of descriptive terms which are highly suggestive – gripping, crushing, squeezing, 'like a vice' and 'like a tight band' (Figure 1.4); similar but less suggestive terms are heavy, tight, 'like a weight' and 'like a pressure'. The nature of the associated arm pain is also helpful since, typically, angina produces a feeling of 'lifelessness' or 'uselessness' in the arm which can be extremely uncomfortable. Tingling in the arm is much less specific and rarely helpful.

The *precipitating* factors are shown in Table 1.2.

Angina is usually *precipitated* by physical exertion, as in this patient. Another important factor in causing angina is strong emotion such as anger or frustration, or great excitement as in sexual intercourse. Cold weather and a heavy meal facilitate the development of angina (Table 1.2).

Table 1.2   Factors precipitating angina

• EXERTION • Emotion • Heavy meal • Cold wind

The *duration* of an anginal attack is usually 5–10 minutes once the causative factor is removed, and this applied to the present case. Angina never lasts a few seconds only. More prolonged pain may be due to myocardial ischaemia which may be progressing to myocardial infarction; alternatively, it may be due to coronary spasm, a particular example of which occurs in Prinzmetal's variant angina which arises characteristically in bed at night and is associated with distinctive S-T elevation in the electrocardiogram. A particularly worrying aspect of this patient's angina is that the pattern was changing and it was starting to occur at rest; this indicates increasing coronary insufficiency and sometimes heralds a myocardial infarction. This transition from typical effort angina to rest angina is designated 'unstable angina' and indicates the need for urgent treatment.

The mode of *relief* of angina is helpful in confirming the nature of the pain.

Angina is relieved rapidly once the precipitating factor such as exertion or emotion is removed.

Table 1.3   Symptoms associated with angina

• Breathlessness • Strangling • Syncope • Belching

The response of anginal pain to nitroglycerine may also be of diagnostic value. Typical angina responds within 1–2 minutes, and this rapid response forms the basis of a useful therapeutic test in doubtful chest pain. If 'relief' is delayed for more than a minute or two, the chest pain is unlikely to be angina.

6

It must also be remembered that the rarer condition of 'oesophageal spasm', with or without associated gastro-oesophageal regurgitation, may also be rapidly relieved by nitro-glycerine.

Finally, useful diagnostic help in angina may be obtained from *other symptoms associated with the chest pain* (Table 1.3). *Breathlessness* may occur due to transient left ventricular failure, though hyperventilation in an anxious patient with functional chest pain must also not be forgotten. A feeling of *strangling or suffocation* in the throat, as described in the classical account of angina by Heberden in 1818, is highly suggestive. *Syncope* is rare, but dizziness may occur, though it is more likely to be due to anxiety than to the angina. *Belching* is an interesting symptom well-documented in angina and usually coinciding with the relief of the pain; the mechanism is unknown.

Functional chest pain

The left-sided chest pain in this patient is very suggestive of the so-called 'functional' pain of cardiac neurosis. This is a very common symptom and important to distinguish from angina. The characteristic features of 'functional' chest pain are shown in Table 1.4. This type of pain is often associated with other symptoms of anxiety, such as excessive fatigue, palpitations and breathing problems, especially inability to take a deep enough breath.

Table 1.4   'Functional chest pain'

- Left mammary or inframmary
- Stabbing or continuous ache
- Lasts seconds or hours
- Unrelated to exertion
- Occurs during quiet introspection
- Associated anxiety symptoms
- Local tenderness may be present

Cervical spondylosis

The patient also has another potential cause of chest pain, cervical spondylosis (Figure 1.5). This is causing the pain in his neck and left shoulder when he is extending his neck in the course of his work. If the upper thoracic vertebrae are affected, pain can occur in the upper chest and be confused with possible angina, though in these circumstances the pain will be related to neck movements and not ordinary physical exertion, and is also frequently associated with pain or paraesthesiae of root distribution down the arm.

Table 1.5   Features of gastro-oesophageal regurgitation

- Burning retrosternal pain
- May get bitter fluid in the mouth
- Occurs soon after eating
- Worse on bending or lying down
- Rapid relief with alkalis

7

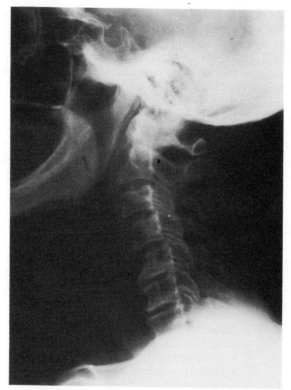

Figure 1.5   X-ray of cervical spondylosis

Gastro-oesophageal regurgitation

The past history of a stomach operation, and the occasional heartburn since, suggest yet another possible cause of chest pain, gastro-oesophageal regurgitation. The characteristic features of this type of pain are shown in Table 1.5. The lack of relationship to meals or posture makes it very unlikely that this patient's pain is due to regurgitation. A simple clinical test of rapid relief of pain with alkalis may be useful in making this diagnosis.

A summary of the important points in the differential diagnosis of the common causes of chest pain is shown in Table 1.6 and Figure 1.6.

Family history

Family history may be relevant in the diagnosis of ischaemic heart disease. Significant factors include a history of *premature* heart attacks in the parents, or ischaemic heart disease in a sibling, also cerebrovascular disease, claudication or diabetes.

In this patient's history, his father's death at 67 years from a heart attack is irrelevant, but his brother's heart trouble may be angina and therefore

8

significant. The mild hypertension in his elderly mother is unlikely to be relevant.

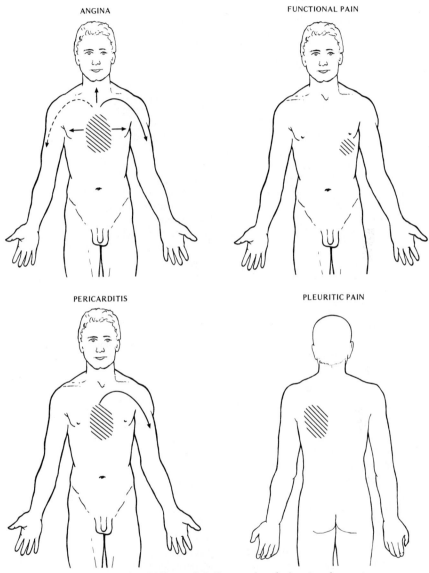

Figure 1.6 Differential diagnosis of chest pain

Personal history

Smoking is a highly relevant coronary risk factor, even though the patient

Table 1.6   Differential diagnosis of chest pain

Site
Restrosternal or across chest	– Angina/infarction
	Pericarditis
Left nipple area	– Anxiety state

Radiation
Left shoulder or arm	– Angina/Infarction
	Pericarditis
	Cervical spondylosis
Lower jaw	– Angina/Infarction
Back of chest	– Dissection of aorta
	Aortic aneurysm
	Angina/infarction – rare

Duration
Few minutes only	– Angina
Less than 30 seconds	– Anxiety state
	Hiatus hernia
Several hours	– Myocardial infarction
	Pericarditis
	Dissection of aorta
	Anxiety state

Precipitating factors
Exertion or emotion	– Angina
Cold air	– Angina
Heavy meal	– Angina
	Oesophagitis
Bending	– Hiatus hernia
	Arthritis of thoracic spine
Neck movement	– Cervical spondylosis
Coughing	– Pericarditis
	Pleurisy
	Nerve root irritation
Exhaustion	– Anxiety state
Arm movements	– Thoracic outlet syndrome

Relief of pain
Within a few minutes of rest	– Angina
Within a few minutes of taking nitroglycerin	– Angina
	Occasionally oesophageal pain
Leaning forward	– Pericarditis
Breath-holding	– Pleuritic pain
Alkalis	– Oesophagitis

Accompanying symptoms
Sweating, nausea, vomiting	– Myocardial infarction
Breathlessness	– 'Strangling' of angina
	Left ventricular failure with angina
	Pulmonary embolism
	Pneumothorax
Haemoptysis	– Pulmonary embolism
	Carcinoma of lung

stopped smoking 2 years previously, since up to 10 years must elapse after stopping smoking before the coronary risk returns to that of the non-smoker. The relationship between *alcohol* and *coronary artery disease* is still controversial, though some work suggests a possible preventive effect of daily alcohol intake. However, its potential beneficial effect on the coronary arteries must be balanced against the harmful effects in causing alcoholic cardiomyopathy and liver disease. In any case, this patients' alcohol consumption was very moderate and therefore very unlikely to cause any clinical disease of the heart or liver.

CONCLUSIONS FROM THE HISTORY

The diagnoses which have emerged clearly from the history are:

- the recent development of angina which is getting progressively worse (unstable angina)
- a longer history of functional left inframammary pain
- symptoms of cervical spondylosis

The main coronary risk factor which has led to the development of his angina is the heavy cigarette smoking which is still relevant after the 2 years' abstinence. A relatively minor factor is the family history of angina in his brother.

ANALYSIS OF THE EXAMINATION

Examination of the patient showed several abnormalities, indicating arteriosclerosis (Table 1.7), though the normal peripheral pulses in the lower limbs show that the change is not yet a generalized one.

Table 1.7 Indications of arteriosclerosis in the patient

- Arcus senilis
- Xanthelasma
- Tortuous brachial artery
- Changes in retinal arterioles

He also has a mild degree of *hypertension*. The significance of this finding will be discussed later.

There was no cardiac abnormality – no cardiac enlargement and no heart failure, which would be indicated by dyspnoea, a gallop rhythm and persistent pulmonary basal or more extensive crepitations.

The sparse crepitations heard over the lung bases which disappeared on coughing are of no clinical significance.

Clinical examination of the heart is often normal in angina unless there is associated hypertension or heart failure.

CONCLUSIONS FROM THE EXAMINATION

- He has evidence of premature arteriosclerosis as indicated by the arcus senilis.
- The arteriosclerosis is manifest in the arteries of the upper limbs and fundi, and is undoubtedly the cause of his coronary artery disease also.
- The examination has revealed two other important coronary risk factors:
  hypertension
  the likelihood of hyperlipidaemia (xanthelasma)

INVESTIGATIONS

There are very few simple investigations which are of value in the diagnosis of angina, and it is important to emphasize that in most cases the diagnosis must be made on the basis of the history.

Electrocardiogram

An electrocardiogram is often recorded but is of very little diagnostic value, since it is likely to be normal unless it is done during an actual anginal attack, when S–T depression might be seen. Of course, it may show evidence of a previous myocardial infarction, and this is claimed to be present in about 25% of patients presenting with angina. This is an important finding in relation to prognosis and it is therefore reasonable to arrange an electrocardiogram for this purpose, but it must be appreciated that electrocardiographic evidence of previous ischaemic damage does not necessarily mean that a current chest pain is due to similar ischaemia and is therefore angina. That decision must be made on the basis of the characteristics of the pain as discussed earlier.

On the other hand, an *exercise electrocardiogram* may be of more value in diagnosing dubious chest pain, especially if similar chest pain is reproduced during the exercise and is accompanied by ischaemic changes in the electrocardiogram, the most reliable and generally accepted being a flat or down-sloping S–T depression of at least 1 mm and lasting at least 0.08 seconds (Figure 1.7). However, if a firm clinical diagnosis of angina can be made on the history, as in this patient's case, an exercise test is superfluous.

More advanced investigations are also available, of which the most valuable is *coronary arteriography*, though *radionuclide studies* with thallium may be helpful at times. These investigations should be reserved for those anginal patients in whom coronary artery bypass surgery is being considered, or for those patients with dubious chest pain in whom it is of considerable importance to establish an accurate diagnosis, e.g. airline pilots.

Chest X-ray

A chest X-ray is useful to show the heart size which, while it is of no diagnostic value, may give some useful prognostic information, since a large heart implies an adverse prognosis. The patient's heart size was normal.

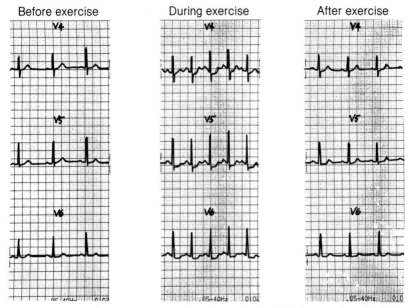

Before exercise During exercise After exercise

Figure 1.7 Exercise test showing ischaemic S–T depression during exercise

Blood lipids

The xanthelasma and arcus senilis in this patient indicate the need for blood lipid estimation since these findings are commonly associated with an increase in cholesterol and β-lipoproteins (Fredrickson's type II hyperlipoprotein-aemia) and the clinical significance of this type of lipid disturbance is that it is often associated with early arterial disease. It should also be remembered, however, that about half the patients with xanthelasma have normal serum lipids.

Routine blood lipid estimation, in the absence of specific clinical indications like xanthelasma or xanthomata, is very much in vogue today but rarely of any real clinical benefit. Although there is considerable evidence relating the development of ischaemic heart disease to abnormal lipid patterns, especially cholesterol, there is still much doubt about the beneficial clinical effects of reducing the abnormal levels once the ischaemic heart disease has become clinically manifest. Lowering blood cholesterol is more likely to be of clinical benefit in a young person in preventing the development of coronary disease, and it is perhaps in these younger symptomatic patients, say in their twenties and thirties, that it might be reasonable to do routine lipid estimation.

The patient's blood lipid levels are shown in Table 1.8. In his case, both the serum cholesterol and serum triglyceride levels were increased, indicating Fredrickson Type IIB pattern, and the ratio of high density to low density lipoproteins was adverse. The significance of this ratio is that it is the low density lipoprotein–cholesterol (LDL) combination which leads to athero-sclerosis, while the high density lipoprotein–cholesterol (HDL) retards its

Table 1.8 Blood lipid levels in the patient

	mmol/l	Normal range mmol/l
Cholesterol	10.4	(3.5–7.0)
Triglyceride	3.8	(0.1–2.1)
HDL–cholesterol	1.8	(0.9–1.9)
LDL–cholesterol	8.6	(2.6–5.1)

development, therefore the HDL/LDL ratio is of more importance than the total cholesterol level.

Urine–sugar

The only other routine test which may be of value in managing angina is a urine check for sugar. If this is present then the *blood sugar* should be estimated to pick up diabetes. Although there is no convincing evidence that control of diabetes benefits the progress of the angina, the diabetic state itself usually requires some sort of treatment, be it diet, oral hypoglycaemic drugs or insulin.

Serum uric acid

Finally, a raised serum uric acid in the absence of gout may be associated with an increased likelihood of coronary disease, but since the significance of this finding is currently not understood there is little point in a routine estimation of serum uric acid.

Neck X-ray

As far as this patient's cervical spondylosis is concerned, the diagnosis could be confirmed by an X-ray of the cervical spine. However, it should be remembered that middle-aged asymptomatic individuals will often show radiological evidence of cervical spondylosis if X-rayed, and so the diagnosis should be made on clinical grounds of cervical nerve root irritation and restricted painful movements of the cervical spine.

MANAGEMENT OF ANGINA PECTORIS

The aims of treatment are shown in Table 1.9.

Relief of the symptom of angina

This may be attained by prevention and by specific treatment. Prevention involves an alteration in life style so that those factors which precipitate the angina are minimized, e.g. avoidance of hurry, reduction of distance, and especially speed, of walking, avoidance of walking in cold weather, especially

Table 1.9 Aims of treatment of
angina pectoris

- To relieve symptoms
- To improve functional capacity
- Prevention of complications

    - myocardial infarction
    - cardiac arrhythmias
    - sudden death

- Prolongation of life

against the wind, reduction of emotional stress as far as possible, moderation in sexual activity. More specific control of angina by drugs such as nitrates, β-adrenergic blocking agents, nifedipine and calcium antagonists will be discussed later.

Improvement in functional capacity

Improvement in functional capacity will improve the quality of life and can be attained by redressing the imbalance between myocardial oxygen demands and myocardial blood flow so that the heart can perform more efficiently and economically. The most important factors determining myocardial oxygen demands are shown in Table 1.10.

Table 1.10 Major determinants
of myocardial oxygen requirements

- Systolic blood pressure
- Heart rate
- Myocardial contractility
- Left ventricular wall tension

Reduction of myocardial oxygen demands

Systolic blood pressure
Control of blood pressure will reduce cardiac work and may be attained by living an equable life with avoidance of emotional stress as far as possible, cessation of smoking (nicotine increases blood pressure and heart rate) and avoidance of obesity. The use of drugs to control hypertension will be discussed later.

Heart rate
Slowing of the heart rate will improve cardiac performance, and may be achieved similarly by avoiding emotional stress, stopping smoking, reducing obesity and, most important, by the use of β-adrenergic blocking drugs.

Myocardial contractility
Myocardial contractility, or the speed of ventricular contraction, may be

modified by controlling conditions which increase the liberation of circulating catecholamines, and, once again, anxiety and smoking are important factors; anaemia and hyperthyroidism may also increase contractility and should be kept in mind.

Left ventricular wall tension
Left ventricular wall tension depends on the left ventricular volume. This may be reduced by drugs such as nitrates and other vasodilators e.g. nifedipine. If heart failure is present, the increased left ventricular volume may be decreased by diuretics.

Improvement in myocardial blood flow

With regard to redressing the balance between myocardial oxygen demands and supply by an improvement in myocardial blood flow, this can be achieved mainly by *surgical measures*, though *nitrates* may help where coronary vasospasm is an important factor, such as rest angina or Prinzmetal's angina.

The place of exercise

One other important way of improving functional capacity is by regular exercise which results in the performance of any given workload at a lower heart rate and blood pressure than in the untrained state. The free prophylactic use of trinitrin will help in allowing regular exercise to be taken.

Prevention of complications

Unlike relief of angina, and improvement in functional capacity, prevention of the major complications in angina – myocardial infarction, major cardiac arrhythmias and sudden death – are goals which modern management has yet to achieve. To date, there are no convincing studies to show that the development of myocardial infarction and/or sudden death in anginal patients in general can be prevented by either medical or surgical means. However, the value of β-adrenergic blocking drugs has been satisfactorily demonstrated in the secondary prevention of both conditions, and there is a reasonable hope and expectation that this may also be the case in anginal patients. Similarly, the value of coronary bypass grafting in those anginal patients with proven multivessel disease has shown some encouraging results in improving the prognosis.

General measures in the management of angina

Before embarking on the specific drug treatment it is important to deal with any more general conditions which may exacerbate the angina (Table 1.11).

Cigarette smoking

Cessation of cigarette smoking is of undoubted benefit since in the short term

Table 1.11   General factors to be considered
in the management of angina

- Smoking
- Hypertension
- Obesity
- Anaemia
- Thyrotoxicosis
- Alteration in lifestyle

it reduces blood pressure and heart rate, and in the long term leads to a reduced risk of sudden death and a non-fatal heart attack. If cigarettes cannot be given up completely, a reduction to the lowest number feasible is indicated. A change to low nicotine cigarettes or pipe smoking is unlikely to be of much benefit since the patient will probably inhale more to maintain the same nicotine-related effects as before.

Hypertension

Control of hypertension will be discussed below, p.24.

Obesity

Obesity is an adverse factor in angina, mainly because of its association with hypertension, hypercholesterolaemia, diabetic tendency and lack of exercise. Control of obesity is, however, a difficult and frustrating exercise for patient and doctor alike. Perhaps the most important concept for the patient to grasp is not that of 'going on a diet' for a period of time to lose weight but of *permanently altering eating habits*. The specific nature of the food intake is less important than the reduction in total calories. It is probably desirable also to reduce the intake of saturated fat – e.g. animal meat, dairy produce – to no more than 30% of the total intake of calories.

Anaemia

Anaemia is a common condition, especially in women. By reducing the oxygen-carrying capacity of the blood and by causing tachycardia, it will exacerbate angina.

Thyrotoxicosis

Thyrotoxicosis increases heart rate, blood pressure and metabolic requirements generally. It is a condition to be kept in mind especially in the elderly anginal patient who may not have overt signs of thyrotoxicosis – unexplained weight loss may be an important clue here.

Life style

Alteration in life style is an important aspect of management of angina, since the patient must learn to 'live with his angina'. Suggested guidelines are shown in Table 1.12.

Table 1.12 Alteration in life style for the anginal patient

* 40 hour week or less
* No weekend work
* Regular vacations
* Pleasant recreation – avoid activity inducing great excitement (e.g. sports matches)
* Regular exercise – walking best (but not in cold winds)
* Avoid heavy lunches followed by exercise
* Avoid emotional crises both at work and in the home

Drug treatment of angina pectoris

Nitrates

Nitrates remain the mainstay of treatment and glyceryl trinitrate (trinitrin) the most useful drug. Their main action is to reduce the workload on the heart, primarily by causing increased venous pooling in the periphery by venodilation (reduced 'preload') and, to a lesser degree, by reducing systemic arterial pressure (reduced 'afterload') (Figure 1.8). In some patients, especially if coronary spasm is present, nitrates may help by coronary vasodilatation.

All anginal patients should be started on sublingual trinitrin both for relief of anginal pain and, more important, for its prevention. The tablets can be used freely as a prophylactic measure and there is no restriction to the number of tablets that can be used throughout the day. It is advisable to warn patients of the possible headache caused by the drug and to encourage them to persist with the treatment if the headache is tolerable since it may diminish in the course of time. If the headache is too severe, an alternative nitrate preparation such as a 5 mg tablet of chewable sorbide nitrate can be tried, which some patients find is less prone to cause headache though the reverse may also be true. It is worth experimenting with both.

If frequent sublingual trinitrin is required during the day, then long acting oral isosorbide nitrate (either dinitrate or mononitrate) can be used in doses from 10 mg to 30 mg (or even more) four times daily. Two recently introduced nitroglycerine preparations may also be of value, especially if oral isosorbide nitrate is not acceptable because of severe headache: (1) a transdermal preparation providing controlled release of nitroglycerine over 24 hours with each patch (Transiderm-Nitro) and (2) a slow release buccal preparation which is held in the cheek pouch for up to 5 hours and slowly releases the nitroglycerine, though on a more erratic basis than the transdermal preparation (Suscard Buccal).

Sublingual tablets of glyceryl trinitrate deteriorate after 8 weeks or so in

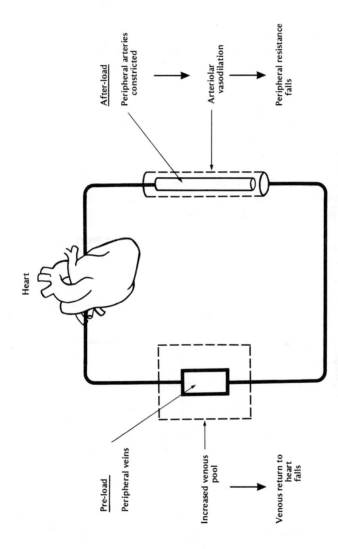

Figure 1.8 Action of nitrates on the peripheral circulation

their container and may therefore be less effective. It is advisable to renew the supply every 6 months or so.

β-Adrenergic blocking drugs

Most anginal patients will also require β-adrenergic blocking drugs. The main action of these drugs in angina is to slow the heart, both at rest and in response to physical and emotional stress, thus reducing cardiac work and so economizing on the limited available coronary blood supply. Another possible benefit, though so far only theoretical, is a reduced likelihood of progression to fatal or non-fatal infarction. To date, however, this benefit has been shown only in the secondary prevention of myocardial infarction, that is after the first heart attack has already occurred.

Contraindications to β-blockade include obstructive lung disease, especially bronchial asthma, heart failure and intermittent claudication. Extra care must also be taken with treated diabetes, since β-blockade may mask warning hypoglycaemic symptoms.

A cardioselective or β-1 receptor blocker, such as metoprolol or atenolol, is better than a non-specific β-1 and β-2 blocker, such as propanolol or timolol, if the treatment is to be used in asthma or intermittent claudication. Table 1.13 shows the different β-adrenergic blockers available with appropriate dosage schedules.

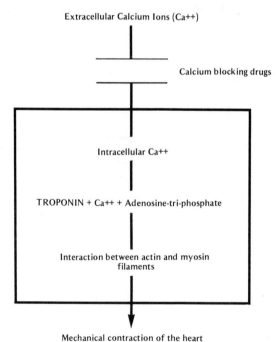

Extracellular Calcium Ions (Ca++)

Calcium blocking drugs

Intracellular Ca++

TROPONIN + Ca++ + Adenosine-tri-phosphate

Interaction between actin and myosin filaments

Mechanical contraction of the heart

Figure 1.9 Simple diagram of role of calcium ion in myocardial contraction and the effect of calcium antagonists

Table 1.13 Pharmacological characteristics of available β-adrenergic blocking drugs

Drug	Non-specific*	Cardioselective*	Intrinsic sympathomimetic activity (ISA)	Equipotent single dose mg	Usual daily dosage range mg
Propranolol	+	−	−	100	120–360
Atenolol†	−	+	−	100	100–200
Metoprolol†	−	+	−	100	100–200
Oxprenolol	+	−	+	100	120–480
Acebutolol	−	+	+	200	300–800
Timolol†	+	−	−	10	15–45
Sotalol	+	−	−	200	160–480
Nadolol	+	−	−	40	40–240
Pindolol	+	−	+	5	7.5–45

*Cardioselective β-blockers are preferred in patients with obstructive airway disease and intermittent claudication. Drugs with ISA are preferred in patients with heart failure
†These drugs have been shown to be of value in the secondary prevention of myocardial infarction

Calcium antagonists

Cardiac contraction is dependent on the free passage of calcium ions ($Ca++$) into the myocardial cells (Figure 1.9).

Calcium antagonists act by interfering with the inflow of calcium ions into the cardiac cell which impairs contractility of the cardiac muscle and so reduces cardiac work.

Nifedipine is the most useful drug of this type for angina and should always be tried if nitrate therapy and β-blocking drugs are ineffective or unacceptable. It is of particular value where the angina is thought to be due to coronary spasm, such as may occur in rest angina or in the much rarer nocturnal Prinzmetal's variant angina. The dose is 10–20 mg three times daily; the main side-effects are flushing due to systemic vasodilatation, postural dizziness due to hypotension, gastrointestinal disorder and leg oedema.

Other calcium antagonists such as verapamil or lidoflazine can be tried, but there is little point in using a combination of different calcium antagonists together in angina if one alone does not work.

Hyperlipidaemia

The beneficial effects of reducing raised blood lipid levels on the clinical course of coronary disease have not yet been convincingly shown in the management of angina, except perhaps in the rare condition of familial hypercholesterolaemia characterized by a very high blood level of low-density lipoprotein–cholesterol and the premature development of extensive atherosclerosis and cutaneous xanthomata.

In common practice, however, coronary disease is more likely to be associated with Fredrickson's Type II or Type IV hyperlipoproteinaemia (Table 1.14), where changes in cholesterol are less marked and reduction of serum cholesterol (and low-density lipoprotein) has yet to be shown to improve clinical progress once coronary disease has become well established, as in an anginal patient.

However, in a younger patient (say under 45 years of age) it is reasonable in these circumstances to try to restrict dietary intake of cholesterol-containing foods, such as dairy produce, eggs and fatty meat, providing this does not mean a radical alteration of eating habits which makes the patient profoundly miserable. It is important also to restrict alcohol intake which can cause hypertriglyceridaemia.

As far as more specific therapy is concerned, cholestyramine (Questran) is a useful and acceptable drug to reduce serum cholesterol, and again it should be reserved for the younger patient since it is unlikely to be of clinical benefit in older ones. Clofibrate has been shown to be associated with long term hazards such as increase in the incidence of gallstones, and, more important, an unexplained increase in mortality, possibly from gastrointestinal neoplasia. Nicotinic acid, in a dose of 1–3 g daily has also been used to lower cholesterol, but has severe side-effects such as flushing, pruritus and gastric irritation.

Table 1.14 Fredrickson's classification of hyperlipidaemia

Type	Cholesterol	Triglyceride	LDL–cholesterol	HDL–cholesterol	Clinical associations
I	↑	Normal (chylomicrons)	Normal	Normal or ↓	Pancreatitis
IIA	↑	Normal	↑	Normal or ↓	Coronary disease Xanthelasma
IIB	↑	↑	↑	Normal or ↓	Coronary disease Xanthelasma
III	↑	↑	↑	Normal or ↓	Coronary disease Xanthomatosis Mild diabetes
IV	Normal	↑ + +	Normal	Normal or ↓	Coronary disease Diabetes Eruptive xanthomas
V	↑	↑ + +	Normal	Normal or ↓	Coronary disease Diabetes Pancreatitis

Hypertension and ischaemic heart disease

Hypertension is one of the three major coronary risk factors (cigarette smoking and a raised serum cholesterol are the other two). The increased risk of coronary disease applies to mild as well as severe hypertension; the arbitrary definition of mild hypertension, usually accepted is a *diastolic* pressure of 90–105 mmHg.

Although the causal relationship between hypertension and coronary disease has been convincingly established, clinical benefits of reducing the diastolic pressure to 90 mmHg or below are much less certain, since the evidence has been lacking.

However, some recent studies carried out in the USA (US Public Health Service Study, US Hypertension Detection and Follow-Up Study) and Australia (Australian National Blood Pressure Study) have demonstrated the benefits of controlling sustained diastolic pressure in this range. It is hoped that the current British Medical Research Council controlled trial in the treatment of mild hypertension may show similar benefits.

What are the implications of these studies for this patient? Since he or she already has angina requiring treatment with β-blocking drugs there is no problem about deciding to treat his or her mild hypertension, as this will be controlled with the β-blocker. In the absence of an associated accepted indication for β-blockade the decision to treat mild hypertension should be made on other criteria such as:

- age – the younger the patient, the worse the prognosis

- sex – females tolerate all degrees of hypertension better than males

- a bad family history of premature death due to hypertension or its complications

- evidence of target organ damage such as cardiac enlargement, heart failure or renal impairment.

- the presence of other coronary risk factors such as cigarette-smoking, raised serum cholesterol, diabetes, and in women, the contraceptive pill.

Although there is convincing evidence that the *prognosis* in hypertension can be related to a single casual blood pressure reading, it is generally considered desirable to take several readings with the patient relaxed over a period of a few weeks before making the decision to commit a patient, perhaps a young asymptomatic patient, to lifelong hypotensive therapy with all the attendant psychological upset and drug side-effects.

The two most widely used drugs in mild hypertension are *thiazide diuretics* and *β-adrenergic blocking drugs*, and it is good practice to try each drug individually before using a combination of both.

β-blockers

Although β-blockers have theoretical advantages of possible protection from sudden death and myocardial infarction, they may have significant longterm side-effects such as exacerbation of bronchospasm, cold extremities, excessive fatigue, insomnia and bad dreams. Consequently, they may be undesirable in patients with chronic obstructive lung disease, intermittent claudication, diabetes and early heart failure.

Thiazides

Thiazides are probably equally effective but also have undesirable side-effects such as potassium deficiency, leading to fatigue and possibly arrhythmias if a heart attack develops, exacerbation of diabetes and gout; a particularly disconcerting side-effect which has emerged from the current British Medical Research Council trial is male impotence.

Systolic hypertension

Systolic hypertension has been found to be equally predictive of the development of coronary disease as the diastolic pressure. So far, however, there have been no satisfactory data on the clinical effects of controlling isolated systolic hypertension.

Coronary artery bypass grafting in angina pectoris

The place of coronary artery bypass grafting (CABG) in the routine manage-

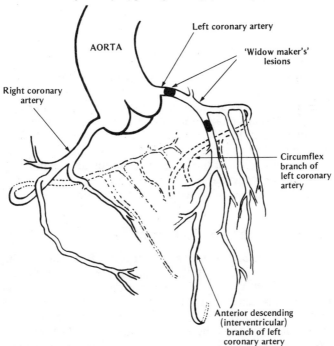

Figure 1.10 'Widow maker's' disease of coronary arteries

ment of angina has not yet been clarified. CABG is currently reserved for anginal patients who remain incapacitated by their angina in spite of adequate medical treatment. It is also becoming increasingly considered in the younger patient with angina – say, arbitrarily, below 45 years of age – even if satisfactorily controlled by medication. The rationale for this view is that the prognosis in angina is very much determined by the presence of single coronary artery disease which carries a good prognosis with medical treatment, or multivessel disease, where the mortality is high (Figure 1.10). The exception to this rule is when the single vessel involved is the main stem of the left coronary artery or its anterior descending interventricular branch, both of which carry a high risk of sudden death ('Widow maker's disease'). If facilities for coronary arteriography become more widely available, it may well be that young anginal patients should be routinely considered for this investigation.

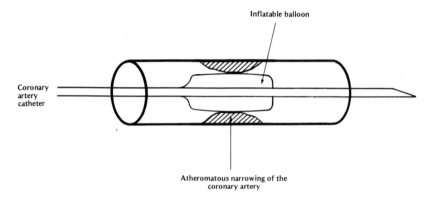

Figure 1.11   Percutaneous transluminal angioplasty

Another potentially useful surgical approach to the management of coronary artery obstruction – percutaneous transluminal angioplasty – has been recently introduced. In this, a balloon is inflated at the end of a coronary artery catheter placed at the site of the coronary obstruction (Figure 1.11). This may result in dilatation of the obstructing lesion and an improvement in coronary flow. The procedure is reserved usually for single vessel disease and carries a lower risk than coronary artery bypass grafting.

NATURAL HISTORY OF ANGINA PECTORIS

The most important feature of the natural history of angina is its unpredictability. Overall, the mortality in stable angina is about 5% each year.

The Framingham (USA) study showed that about 25% of the males with angina will have a myocardial infarction within 5 years, while women have half this incidence. Furthermore, the study also showed that one third of all patients with stable angina will die within 8 years and half of these deaths will be sudden. A more meaningful survey of the natural history of angina in terms of British general practice has been carried out by Dr John Fry (Figure 1.12).

He found that approximately a quarter of 200 anginal patients lost their pain altogether, while in another quarter the angina was mild and easily controlled, and 6% were severely disabled by their angina; overall, 45% died over a 25 year period, most from subsequent myocardial infarction or heart failure.

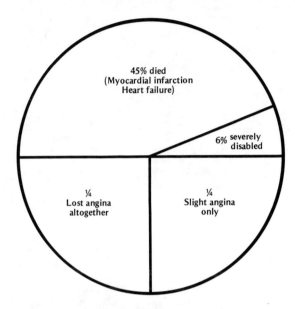

Figure 1.12   Natural history of angina (from survey over 25 years in general practice by Dr John Fry)

The prognosis in angina is influenced adversely by previous myocardial infarction or heart failure, by associated hypertension, by cardiac enlargement and also by electrocardiographic evidence of left ventricular hypertrophy.

The other important, perhaps the most important, prognostic influence in angina is the presence of single vessel, double vessel or triple vessel disease (Figure 1.13). A typical study has shown an annual mortality of 2% with single vessel disease (unless it is the left main coronary artery or its anterior interventricular branch), 7% with two vessel disease and 11% with all three vessels involved. The evidence so far also suggests that coronary artery bypass grafting leads to a better prognosis in triple vessel disease than does medical treatment, and it is on this basis that the more extensive use of coronary arteriography, especially in the young patients, should be encouraged. It is as well to remember also that the procedure of coronary arteriography itself carries a very slight risk of morbidity, e.g. myocardial infarction and even death.

As far as standard treatment of angina with nitrates, β-blockers, nifedipine etc. is concerned, there is no convincing evidence as yet that the treatment prolongs life. However, the quality of life may be substantially improved and wholly justifies the continued use of medical treatment of angina.

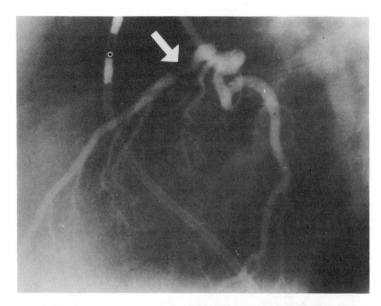

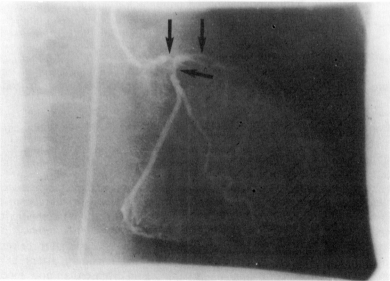

Figure 1.13   Multivessel disease

CAN WE INFLUENCE THE NATURAL HISTORY OF CORONARY DISEASE?

Since coronary arteriosclerosis can start early in life it is prudent to consider what can be done to delay its onset and modify its degree, thereby favourably influencing its bad prognosis in later life.

Essentially, this implies establishing good health habits and a life style which avoids, in early adult life and even in childhood, adverse risk factors. The most important intervention is *prevention of smoking* in childhood and adolescence; also vigorous sport can be encouraged and obesity prevented by reduction of calorie intake, and at the same time the intake of saturated fat (animal fat) could be reduced.

Measures to influence prognosis

Once coronary disease has become established, measures to influence prognosis are much more difficult.

Stopping cigarette smoking

From the therapeutic point of view, this is the most important coronary risk factor of all, since stopping smoking has been shown clearly to result in a progressive reduction over a period of 10 years of the risk of myocardial infarction and sudden death.

Control of hypertension

Recent evidence suggests that this is likely also to reduce the risk of fatal and non-fatal infarctions. The evidence also points towards the desirability of controlling mild hypertension.

Reduction of blood cholesterol

The clinical benefits have not yet been established clearly. However, it is advisable to reduce the serum cholesterol in young patients.

Control of obesity

This is a desirable measure, and in controlling the obesity other beneficial effects may occur, such as reducing the tendency to hypertension, hyperlipidaemia and carbohydrate intolerance as well as increasing the likelihood of adequate exercise. The reduction in calories should be accompanied by a reduction also in the intake of saturated animal fat.

Control of diabetes

The clinical benefits in relation to coronary disease have not been shown.

Stress

Although there is good evidence that acute psychological stress can precipitate an acute myocardial infarction in a patient with established coronary disease, there is no convincing evidence that chronic psychological stress actually leads to the development of coronary artery disease. However, it would be common sense to reduce mental and emotional stress in a patient with angina, though this may be easier said than done, since it is the patient's personality which decides the response to stress, rather than the external stress itself.

SUMMARY OF USEFUL PRACTICAL POINTS IN THE MANAGEMENT OF ANGINA PECTORIS

- The diagnosis of angina is made primarily on the basis of a good clinical history. Examination and investigation are of limited diagnostic value.

- It is important to look for, and treat if possible, associated coronary risk factors which may worsen the prognosis, such as cigarette-smoking, hypertension, hypercholesterolaemia (in younger patients), diabetes and obesity, and remember the contraceptive pill in women.

- Encourage the free prophylactic use of sublingual trinitrin. For additional nitrate therapy, use oral sorbide nitrate, transdermal nitro-glycerine or buccal nitroglycerine. β-Blockers may improve prognosis as well as control angina. Calcium antagonists also have a valuable place in treatment.

- Coronary arteriography, with a view to surgical treatment, should be considered in younger patients with angina (arbitrarily, under 45 years of age) and for patients of any age incapacitated by angina which is resistant to medical treatment.

2

Breathlessness

PRESENT HISTORY

A 62-year-old male patient was admitted to hospital as an emergency with severe breathlessness, wheezing and a cough productive of yellow sputum for the previous 4 or 5 days.

Recurrent bronchitis

He had suffered with recurrent bronchitis for 15–20 years. Initially this occurred only during the winter, but over the past few years it had troubled him all the year round, resulting in increasing breathlessness on exertion, attacks of wheezing and a continuous cough, usually with thick grey sputum but this would frequently change to green or yellow when his bronchitis was bad. He had never coughed up any blood. As a result of his severe breathlessness he had to take early retirement on medical grounds from his work as a miner which he had carried out since adolescence. His breathlessness was now such that he was unable to climb the stairs to his bedroom without stopping several times.

Nocturnal dyspnoea

Over the past year he had developed attacks of awakening at variable times in the middle of the night gasping for breath. He volunteered that he always had to get out of bed and stand by an open window (Figure 2.1); the breathlessness would then subside within 10–15 minutes. When asked whether he coughed during these attacks, he said he would sometimes have a dry cough and sometimes bring up frothy sputum unlike the thick gelatinous sputum he usually brought up; he had not noticed any blood in the frothy sputum. These attacks were getting more frequent and were now averaging two a week. Over the same period he had increased the number of pillows he used from two to four, since his breathing was worse if he lay flat in bed.

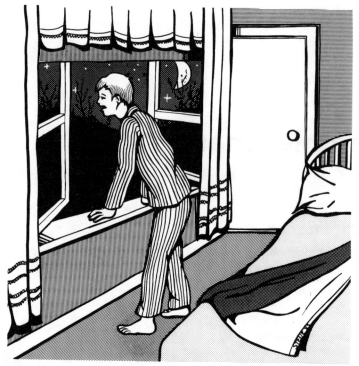

Figure 2.1 The patient in an attack of nocturnal breathlessness
(illustration by Steven Hurst)

Other relevant facts on direct enquiry

Ankle swelling

He admitted to recurrent swelling of both ankles and feet over the past few months. This seemed to occur usually when he had a flare-up of his bronchitis.

Headache

He had noticed some rather severe early morning headaches during the last month or two, and also thought his eyesight was getting rather poor over the same period.

PAST HISTORY

He had a heart attack 10 years earlier and had two further admissions for suspected heart attacks since. He had suffered with chest pain on exertion since the first heart attack but this had become less frequent over the past year, and he thought this was due to not being able to exert himself to any significant extent because of his breathlessness.

FAMILY HISTORY

There was no relevant family history and, in particular, no familial predisposition to chronic bronchitis.

PERSONAL HISTORY

He had been a heavy smoker, 40 cigarettes per day, most of his life, but gave up about 4 years ago when his breathing became really bad. He also used to drink quite heavily for a number of years, 7 or 8 pints (4–4.5 litres) per day, but over the last few years had drunk very little since he has had difficulty getting to the 'pub'.

EXAMINATION

The abnormal physical signs are shown in Figure 2.2.

General

He was apyrexial and overweight. He was not unduly breathless sitting propped up in bed. He had central cyanosis and early finger clubbing. There was no palmar erythema in the hands ('liver palms').

The external jugular veins were distended but not pulsatile and the veins did not collapse in inspiration. There was pitting oedema over both ankles and feet. The liver edge was not palpable but percussion showed dullness extending to about a handbreadth below the right costal margin, and there was tenderness over the dull area.

Respiratory system

The chest was not 'barrel-shaped' but expansion was very poor generally, only $\frac{3}{4}$-inch (2 cm) at midsternal level. The trachea was central. Vocal fremitus was generally reduced. The percussion note seemed normal except over both lung bases where it was dull; there was no reduction of cardiac or hepatic dullness. Breath sounds were poor generally, and harsh at the lung bases. There were widespread high-pitched inspiratory and expiratory rhonchi over both lungs, front and back. There were also scattered medium crepitations posteriorly. There was no gynaecomastia.

Cardiovascular system

The pulse was 90/min and regular and the blood pressure 120/60 (lying). The apex could not be localized but there was a definite left parasternal lift. The heart sounds were difficult to hear because of the widespread rhonchi, but a protodiastolic gallop rhythm could just be heard and the pulmonary second sound was increased. There was a blowing midsystolic murmur over the lower sternal area and apex, where it was loudest, and it was clearly conducted out to the left axilla; it did not radiate downwards over the liver and was not louder on inspiration.

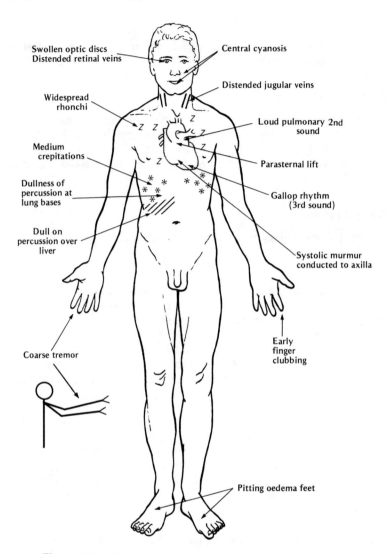

Figure 2.2 Abnormal physical signs in the patient

Abdomen

There were no distended superficial abdominal veins, no splenic enlargement and no ascites.

Central nervous system

He was rather drowsy and slightly confused. He had a coarse tremor affecting both hands accentuated on stretching them out. Fundal examination showed blurring of the margins of both optic discs, which seemed slightly swollen; the retinal veins were distended and the arterioles rather narrow and tortuous with some arteriovenous nipping; there were no retinal haemorrhages or exudates. The cranial nerves were otherwise normal, and no other abnormality was detected in the motor system, sensory system or cerebellar system.

ANALYSIS OF THE HISTORY

Breathlessness

On exertion

The major symptom in this patient was his breathlessness. The main causes of breathlessness are shown in Table 2.1. In clinical practice, the important differentiation usually required is between heart disease and lung disease and some helpful distinguishing features are shown in Table 2.2. The types of pulmonary disease leading to breathlessness are shown in Table 2.3. The timing of the onset of the breathlessness may help in diagnosing the cause (Table 2.4).

Table 2.1   Causes of breathlessness

- Lung disease
- Heart disease
- Anaemia – tissue anoxia
- Obesity – increased work of breathing
             restricted movement of chest wall
- Thyrotoxicosis – increased oxygen requirements
- Anxiety state

Table 2.2   Distinguishing features between dyspnoea due to heart disease and to lung disease

Lung disease	Heart disease
History of respiratory disease	History of hypertension, cardiac ischaemia or valvular heart disease
Slow development	Rapid development
Present at rest	Mainly on exertion
Productive cough common	Cough uncommon, and then 'dry'
Aggravated by respiratory infection	Unaffected by respiratory infection

In this patient, the history of recurrent bronchitis with a chronic productive cough, often with purulent sputum, clearly indicates that his main problem is *chronic bronchitis*. The epidemiological definition of this condition is *a productive cough on most days in a 2 month period per year for at least 2 years*, and on this basis the patient certainly fits in. In the early stages of the disease he was only significantly incapacitated when he had an acute flare-up of his bronchitis, to which these patients are highly susceptible. However, the

Table 2.3   The common pulmonary causes of breathlessness

• Obstructive disease	• Chronic bronchitis
	• Asthma
• Restrictive disease	• Fibrosis
	• Collapse
	• Pleural effusion
	• Pneumothorax
• Neuromuscular disease affecting respiratory muscles	• Poliomyelitis
	• Infective polyneuritis

Table 2.4   The onset of breathlessness as a diagnostic help

• Acute	• Spontaneous pneumothorax
	• Pulmonary collapse
	• Pleural effusion
	• Pulmonary embolus
• Paroxysmal	• Bronchial asthma
	• Recurrent pulmonary emboli
• Over a few months	• Tuberculosis
	• Carcinoma
	• Pleural effusion
	• Infiltrations
• Over many months	• Chronic bronchitis
	• Pulmonary fibrosis
	• Pneumoconiosis

steady progress of his disease has led to permanent year-round disability due to the breathlessness.

Paroxysmal nocturnal dyspnoea

There is another cause of breathlessness in this patient – *left ventricular failure*. This is indicated by the attacks of paroxysmal nocturnal dyspnoea which necessitate his getting up and standing by an open window. Paroxysmal nocturnal dyspnoea commonly results from left ventricular failure (cardiac asthma) but may also occur in lung disease, especially bronchial asthma and less commonly in chronic bronchitis, thought mainly to be due to pooling of secretions in the lungs during sleep. The differentiation between cardiac and bronchial paroxysmal nocturnal dyspnoea is shown in Table 2.5. Wheezing is not a very helpful differentiating symptom: although it is usually more marked in bronchial asthma it can also occur in cardiac asthma due to oedema of the bronchial mucosa.

Table 2.5   Differentiation between 'cardiac' asthma and bronchial asthma

	Cardiac	*Bronchial*
Past history	Hypertension	Asthma
	Cardiac ischaemia	Chronic bronchitis
	Valvular disease	
Timing	Any time	Early morning
Dyspnoea	Mainly inspiratory	Mainly expiratory
Cough	Follows dyspnoea	Precedes dyspnoea
Sputum	Pink and frothy	Thick and gelatinous
Relief	Standing up	Coughing up sputum
	(by open window)	
	Intravenous diuretic	Bronchodilator
Lung signs	Mainly crepitations	Mainly rhonchi
Cardiac signs	Gallop rhythm	—

In this patient the diagnosis of left ventricular failure is based mainly on the coughing up of frothy sputum, though the necessity to stand by the open window is also very suggestive. Additionally, the past history of ischaemic heart disease establishes the cause for the left ventricular failure.

Sputum

The nature of the sputum is often helpful in indicating its cause (Table 2.6). The history of chronic production of thick grey sputum in this patient indicates chronic bronchitis, and the frequent change to yellow or green sputum is due to super-added acute bronchitis caused by acute bacterial infection.

Table 2.6   Diagnostic value of sputum

• Clear white or grey	– Uninfected bronchitis
• Green or yellow	– Bacterial infection
• 'Rusty' sputum	– Lobar pneumonia (pneumococcal)
• Thin white mucoid	– Viral bronchitis
• Thick and sticky	– Bronchial asthma
• Large amount watery	– Alveolar cell carcinoma
• 'Redcurrant jelly'	– Bronchial carcinoma
• Large amount purulent and offensive	– Bronchiectasis Lung abcess
• Pink and frothy	– Left ventricular failure Mitral stenosis

Swelling of the ankles

Swelling of the feet and ankles in a patient with longstanding chronic bronchitis strongly suggests *right ventricular failure*. The term *'cor pulmonale'* is strictly defined by the World Health Organization as right ventricular hypertrophy due to primary lung disease. In practice, however, the term 'cor pulmonale' is used more commonly to describe right ventricular failure due to chronic lung disease. The failure of the right ventricle in chronic obstructive lung disease is due mainly to the associated pulmonary hypertension, and the factors responsible for the pulmonary hypertension are shown in Table 2.7.

The relationship between the oedema and the flare-ups of the bronchitis in this patient is due to the increased pulmonary hypertension resulting from the extra anoxia caused by the lung infection.

Table 2.7   Causes of pulmonary hypertension in chronic lung disease

- Reduced pulmonary vascular bed due to lung damage
- Hypoxia
- Increased cardiac output
- Secondary polycythaemia increasing blood viscocity
- Sometimes left ventricular failure

Headache

The development of headaches in a chronic bronchitic is an ominous symptom and suggests increasing carbon dioxide retention due to *respiratory failure*. The cause of the headache is probably the cerebral vasodilatation caused by the hypercapnia. Increasing hypercapnia will progressively affect the central nervous system leading to confusion, drowsiness, muscular twitches or tremors, coma and even death.

Past history

The significant feature here is the ischaemic heart disease which provides the basis for his nocturnal attacks of left ventricular failure.

Left ventricular involvement may occur as a result of chronic lung disease itself, although the reasons are not always clear. Both left ventricular enlargement and left ventricular failure may develop. Some of the suggested mechanisms are shown in Table 2.8. In this patient, however, there is no need to suggest any cause for the left ventricular failure other than the ischaemic heart disease.

Table 2.8   Suggested mechanisms for left ventricular involvement in chronic obstructive lung disease

- Bronchial artery – pulmonary artery shunts
- Chronic hypoxia impairing left ventricular function
- Secondary polycythaemia reducing coronary perfusion
- Common cardiac muscle bundles between both ventricles

Occupational history

His work as a coalminer may be relevant in the aetiology of his chronic lung disease. His lungs may be affected in two ways – from the development of pneumoconiosis, or from the chronic irritation of the coal dust in the absence of any radiological evidence of pneumoconiosis. Early stages of pneumoconiosis, diagnosed by a generalized reticular or small nodular pattern on chest X-ray, are not usually associated with significant respiratory impairment, but the later stages, showing as substantial fibrotic and large nodular areas in the chest X-ray, do lead to breathlessness. The correlation between the X-ray findings and lung function and disability is a poor one, and in the UK often forms the basis of dispute between the patient and the Government Pneumoconiosis Panel.

Cigarette smoking

Cigarette smoking is the single most important factor contributing to the development of chronic bronchitis. The adverse effects of smoking on lung function are shown in Table 2.9. Although smoking is harmful to all patients with chronic bronchitis, there appears to be a particularly susceptible group in whom all the adverse effects of smoking are particularly marked. Although all the factors determining this susceptibility have not been clearly identified, Table 2.10 shows some of those involved.

Table 2.9   Adverse effects of smoking on lung function

- Impairment of bronchial ciliary movement
- Increase in bronchial mucus-secreting glands
- Increase in stickiness of the mucus
- Increase in airway resistance
- Increase in pulmonary proteolytic enzymes → emphysema
- Inhibition of alveolar macrophages → increased susceptibility to bacterial infection

Table 2.10   Factors increasing susceptibility to the harmful effects of smoking on the lungs

- Recurrent respiratory disorders in childhood
- Intercurrent respiratory infections
- Familial (genetic) predisposition
- Deficiency in plasma antiproteolytic activity (α-1 antitrypsin deficiency)

CONCLUSIONS FROM THE HISTORY

- The patient has a history of chronic bronchitis.

- The more recent episodes of ankle swelling with the acute exacerbations of his bronchitis indicate attacks of cor pulmonale.

- The most important predisposing factor in the chronic bronchitis is the long history of cigarette smoking. His occupation as a miner also suggests the possibility of an additional contributory cause, pneumoconiosis.

- The paroxysmal nocturnal dyspnoea associated with frothy sputum indicates that he also has left ventricular failure.

- The previous heart attacks are the likely basis of these attacks of left ventricular failure.

- The recent headache may suggest the development of respiratory failure with carbon dioxide retention.

ANALYSIS OF THE EXAMINATION

This patient shows the clinical features of the '*blue bloater*', in which the predominant pulmonary pathology is chronic bronchitis. This contrasts with the '*pink puffer*', where the pathological changes are those of emphysema. The main distinguishing features between the 'pink puffer' and the 'blue bloater' are shown in Table 2.11. The hyperventilation in the 'pink puffer' maintains oxygenation of the blood, producing pinkness, while the congestive cardiac failure and respiratory failure in the 'blue bloater' lead to the blueness of the cyanosis.

Table 2.11 Differentiation between the 'pink puffer' and the 'blue bloater'

	'*Pink puffer*'	'*Blue bloater*'
Colour	Pink (well-oxygenated)	Blue (cyanosed)
Breathing	Hyperventilation	Quiet
Sputum	Scanty	Profuse, often purulent
Chest examination	Barrel-shaped	Not overinflated
	Quiet chest	Noisy chest (rhonchi)
Right heart failure	Uncommon	Frequent
Chest X-ray	Overinflated lungs	Normal translucency
	Attenuated peripheral vessels	Normal peripheral vessels
Arterial P_{CO_2}	Normal or low	Increased
Diffusing capacity	Reduced	Normal

The cyanosis, distended neck veins, oedema and tender liver indicate *cor pulmonale* in this patient (Figure 2.3). Although the liver appeared enlarged on percussion, emphysema itself may cause downward displacement of the liver which may simulate enlargement. However, the tenderness over this patient's liver suggests congestion.

Finger clubbing is unusual in uncomplicated chronic bronchitis and so some other cause must be sought in this patient. The causes of finger clubbing are shown in Table 2.12. A possible cause in this patient, in view of the occupational history, is pneumoconiosis.

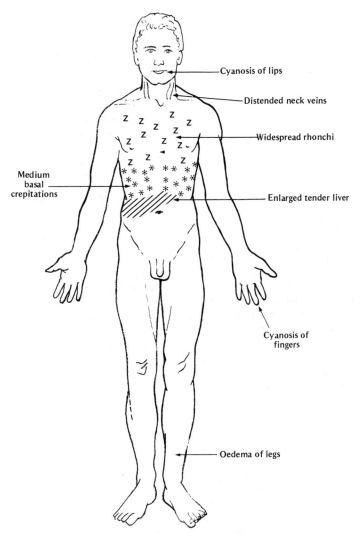

Cyanosis of lips

Distended neck veins

Widespread rhonchi

Medium basal crepitations

Enlarged tender liver

Cyanosis of fingers

Oedema of legs

Figure 2.3   Signs of cor pulmonale in the patient

The widespread rhonchi in his lungs indicate bronchitis. Crepitations are unusual in bronchitis unless there is associated bronchopneumonia. In this patient, the scattered crepitations might be due to pulmonary congestion associated with left ventricular failure.

The *parasternal lift* indicates right ventricular hypertrophy and the *loud pulmonary second sound* is caused by pulmonary hypertension. The *protodiastolic triple rhythm* is due to an audible third heart sound and is commonly found in right ventricular failure. A presystolic gallop rhythm due to a fourth (atrial) heart sound is usually found in conditions causing left ventricular strain or failure, such as hypertension. The blowing systolic murmur conducted out to the axilla suggests *mitral incompetence* which may be due to

Table 2.12   Causes of finger clubbing

• Pulmonary	• Chronic suppuration 　　tuberculosis 　　bronchiectasis 　　lung abscess 　　emphysema • Carcinoma of bronchus • Pneumoconiosis
• Heart disease	• Infective endocarditis • Congenital cyanotic
• Gastrointestinal disease	• Ulcerative colitis • Crohn's disease • Idiopathic steatorrhoea • Cirrhosis
• Familial	

stretching of the mitral valve ring by the left ventricular failure. A systolic murmur in the lower sternal area may also be due to tricuspid incompetence occurring in severe cor pulmonale: in these circumstances the murmur would be conducted down over the liver and would be louder with inspiration, and sometimes there would be associated expansile pulsation of the liver and giant 'V' waves seen in the jugular veins.

The findings in the nervous sytem of drowsiness, tremor and papilloedema are probably due to carbon dioxide retention resulting from respiratory failure. However, other causes of papilloedema should always be considered and excluded (Table 2.13).

Table 2.13   Causes of papilloedema

• Brain tumour
• Malignant hypertension
• Subarachnoid haemorrhage
• Benign intracranial hypertension
• Cerebral vein thrombosis
• Hypercapnia
• Hypocalcaemia

His excessive past alcohol consumption always raises the possibility of cirrhosis. However, there were none of the usual classical features (Figure 2.4).

CONCLUSIONS FROM THE EXAMINATION

- The chest examination shows the features of chronic bronchitis rather than emphysema.
- He has evidence of cor pulmonale.

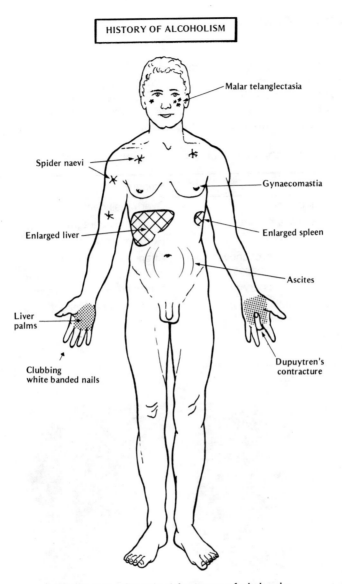

HISTORY OF ALCOHOLISM

Malar telanglectasia

Spider naevi

Gynaecomastia

Enlarged liver

Enlarged spleen

Ascites

Liver palms

Dupuytren's contracture

Clubbing white banded nails

Figure 2.4   Classical features of cirrhosis

- He also has signs of left ventricular failure associated with mitral incompetence which is probably functional due to stretching of the mitral valve ring.

- Neurological examination has confirmed respiratory failure with carbon dioxide retention leading to drowsiness, tremor and papilloedema.

43

INVESTIGATIONS

Chest X-ray

This is a very helpful test in the diagnosis of chronic obstructive lung disease. The diagnostic features of chronic bronchitis and of emphysema are shown in Table 2.14. The patient's X-ray (Figure 2.5) shows the features of chronic bronchitis but there is also a generalized nodulation attributable to an early stage of pneumoconiosis. This would account for his finger clubbing.

Table 2.14 X-ray changes in chronic bronchitis and emphysema

Chronic bronchitis	Emphysema
Normal translucency	Overtranslucent
Normal ribs and diaphragm	Low flat diaphragm
	Horizontal ribs
Increased peripheral bronchovascular markings especially at bases	Attenuated peripheral arteries
Prominent main pulmonary artery	Normal main pulmonary artery
No bullae but old inflammatory disease may be evident	Bullae may be present
Large heart due to right ventricular dilation	Narrow heart

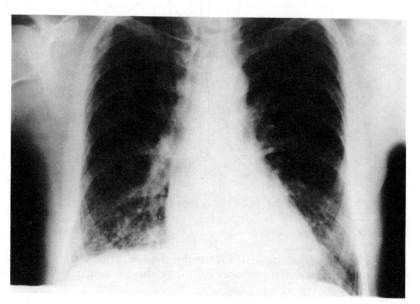

Figure 2.5 Patient's chest X-ray showing chronic bronchitis and early pneumoconiosis

One other important function of the chest X-ray in chronic obstructive lung disease is to identify treatable lesions which might contribute to respiratory failure such as lung collapse due to bronchial obstruction, pneumothorax or pleural effusion.

Figure 2.6 offers an example of a typical chest X-ray in emphysema.

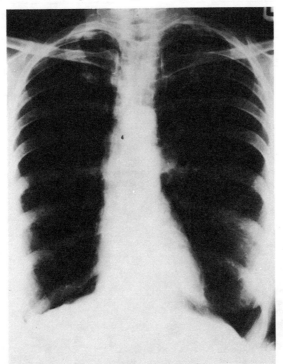

Figure 2.6 Typical X-ray appearances in emphysema with horizontal ribs, flat diaphragm and translucent lungs

Lung function tests

Spirometry is another important test in the diagnosis of chronic lung disease. The results will depend on whether bronchitis or emphysema predominates; the comparison is shown in Table 2.15.

Table 2.15 Lung function tests in chronic bronchitis and emphysema

	Chronic bronchitis	*Emphysema*
Forced vital capacity (FVC)	↓ (slight)	↓ (marked)
One second forced expiratory volume (FEV₁)	↓	normal
FEV₁/FVC ratio	↓ (<70%)	normal or ↑ (>70%)

This patient's own result is shown in Table 2.16 and clearly indicates an obstructive picture due to chronic bronchitis.

Table 2.16 Patient's lung function test result showing an obstructive picture

	Result	Ratio	Predicted normal (litres/second)
FEV$_1$ litres/sec	1.55		(3.54)
FVC litres/sec	3.50		(4.58)
FEV^1/FVC ratio		45%	

A simpler assessment of lung function can be carried out in general practice with a Wright Peak Flow Meter (Figure 2.7), since the peak expiratory flow rate (normal 400–500 litres/minute) is directly related to the degree of small airway obstruction.

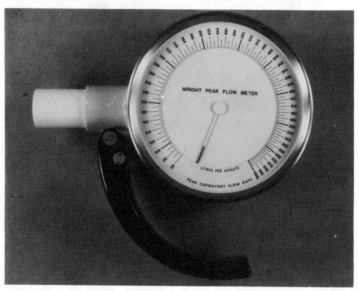

Figure 2.7 Wright Peak Flow Meter

The simplest test of all is with a stethoscope and watch, by which the duration of expiration (auscultated over the trachea) can be timed and should not normally exceed 4 seconds.

An additional use of expiratory duration or a flow rate test is to repeat the test after bronchodilatation, say with an aerosol bronchodilator, when improvement indicates that the small airway obstruction is reversible. This repeat testing can also be used as a simple objective measure of the efficacy of long term treatment in relieving small airway obstruction.

More complex respiratory tests can be done in a respiratory laboratory but are rarely of value in the management of chronic bronchitis or emphysema.

Blood gas measurement

This is an important objective test to detect respiratory failure, but is mainly used in hospital patients. Oxygen and carbon dioxide pressure are measured, as well as the pH of the blood. Respiratory failure leads to acidosis, carbon dioxide retention and anoxaemia. Changes in these levels with treatment form the most reliable measures of response to treatment.

The results in this patient are shown in Table 2.17, indicating anoxaemia, carbon dioxide retention and a mild acidosis. An increasing $P\text{CO}_2$ would suggest an urgent need for positive pressure ventilation.

Table 2.17 Patient's blood gas results showing acidosis, anoxaemia and carbon dioxide retention

	Result	Normal range
$P\text{O}_2$	6.0 kPa	12–15 kPa)
$P\text{CO}_2$	8.5 kPa	4.5–6 kPa)
pH	7.30	(7.35–7.45)

Blood count

Red cells

Chronic obstructive lung disease frequently leads to an increase in red cells secondary to hypoxaemia (secondary polycythaemia). This finding may be clinically relevant in two ways.

(1) It may increase blood viscosity and therefore impair perfusion of coronary, cerebral or peripheral blood vessels.

(2) It may be a therapeutic target in cor pulmonale when venesection would be of value.

White cells

There may be a *polymorph leukocytosis* with acute respiratory infection. If bronchial asthma is an important factor there may also be an *eosinophilia*.

Results

The patient's blood count is shown in Table 2.18 and indicates secondary polycythaemia with an increase in haemoglobin and packed cell volume, as well as a polymorph leukocytosis due to active infection.

Table 2.18 Patient's blood count showing secondary polycythaemia and polymorph leukocytosis

	Patient	Normal range
Hb	18.3	(12–16 g/dl)
Packed cell volume	53%	(45–50%)
WBC	12.7	($4–11 \times 10^9$/l)
polymorphs	83%	(40–75%)
Platelets	247	($150–400 \times 10^9$/l)

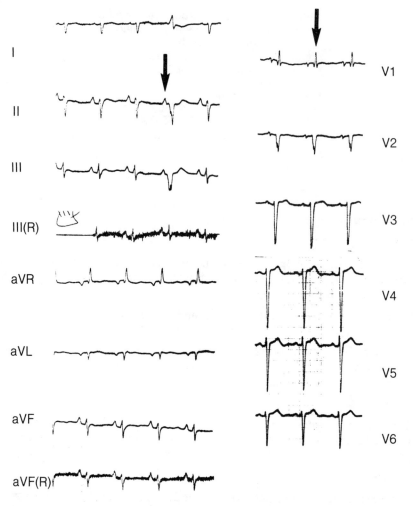

Figure 2.8 Patient's electrocardiogram showing right atrial and right ventricular hypertrophy

Sputum examination for pathogens

This is rarely of practical clinical value. Often no pathogens are found, but even if they are, the result becomes available too late for the start of treatment though it may help in its modification.

Electrocardiogram

This is of little diagnostic help. It is often normal in the early stages of chronic bronchitis. When pulmonary hypertension develops, tall peaked 'P' waves may be seen (P pulmonale) due to right atrial hypertrophy, and a tall R wave in lead VI may indicate right ventricular hypertrophy: this may be accompanied by S–T depression and T inversion in advanced right ventricular strain.

The patient's e.c.g. is shown in Figure 2.8 and indicates right atrial and right ventricular hypertrophy.

Another useful function of the e.c.g. is to detect a treatable arrhythmia, such as atrial fibrillation, which might improve cardiac function.

MANAGEMENT

The principles of management of chronic obstructive lung disease are listed in Table 2.19.

Table 2.19 Management of chronic bronchitis

• General measures	
• Specific measures	• infection
	• airway obstruction
	• anoxaemia
	• heart failure
• Rehabilitation	

General measures

Smoking

The most important single preventive measure is *complete abstinence from smoking*. Unfortunately, as every smoker, and every doctor, knows this is far easier said than done! Some practical suggestions which might help are given in Table 2.20. Although it is more effective, albeit more difficult, to stop smoking completely, sometimes this is beyond the ability and will-power of the patient. Other means of limiting the harmful effects of smoking are shown in Table 2.21.

Abstinence from smoking is equally important in primary and secondary prevention. Child smokers come from parent smokers and this relationship should be continually emphasized with the family.

There are other important factors which may aggravate the disease and therefore should be avoided as far as possible (Table 2.22).

Table 2.20   The role of the doctor and the patient in giving up smoking

Action by the doctor
- Explain the health risks in a simple and personally-relevant manner
- Emphasize the health, *and financial*, benefits of stopping
- Advise the patient on methods to stop smoking
- Constant reassurance that the health is improving
- Allay anxiety about subsequent gain in weight

Action by the patient
- Think about and accept reasons for stopping
- Decide to stop – then stop
- Get rid of cigarettes, lighters, ashtrays
- Change routine – do something else when craving occurs, e.g. washing up
- Ask help from family and friends to give up smoking also and not to offer temptations
- Chewing gum may help
- Constant self-reassurance about being less breathless, having less cough and having more money

Table 2.21   Helpful measures for smokers who cannot stop smoking

- Low tar/low nicotine cigarettes
- Smoking fewer cigarettes
- Less inhalation
- Fewer puffs
- Leaving a longer stub

Table 2.22   Factors other than smoking causing exacerbations of chronic bronchitis

- Contact with others in the 'flu' season
- Going out in cold, damp weather
- Fogs and smogs
- Sedatives and hypnotics
- Unnecessary operations involving anaesthetics

Obesity

Obesity may compromise an already deficient cardiorespiratory system. Like smoking, obesity is easy to give advice about but very difficult to control. High protein, low fat, low carbohydrate diets may be therapeutically desirable but are often too expensive for the chronically disabled out-of-work patient to buy. Perhaps all that the doctor can hope to achieve is to encourage the patient to reduce the overall intake of whatever food he is able to afford. The most important goal is not to put the patient on a temporary 'diet' but to alter the eating habits permanently.

Depression

The severe and frustrating disability in these patients may understandably lead to *depressive state*. An optimistic outlook from the doctor may do more good than psychotropic drugs which should anyway be avoided because of the possibility of respiratory depression.

Medical supervision

Periodic supervision by the family doctor may be of value. It offers the opportunity of detecting early signs of cor pulmonale, which could be treated with diuretics, as well as checking for infected sputum necessitating a further course of antibiotics, since many patients with chronic bronchitis are very remiss in seeking medical aid on the basis of sputum colour change alone. Additionally, an encouraging and optimistic expression of progress may be of considerable value to the patient and his family.

Home Nursing Service

The home nursing service may also be helpful to the housebound patient and his family (Table 2.23).

Table 2.23   Help offered by home nursing service

- Bathing or washing
- Check correct medication taken, give injections if necessary
- Show correct use and hazards of oxygen administration
- Breathing exercises and postural drainage at request of the doctor
- Assess chiropody needs and arrange provision of aids, e.g. back-rests, walking sticks, commodes
- Enlist help of other required services, e.g. for adaptation of bathroom or toilet

Social services

A social services worker also has a part to play in home management of these patients and can offer useful advice and help (Table 2.24).

Table 2.24   Help offered by social services worker

- Finance counselling with limited budget
- Advice on welfare rights

    attendance allowance
    mobility allowance
    heating allowances

- Arrange for home-help
- Arrange meals-on-wheels or attendance at a luncheon club
- Attendance at a day care centre with appropriate transport
- Arrange 'night-sitters' if necessary
- Assess housing facilities and investigate rehousing if necessary

Specific treatment

Infection

The most frequent pathogens causing an acute on chronic bronchitis are *Haemophilus influenzae* and *Streptococcus pneumoniae*. Therefore, a broad-spectrum antibiotic such as *ampicillin* or *tetracycline* should be started promptly. If this fails to clear the infection within 4 or 5 days, as indicated by change from green or yellow sputum to white or grey, a change to *co-trimoxazole* (Septrin) is often helpful. Continued failure to respond would suggest the need for sputum examination for more specific guidance on choice of subsequent antibiotic.

Small airway obstruction

The obstruction to the bronchioles in chronic bronchitis is due to several factors, some of which are reversible and some not (Table 2.25).

Table 2.25   Small airway obstruction in chronic bronchitis

• Reversible	• mucosal oedema and inflammation
	• mucus
	• bronchospasm
• Irreversible	• loss of lung elasticity (emphysema)
	• bronchiolar fibrosis and stenosis

Mucosal inflammation and oedema are best controlled with antibiotics.

Obstruction by *mucus* may be helped by deep breathing exercise and some gentle tapping over the lung bases by a spouse or other relative.

Cough mixtures are widely used. These are of two types – *expectorants* to encourage the production of sputum and *linctuses* to suppress the cough.

Although there is no scientific evidence that an expectorant mixture increases the production of sputum, the belief among patients that it is effective in bronchitis is very strong. It may therefore be useful to prescribe a harmless expectorant mixture for its role as a placebo. Some of the cough medicines in current use in the British National Formulary (BNF) are shown in Table 2.26. There is also a very large variety of compound proprietary medicines, often based on the preparations shown in Table 2.26.

Table 2.26   Common expectorant cough medicines in the BNF

• Ammonium chloride mixture
• Guaiphenesin
• Ipecacuanha
• Squill

Cough suppressants are often based on a belief in the demulcent effect of a linctus containing syrup or glycerol in relieving a dry irritating cough. A simple linctus is both harmless and inexpensive and may also have a useful role as a placebo. More potent and effective cough suppressants such as codeine and pholcodine are commonly prescribed for suppression of cough in acute and chronic bronchitis. Such treatment is seldom necessary if antibacterial therapy is started promptly. Perhaps the use of a cough suppressant may be justified when sleep is constantly disturbed by a dry irritant cough. An unfortunate side-effect with these drugs is constipation. Like expectorant mixtures, there are many proprietary linctuses from which to choose.

One of the simplest measures, and perhaps one of the most effective, in loosening sputum is inhalation of steam using a jug of hot water and towel. Some added compound benzoin tincture may be of value, not least as a placebo.

Some degree of *bronchospasm* is often present and it is always worth trying a *bronchodilator*. The most effective preparations are the *aerosol inhalations* (Table 2.27). Isoprenaline should be avoided because of a potential fatal reaction if used excessively.

Table 2.27 Bronchodilator aerosols

• β-Receptor stimulants	• salbutamol
	• terbutaline
	• rimiterol
	• fenoterol
• Sympathomimetic	• isoprenaline
	• orciprenaline
• Anticholinergic	• ipratropium

Oral bronchodilator preparations are also widely used but less effective than the aerosols (Table 2.28).

Table 2.28 Oral bronchodilators

• Aminophylline tablets	100–300 mg repeated as necessary
• Choline theophyllinate	200 mg t.d.s.
• Proxyphylline	300 mg t.d.s.
	600 mg at night
• Theophylline	60–200 mg t.d.s.

In a chronic bronchitic patient with resistant small airway obstruction shown by persistent rhonchi, it may be worth trying a *steroid preparation* since it sometimes produces an unexpected improvement. It may do this either by relaxing bronchospasm or by aiding the resolution of mucosal oedema. Steroids may be given either in *aerosol form* which is associated with minimal systemic absorption and therefore side-effects, or as oral tablets in the more severe case (Table 2.29).

Table 2.29 Steroid use in chronic bronchitis

• Aerosol	• beclomethasone	100 μg (2 puffs) q.d.s.
	• betamethasone	100 μg (1 puff) q.d.s.
• Oral prednisolone		10 mg t.d.s. to start
		Reduce by 5 mg each day

Cromoglycate (Intal), an antiallergic drug, is sometimes tried in patients in whom the small airway obstruction is completely resistant to all other measures. It is rarely of value.

Anoxaemia

Oxygen administration is of considerable value in severe anoxaemia. Inspired oxygen concentration must be kept at no more than 24–28%, otherwise the anoxic stimulus which keeps the respiratory centre functioning is removed and respiratory failure follows. This is achieved by using a Venturi mask to give the oxygen.

Domiciliary oxygen is available and of considerable benefit to the severely dyspnoeic patient. Portable oxygen equipment is being developed to allow increased mobility but is, as yet, not wholly satisfactory. Although continuous administration of oxygen for at least 15 hours each 24 hours has been shown to retard the development of pulmonary hypertension and therefore overt right heart failure, the practical aspects of achieving this make it unlikely to be of significant clinical benefit to the patient.

Heart failure

Diuretic treatment
The mainstay of treatment in cor pulmonale is diuretics. A mild diuretic, such as a thiazide, is unlikely to be of value in florid right ventricular failure so it is advisable to use a *loop diuretic* such as frusemide or ethacrynic acid (Figure 2.9). Particular attention should be paid to *hypokalaemia* induced by these potent diuretics, and it is usually best to give supplementary potassium, in the form of 'Slow K' or effervescent potassium, or use an additional potassium-retaining diuretic, such as amiloride or triamterene. Hypokalaemia may be recognized clinically by excessive fatigue or by cardiac arrhythmia, especially if the patient is also being treated with digoxin.

The best simple objective test of response of heart failure to diuretic treatment is progressive loss of body weight.

Digoxin
Digoxin is of limited value in the treatment of cor pulmonale with sinus rhythm. This is probably because the cardiac output is usually normal or high in spite of the heart failure. There is also a potential hazard in using digoxin: with the improvement in the respiratory acidosis with treatment of the cor pulmonale and the effects of the diuretic used in that treatment, the serum

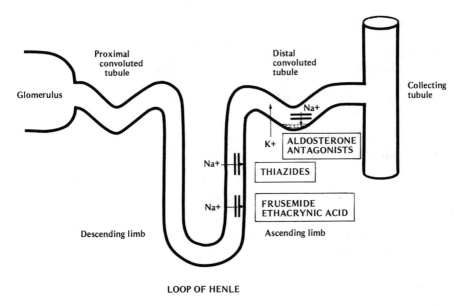

LOOP OF HENLE

THIAZIDES PREVENT Na+ ABSORPTION IN ASCENDING LIMB
FRUSEMIDE AND ETHACRYNIC ACID PREVENT Na+ ABSORPTION IN ASCENDING LIMB
ALDOSTERONE ANTAGONISTS ACT ON DISTAL TUBULE AND PREVENT K+ EXCRETION.

Figure 2.9   Site of action of various diuretics in the kidney

potassium tends to fall and facilitate the development of arrhythmias.

The only real indication for digoxin in cor pulmonale is when there is an associated atrial fibrillation requiring control of the ventricular rate.

Salt restriction
Dietary salt restriction should always be tried in cor pulmonale. At the least, this means no added salt with the cooked food, which reduces daily salt intake to 3–5 g. Avoiding salt altogether in the cooking reduces salt intake to 0.5–1 g daily, but the food is unpalatable and this measure is therefore unlikely to be of much practical value.

Venesection
This is only useful as an emergency measure in the acute treatment of severe cor pulmonale when the patient is polycythaemic with a high haemoglobin and packed cell volume.

One or 2 pints (0.5–1.0 litres) of blood may be removed, and can result in immediate relief of the heart failure. The procedure is of no significant value in the long term management of the condition since secondary polycythaemia in these patients is a compensatory mechanism for the hypoxaemia; venesection would therefore be counterproductive.

Left ventricular failure

Diuretic treatment is the most important factor in managing the patient's left ventricular failure, and salt restriction may help here also. The place of digoxin in the long term treatment of left ventricular failure with sinus rhythm remains controversial. It is, however, always worth trying in those patients who fail to respond adequately to diuretics alone.

REHABILITATION

Retraining

Retraining a severely incapacitated chronic bronchitic patient unable to continue his work because of the physical effort involved is possible with the help of government retraining courses. However, the likelihood of return to suitable alternative gainful work is small. Demoralization is therefore common in these patients and leads to depression. This requires constant encouragement and maintenance of interest by the doctor.

Exercise

A programme of gradually increasing exercise, mainly walking, may be of some value in the less-disabled patients. Although exercise does not improve lung function, it may train skeletal muscle to function more efficiently and so improve exercise tolerance. Supplementary oxygen may be of help during the exercise programme to allow it to continue.

Breathing exercises

Regular breathing exercises, using diaphragmatic muscles, may also be beneficial by averting bronchiolar blockage by retained secretions.

NATURAL HISTORY OF CHRONIC BRONCHITIS

Prevalence

Chronic bronchitis is a common condition in the United Kingdom and affects about 20% of adults over 45 years of age.

Age incidence

Symptoms of chronic bronchitis usually begin in the 40s and 50s, and the condition is characterized by a long and chronic course which may span 20–40 years. Some 30000 patients die of this disease annually in the UK, most over the age of 65 years.

Disability

The degree of disability is variable (Figure 2.10); approximately one half of the patients will be minimally affected, with very little functional disability;

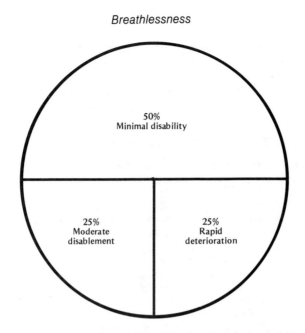

Breathlessness

50%
Minimal disability

25%
Moderate
disablement

25%
Rapid
deterioration

Figure 2.10   Degree of disability in chronic bronchitis

one quarter will be *moderately disabled* with restriction of work and leisure activities; one quarter will deteriorate rapidly and die within 5–10 years of the onset of symptoms.

Prognosis

The prognosis and the amount of incapacity depend very much on the degree of impairment of respiratory function, and the FEV_1 is a good and simple objective guide (Table 2.30).

Table 2.30 FEV_1 related to disability and prognosis

FEV_1	Disability	Median survival (years)
> 1.5 litres	Little	> 10
1.25–1.5 litres	Dyspnoea on moderate exertion	10
1 litre	Sedentary existence	5
500 ml or less	Severely immobilized	2

Patients with predominant emphysema ('pink-puffers') are less prone to recurrent acute respiratory infections than those with predominant chronic bronchitis ('blue-bloaters'), but when infections do occur, they are more likely to lead to respiratory failure and even death. In contrast, patients with predominant chronic bronchitis experience many episodes of acute respiratory infection, often with respiratory failure, and have a striking ability to recover.

The occurrence of cor pulmonale will have a very adverse effect on the prognosis and most patients will die within 2–3 years of its onset.

CAN WE MODIFY THE NATURAL HISTORY?

The relevant factors contributing to the development of chronic bronchitis and emphysema are shown in Table 2.31.

Table 2.31 Contributory factors in the development of chronic obstructive lung disease

- Age – 40s and over
- Sex – more frequent in males
- Familial predisposition
- Social class – more frequent in Class V
- Cigarette smoking
- Recurrent respiratory infection
- Air pollution
- Occupation
- Climatic factors

Age, sex, family

Age, sex and familial predisposition cannot be altered.

Social class

It is possible to improve social class – e.g. the unskilled labourer in Class V may move upwards – but it is difficult, and it remains to be convincingly demonstrated that an improvement in social class leads to a reduced incidence of chronic bronchitis.

Smoking

The most important remediable factor is cigarette smoking, both for primary prevention of the disease and in retarding the deterioration of the established disease.

Respiratory infection

Rapid control of the repeated acute respiratory infections with antibiotics will do much to reduce progressive lung damage. It may well be desirable to give an advance supply of an appropriate antibiotic to patients with instructions to use immediately on their own initiative whenever they suspect an acute respiratory tract infection; the best indication of this is a change of sputum colour from white or grey to green or yellow.

There is little evidence that continuous prophylactic long term antibiotics are of much value in preventing recurrent respiratory infections.

Air pollution

Air pollution is probably an important factor in chronic bronchitis and includes pollution from domestic fuel as well as that from industrial effluents and car exhausts. Additionally, pollution can occur in the occupational environment such as the coal mine. Control of these types of pollution are best achieved by statutory measures such as a Clean Air Act, effective control of car emission fumes, efficient dust exhaust and collection systems and the use of masks in dusty occupations. Regular monitoring of the contamination in the environmental air is also highly desirable.

Occupation

Although occupations can be changed, financial pressures to continue may be a paramount factor.

Climatic factors

Although a climate with damp, fogs and smogs is adverse to the chronic bronchitic, any move to a more suitable climate is for the vast majority of patients more likely to be in the realms of fantasy than of fact.

USEFUL PRACTICAL POINTS IN CHRONIC BRONCHITIS

- The most important single factor in both primary and secondary prevention of chronic bronchitis is abstinence from cigarette smoking.

- The 'Pink Puffer' (predominant emphysema) is less likely to develop recurrent respiratory infections, respiratory failure and right heart failure, than the 'Blue Bloater' (predominant chronic bronchitis), and therefore has a better prognosis.

- Patients with chronic bronchitis may develop attacks of paroxysmal nocturnal dyspnoea which can be distinguished from left ventricular failure by the symptoms and signs as well as the rapid response to bronchodilatation. The two conditions may exist together.

- The basic principles of treatment of chronic bronchitis are stopping smoking, control of infection with antibiotics, control of small airway obstruction with bronchodilators and steroids, improvement in anoxaemia with 24–28% oxygen, and treatment of right ventricular failure (cor pulmonale) with diuretics.

- Any hypnotic or respiratory depressant drug can cause lethal respiratory failure in a 'Blue Bloater'.

3

High blood pressure

PRESENT HISTORY

A 51-year old male electrician was referred to hospital by his general practitioner with a 12 month history of high blood pressure poorly controlled on treatment.

High blood pressure

The high blood pressure apparently started when he had 'nephritis' 20 years previously. He had received intermittent treatment for the blood pressure since then, but he admitted he had not bothered much with seeing his doctor.

About 1 year ago, he began to get severe throbbing *headache* at the back of his head especially on waking in the morning. He had not noticed any visual disturbance or vomiting with the headache. His doctor had found his blood pressure high again, at 200/130, and treated him first with methyldopa and subsequently added atenolol.

His headaches improved somewhat with treatment, but his blood pressure control had remained unsatisfactory and he was therefore referred to hospital for specialist advice.

Other relevant facts on direct enquiry

Chest pain

He admitted to occasional attacks of stabbing pain around the left breast which had been present for about a year – in fact since he had been told that his blood pressure was high again. There was no relation to exertion, meals or posture. The discomfort would last for a few seconds and was usually accompanied by a 'flutter over his heart', by which he meant several forceful heart beats.

Breathlessness

He thought that he was becoming rather breathless on exertion for the past few months. He was able, however, to sleep comfortably on two pillows and never awakened with acute breathlessness in the night.

Dizziness

He had occasional dizziness for the past year. This would consist of a feeling of faintness or lightheadedness which usually occurred on getting out of bed. He did not have any feeling of rotation of his surrounding, or himself, and there was no 'ringing' in his ears when he felt dizzy. He had also noticed that sudden movements of his head could result in transitory dizziness. He denied any neck pain.

Pain in the legs

For the previous 6 months he had experienced pain in the calves on walking. The right leg was worse than the left. Initially, the pain had occurred only on going uphill, but more recently it had developed while walking on the level, especially if he was hurrying.

Urinary symptoms

The only symptom was occasional discomfort in the left loin when he drank more fluid than usual, especially at weekends when he would go out for a few pints of beer.

He had not had any swelling of his feet or ankles since his attack of 'nephritis'.

Cough

He had a 'smoker's cough' with white or grey phlegm most mornings. This had been present for at least 20 years.

He also admitted frequent 'chest colds' in the winter, and often had to have antibiotic treatment.

Past history

He had suffered *sore throats* as a child.

He had an attack of 'nephritis' when he was about 31 years old. During the attack he was 'swollen all over'. He could not remember passing blood in his urine.

He was admitted to hospital for about 6 weeks, and his blood pressure had been found high during his inpatient stay. He subsequently attended the medical outpatient department for about 1 year. He was then told that his kidneys had settled down and his blood pressure had become normal. He was discharged and advised to keep in touch with his GP.

Family history

His father had high blood pressure and died of a stroke when he was 73 years old. His mother, aged 72 years, suffers from mild Parkinson's disease. He had two brothers and one sister, all of whom were well.

Personal history

He smoked 25–30 cigarettes daily for the past 30 years. He drank moderately, usually at weekends – 5–6 pints (3–3.5 litres) of beer.

Drug history

His current treatment comprised methyldopa 500 mg q.d.s. and atenolol 100 mg once daily, which he had taken for 1 year. He admitted that over the years he had been given various drugs for his blood pressure but had not been very good at taking the tablets as he felt so well and did not think that the tablets were necessary.

EXAMINATION

General

The abnormal signs are shown in Figure 3.1.
The patient had a plethoric appearance but he was not overweight.
There was no arcus senilis or xanthelasma.

Cardiovascular system

He was not dyspnoeic. The neck veins were not distended and there was no oedema of the legs.

The pulse was 56/min and regular. The radial artery was thickened but the brachial artery was not tortuous.

The blood pressure was 190/130 (lying) and 180/125 (standing). There was no difference between the two arms.

The apex beat was displaced to the left in the anterior axillary line, and was a sustained forceful thrust. There was no parasternal lift. The heart sounds were not palpable and there were no thrills.

There was a presystolic (fourth heart sound) triple rhythm at the apex, and a blowing midsystolic murmur conducted out to the axilla. The aortic second sound was loud.

The arterial pulses in the lower limbs are shown in Table 3.1.

The right foot was colder than the left. There were no ulcers and no obvious loss of hair in the right leg.

Respiratory system

There were persistent fine crepitations at both lung bases which did not clear on coughing.

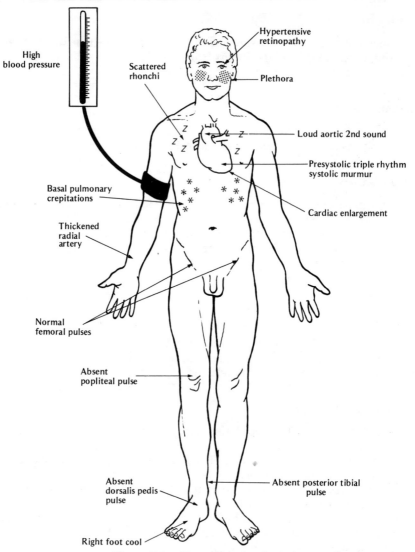

Figure 3.1 Abnormal physical signs

Table 3.1 The patient's arterial pulses

	Right	Left
Femoral	+	+
Popliteal	−	+
Posterior tibial	−	+
Dorsalis pedis	−	+

There were occasional scattered high-pitched rhonchi during inspiration and expiration.

Abdomen

No abnormality was detected. In particular, the kidneys were not palpable and there were no renal murmurs.

Central nervous system

Fundal examination showed that the arterioles were narrowed with well-marked arteriovenous nipping.

There were no haemorrhages or exudates.

No other abnormality was found in the nervous system.

There were no carotid murmurs.

Cervical spine

There was restriction of lateral flexion of the neck in both directions. The other movements were free and painless.

ANALYSIS OF THE HISTORY

Hypertension

This was the main presenting problem.

The first consideration is whether the hypertension is primary (essential) or secondary to some other cause.

Essential hypertension

In 90–95% of patients presenting with hypertension, the cause is unknown.

The most useful clue in the aetiology of essential hypertension is a positive family history. If both parents are hypertensive, the incidence in the offspring is 50%; if one parent is affected, the incidence is 25%.

The patient's father had hypertension. Essential hypertension remains, therefore, a possible diagnosis.

Secondary hypertension

An underlying cause for the hypertension is more likely in younger patients. The causes of secondary hypertension are shown in Figure 3.2.

Table 3.2 Features of acute glomerulo-tubular nephritis

• Previous sore throat
• Hypertension
• Generalized oedema
• Haematuria
• Oliguria

Renal disease

This is the most frequent cause of secondary hypertension.

The features of acute *glomerulo-tubular nephritis* are shown in Table 3.2.

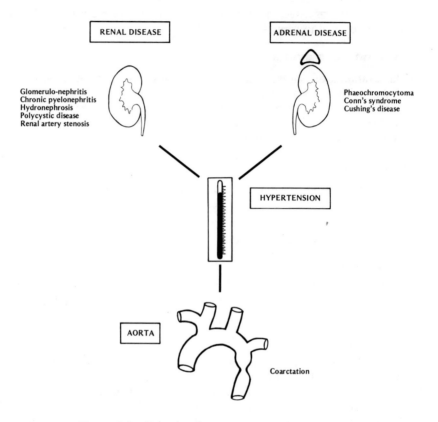

Figure 3.2 Causes of secondary hypertension

The patient's past history of sore throat, generalized oedema and hypertension strongly suggests this diagnosis. In 10% of patients with acute nephritis, proteinuria persists and after some years chronic glomerulo-tubular nephritis, hypertension and renal failure develop. This may be the case in this patient.

Chronic pyelonephritis is the renal disease found most often to be associated with secondary hypertension. The history is usually of repeated attacks of frequency, dysuria and loin pain. Sometimes these symptoms are minimal though chronic pyelonephritis is developing.

There were no symptoms of pyelonephritis in the patient.

Hydronephrosis due to obstructive uropathy may present in various ways (Table 3.3).

Table 3.3 Symptoms of hydronephrosis

- Recurrent urinary tract infection
- Difficulty in micturition
- Colicky pain from loin to groin
- Constant dull ache in renal angle
- Symptoms of uraemia

The only symptom experienced by the patient, which might be relevant, is the mild discomfort in the left loin when his fluid intake was high.

Polycystic disease may also present in various ways (Table 3.4).

Table 3.4 Presentation of polycystic disease

• Usual	• Hypertension
	• Haematuria
	• Uraemia
• Unusual	• Pain in renal angles
	• Abdominal swelling

The lack of a family history of polycystic disease, and the absence of the other symptoms, apart from hypertension, makes this diagnosis unlikely, though abdominal examination is necessary to exclude the diagnosis.

Renal artery stenosis does not cause any symptoms directly, and diagnosis is suggested on auscultation of the renal arteries.

Endocrine disease

All the endocrine disorders that may cause secondary hypertension are rare.

Pheochromocytoma is due to a tumour of the adrenal medulla resulting in excessive secretion of adrenaline and noradrenaline. The typical features of this are shown in Table 3.5. These symptoms occur in attacks and are associated with paroxysmal or sustained hypertension.

None of these symptoms was evident in the patient.

Conn's syndrome (primary hyperaldosteronism) is due to a tumour of the

Table 3.5 Clinical features of pheochromocytoma

- Throbbing headache
- Excessive sweating
- Palpitations
- Tremor
- Pallor
- Feeling of apprehension
- Angina may occur

adrenal cortex producing an excess of aldosterone. The features are shown in Table 3.6.

Table 3.6 Clinical features of Conn's syndrome

- Episode of weakness due to hypokalaemia
- Polyuria
- Polydipsia
- Oedema – rare
- Tetany – rare (due to hypokalaemic alkalosis)

Cushing's syndrome may be due either to a pituitary basophil adenoma or to primary adrenal disease (hyperplasia or carcinoma). The symptoms which occur as a result of the various disorders in Cushing's syndrome are shown in Table 3.7. There were no symptoms to suggest Cushing's syndrome.

Table 3.7 Clinical features of Cushing's syndrome

- Obesity
- Muscle weakness
- Backache
- Spontaneous bruising
- Mental   – depression
- Females   – hirsuties
                       acne
                       baldness
                       amenorrhoea
- Diabetes – thirst
                       polyuria
                       loss of weight

Coarctation of the aorta

This does not produce any symptoms. Diagnosis is made primarily by clinical examination.

Headache

Headache is frequent in patients with hypertension. It often begins after the patient has been told that his blood pressure is high, and is then undoubtedly due to anxiety. For hypertension to cause a headache, the level of blood pressure must be very high (diastolic pressure at least 125 mmHg), and therefore a true hypertensive headache is most commonly seen in malignant hypertension and hypertensive encephalopathy.

The distinction between a hypertensive headache and an anxiety headache is shown in Table 3.8.

The features of the patient's headache indicate a true hypertensive headache.

Table 3.8 Distinction between a hypertensive headache and a functional headache

	Hypertension	Functional
Type	Throbbing	'Band-like', pressure fullness, bursting
Site	Occipital	Often at vertex
		Occasionally occipital
Timing	Early in morning	Any time
		Often with emotional stress
Duration	Several hours	Hours, days, weeks or months

Another important cause of a throbbing vascular headache is migraine, but this is often associated with visual disturbances (fortification spectra, visual field defects) and nausea or vomiting.

Chest pain

The characteristics of the patient's chest pain indicate a functional origin associated with anxiety. The 'flutter' associated with the pain suggests ectopic beats, which are also common in anxiety.

Breathlessness

The recent breathlessness could be due to left ventricular failure or to chronic bronchitis, or to both conditions.

The distinction between these two causes of breathlessness can be difficult and Table 3.9 shows some helpful distinguishing features.

Table 3.9 Differentiation between cardiac and pulmonary dyspnoea

Cardiac	Pulmonary
More on exertion	More at rest
No wheezing	Wheezing common
(unless acute pulmonary oedema)	
Chest infection uncommon	Chest infection frequent

Dizziness

The occurrence of the dizziness on getting out of bed suggests postural hypotension due to antihypertensive treatment.

The timing of the dizziness is related to the reduction of circulating blood volume, a normal physiological change in the morning. The lowered blood volume will enhance the hypotensive effect of any hypotensive drug, and not just the peripheral vasodilators.

The relationship of the dizziness to sudden head movement indicates

69

cervical spondylosis, with compression of the vertebral arteries in the vertebral canal with movement of the cervical spine.

The absence of vertigo, tinnitus and a past history of deafness excludes a labyrinthine cause for the dizziness.

Calf pain on walking

This indicates intermittent claudication due to peripheral arterial disease.

In addition to the hypertension the heavy cigarette smoking is an important contributory factor in causing the peripheral arteriosclerosis.

Cough

The chronic morning cough with white or grey sputum indicates chronic bronchitis. This is defined for epidemiological purposes as a chronic productive cough on consecutive days for 2 months for at least 2 years.

Past history

The patient had features suggesting acute glomerulo-tubular nephritis (Table 3.2). This has already been discussed.

Although complete recovery occurs in the majority of patients with loss of the hypertension, 10% will go on to chronic nephritis with hypertension.

This remains a likely diagnosis.

Family history

The only relevant factor was his father's hypertension which suggests the possibility of the patient inheriting essential hypertension.

Personal history

The cigarette smoking is a highly relevant factor in the development of intermittent claudication. Possible mechanisms are shown in Table 3.10.

Table 3.10   Possible mechanisms of arterial damage caused by cigarettes

• Damage to arterial wall by carbon monoxide
• Reduced levels of 'protective' circulating high-density lipoproteins
• Release of catecholamines – increase in blood pressure   increased platelet aggregation

CONCLUSIONS FROM THE HISTORY

- He has severe hypertension.

- The origin may be either essential (positive family history) or secondary to renal disease (chronic nephritis or hydronephrosis).

- He has chronic bronchitis due to smoking.

- He has intermittent claudication due to smoking.

- His chest pain is functional.

- His breathlessness may be due to the chronic bronchitis or left ventricular failure secondary to hypertension, or both.

- He has vertebrobasilar insufficiency associated with cervical spondylosis.

ANALYSIS OF THE EXAMINATION

Plethoric appearance

There may be several possible associations between hypertension and a plethoric appearance (Table 3.11)

Table 3.11   Plethoric appearance in hypertension

• Cushing's syndrome	
• Polycythaemia	– primary
	secondary
• Steroid treatment	
• Renal disease	– hydronephrosis
• Hepatic disease	– hepatoma

Cushing's syndrome is rare in males. Also, the patient had none of the other typical signs of Cushing's syndrome (Figure 3.3).

The features of primary *polycythaemia rubra vera* are shown in Figure 3.4. Apart from the hypertension and plethoric face no features were present in the patient to suggest primary polycythaemia.

Secondary polycythaemia can result from chronic bronchitis, but the degree of disability in the patient appears inadequate to lead to secondary polycythaemia. A blood count will decide.

The patient had not been taking *steroids*.

Secondary polycythaemia is a rare complication of *hydronephrosis*.

The only symptom which may give some support to this diagnosis is the loin discomfort after excessive fluid intake. This diagnosis therefore remains possible.

Hepatoma is usually preceeded by cirrhosis, and there was nothing in the history or on examination to suggest this diagnosis in the patient. Liver enlargement also results from malignant change and this was not found in the patient.

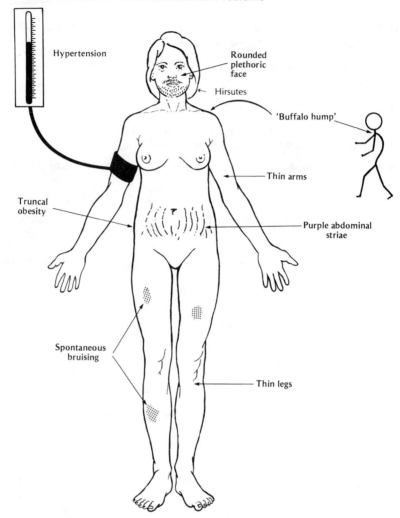

Hypertension

Rounded
plethoric
face

Hirsutes

'Buffalo hump'

Thin arms

Truncal
obesity

Purple abdominal
striae

Spontaneous
bruising

Thin legs

Figure 3.3 Typical signs of Cushing's disease

Cardiovascular system

The slow pulse indicates adequate β-blockade by the atenolol.

The patient has a severe degree of hypertension. The equality of the blood pressure levels in both arms excludes unilateral arterial obstruction affecting the subclavian artery; it will also exclude the less common types of coarctation of the aorta in which the narrowing occurs between the left common carotid artery and the left subclavian artery (Figure 3.5).

The displaced sustained forceful apex beat indicates left ventricular hypertrophy due to the hypertension.

The presystolic triple rhythm is due to the addition of the fourth heart sound.

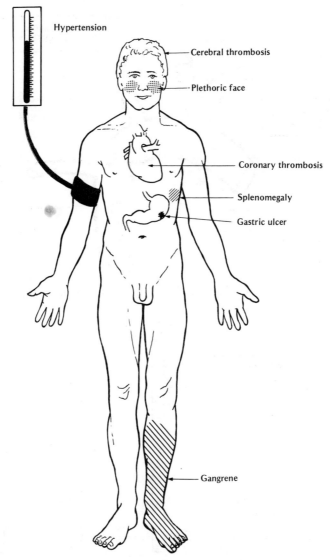

Figure 3.4 Features of polycythaemia rubra vera

The other types of gallop rhythm are shown in Figure 3.6. The causes of gallop rhythm are shown in Table 3.12.

In the patient's case the presystolic gallop is due to left ventricular strain, caused by the hypertension.

The loud aortic second sound is due to the hypertension.

The apical systolic murmur conducted to the axilla suggests mitral incompetence, the causes of which are shown in Table 3.13. The likely cause in

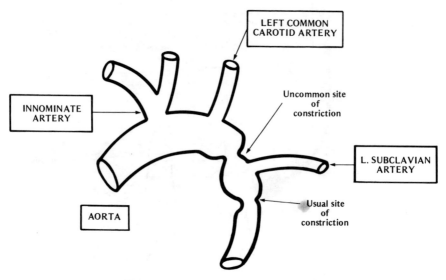

Figure 3.5 Sites of coarctation of the aorta

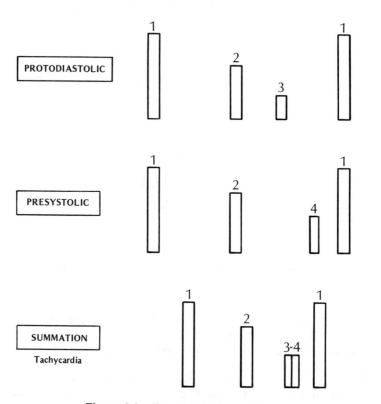

Figure 3.6 Types of gallop rhythm

Table 3.12 Causes of gallop rhythm

• Protodiastolic (3rd heart sound)	• Normal in young people • Left to right shunts • Mitral regurgitation • Left or right heart failure
• Presystolic (4th heart sound)	• Hypertension • Aortic or pulmonary stenosis • Anginal attack

Table 3.13 Causes of mitral regurgitation

• Organic	– Rheumatic heart disease Rupture of papillary muscle Infective endocarditis
• Functional	– Dilatation of mitral valve ring

the patient is dilatation of the mitral valve ring as a result of the hypertensive left ventricular enlargement and early heart failure.

Respiratory system

The fine crepitations at the lung bases suggest pulmonary congestion due to early left ventricular failure. The scattered rhonchi are caused by the chronic bronchitis.

Arteriosclerotic changes

The diagnosis of arteriosclerosis is based on the changes shown in Table 3.14.

Table 3.14 Diagnosis of arteriosclerosis in the patient

• Thickened radial artery
• Absent peripheral pulses in the right leg
• Changes in fundal arterioles

The absence of arterial pulsation in the right leg from the popliteal artery downwards indicates that the obstructive lesion is likely to be in the femoral canal, a common site of atherosclerosis leading to intermittent claudication.

Fundi

Four grades of retinopathy due to hypertension are usually recognized (Figure 3.7).

75

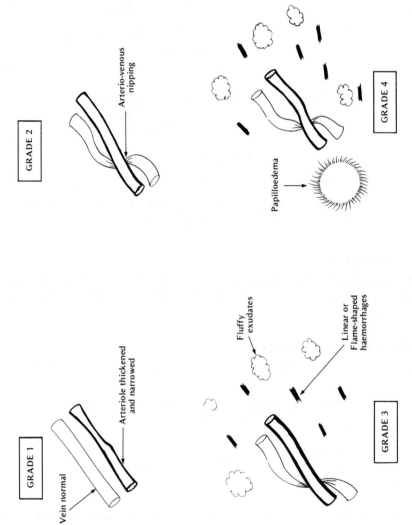

Figure 3.7 Grades of hypertensive retinopathy

The patient had narrowed arterioles with arteriovenous nipping, which indicates Grade 2 *hypertensive retinopathy*.

CONCLUSIONS FROM THE EXAMINATION

- The severe hypertension was confirmed.

- The absence of grade III or IV fundal changes excludes malignant hypertension.

- He had left ventricular strain associated with mitral incompetence, probably functional.

- He has arterial obstruction in the right leg, probably in the femoral artery or its deep branch.

- The lung signs indicate chronic bronchitis and mild left ventricular failure.

- The cause of his plethoric appearance was not evident from the examination.

- There were no other signs to suggest a renal or other primary cause for his high blood pressure.

INVESTIGATIONS

Chest X-ray

This is an important and necessary test in hypertension, primarily to detect cardiac enlargement which has an adverse effect on prognosis.

The typical picture of left ventricular enlargement is shown in the patient's chest X-ray in Figure 3.8.

The chest X-ray may also help in the diagnosis of coarctation of the aorta. The typical change is notching along the inferior margins of the ribs due to the erosive effect of the enlarged pulsating anastomotic intercostal arteries (Figure 3.9).

One other important finding in the chest X-ray in a hypertensive patient is pulmonary venous congestion as a result of left ventricular failure (Figure 3.10).

Electrocardiogram

The e.c.g. gives an accurate indication of left ventricular hypertrophy with or without strain. This is also very relevant in assessing the prognosis in a hypertensive patient.

The changes in hypertension are listed in Table 3.15. The most reliable guide to left ventricular hypertrophy is to add the R wave in V5–V6 (whichever is larger) to the S wave in V1 – if the sum exceeds 35 mm in a middle-aged or elderly patient, then left ventricular hypertrophy is present.

With more serious cardiac enlargement due to hypertension, S–T

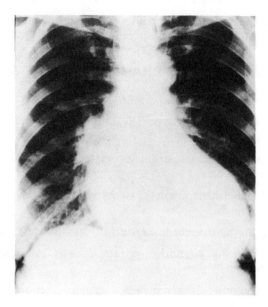

Figure 3.8   Chest X-ray showing left ventricular enlargement

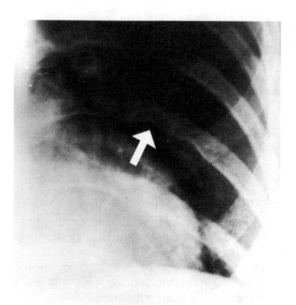

Figure 3.9   Chest X-ray showing rib notching in coarctation of aorta

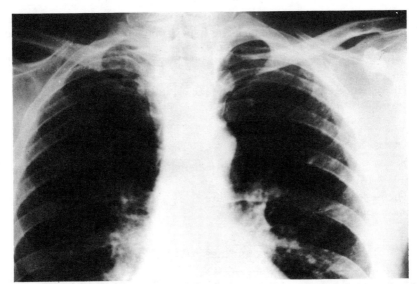

Figure 3.10 Chest X-ray showing congestion of the upper lobe veins in early left ventricular failure

Table 3.15 Electrocardiogram changes in hypertension

- Left axis deviation
- Tall R waves in V5–V6
- Deep S waves in V1
- S–T depression and T inversion V5–V6 (strain pattern)
- Bifid P wave – left atrial hypertrophy

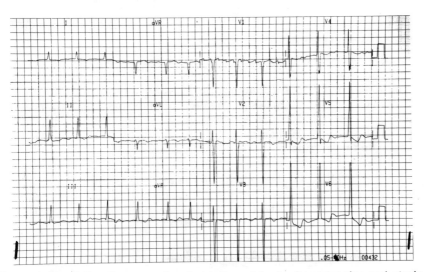

Figure 3.11 Patient's e.c.g. showing left ventricular hypertrophy and strain

79

depression and T inversion occur in the anterior leads (I, aV1, V5–V6). This probably represents ischaemia in the hypertrophied left ventricular muscle which has outstripped its blood supply.

Left atrial hypertrophy occurs only with marked left ventricular hypertrophy.

The patient's e.c.g., shown in Figure 3.11, indicates left ventricular hypertrophy and strain.

Urine examination

This is a useful test in hypertensive patients and may help in various ways (Table 3.16).

The patient's e.c.g., shown in Figure 3.11, indicates left ventricular hyper-disease, but no red cells or casts.

Table 3.16   Urine abnormalities in relation to the hypertension

• Proteinuria	– parenchymal renal disease
• Casts	
• Hyaline	– normal
	chronic glomero-tubular nephritis
• Granular	– degeneration of renal tubules
• Red cells	– acute glomerulo-tubular nephritis
	malignant hypertension
	polycystic disease
• Pus cells	– pyelonephritis
• Pathogenic bacteria	– pyelonephritis

Intravenous pyelogram

There is no place for a routine intravenous pyelogram (ivp) in the management of hypertension.

The specific indications for an ivp are shown in Table 3.17.

An ivp was carried out in this patient because of the past history of nephritis and the discomfort in the left loin with excessive fluid intake. The result is shown in Figure 3.12. He had gross hydronephrosis, hydro-ureter and cortical atrophy on the left side.

Table 3.17   Indications for an i.v.p in hypertension

• Young patient – ?secondary hypertension
• Past history of kidney disease
• Current urinary symptoms
• Examination – large kidney(s)
• Resistant to treatment

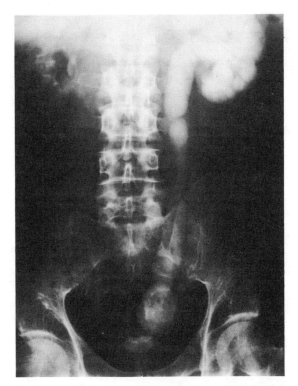

Figure 3.12   Patient's i.v.p. showing gross left-sided hydronephrosis

The renal disease could certainly account for the patient's hypertension by activation of the renin–angiotensin–aldosterone system (Figure 3.13).

Hydronephrosis can also cause polycythaemia by increasing the output of erythropoietin from the diseased kidney.

Biochemical tests

Blood urea, serum creatinine

These are the simplest measures of renal function and therefore useful in hypertensive patients for two reasons – to detect renal disease as a cause of the hypertension, and also to assess how much renal damage has resulted from the high blood pressure.

The serum creatinine is a more sensitive index of renal dysfunction than the blood urea: it will increase early in renal failure while the blood urea is raised only when the failure has become well established.

The patient's results were both abnormal, indicating definite renal failure (Table 3.18).

Routine testing of blood urea and creatinine is not necessary in patients with mild hypertension unless renal disease is suspected clinically.

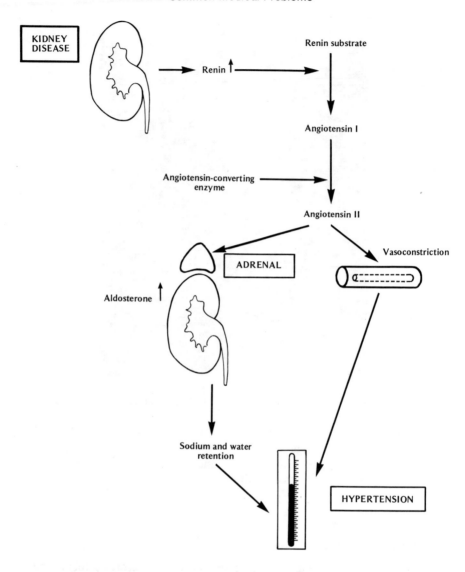

Figure 3.13 Renin–angiotensin–aldosterone system causing 'renal' hypertension

Table 3.18 Patient's blood urea and creatinine results

	Result	Normal range
Creatinine	192 μmol/l	(60–120 μmol/l)
Urea	11.6 mmol/l	(3.3–6.6 mmol/l)

Serum potassium

This is an important electrolyte to measure in hypertensive patients. The relevance of the serum potassium level in the hypertensive patient is shown in Table 3.19.

Table 3.19 The relevance of the serum potassium level in hypertension

---

• Low serum K – Hyperaldosteronism – primary (Conn's syndrome)
                                           – secondary   – malignant hypertension
                                                           – renal ischaemia
                      Thiazide treatment
• High serum K– Renal failure

The patient's result was normal.

The other electrolytes are of little help in the diagnosis or management of hypertension.

Creatinine clearance

This test is a measure of the glomerular filtration rate, and therefore a more sensitive index of renal dysfunction than the blood urea level.

It is a time-consuming test and is rarely necessary in the management of hypertension. A simple estimation of the serum creatinine level is almost as good and usually suffices for clinical purposes.

Blood count

This is of no value in the routine diagnosis or management of hypertension.

It was, however, carried out in this patient because of the plethoric appearance. The result is shown in Table 3.20, and confirms polycythaemia. The normal white cell count and platelet count exclude primary polycythaemia vera.

Table 3.20 Patient's blood count showing secondary polycythaemia

		Normal
Hb	$17.6 \times$ g/dl	(12–16)
Red cell count	7.5×10^{12}/l	(4–6)
Packed cell volume	52%	(45)
White cell count	6.8×10^{9}/l	(5–10)
Platelet count	273×10^{9}/l	(150–400)

Investigations for special types of hypertension

More complex investigations may be necessary in special types of hypertension. They are listed in Table 3.21.

Table 3.21   Special investigations in secondary hypertension

• Pheochromocytoma	– Urinary catecholamine excretion
	Adrenal angiogram
	Computerized axial tomography (CAT) scan
• Conn's syndrome	– Aldosterone assay
	Adrenal angiogram
	CAT scan
• Renal artery stenosis	– Renin level in renal veins
	Renal arteriogram
	Isotope renogram
• Cushing's disease	– Serum cortisol levels
	Urinary steroid excretion
	Adrenal angiogram
	(Plasma ACTH level is possible)

Investigation of intermittent claudication

The most useful investigation is arteriography. The purpose is twofold – to establish the site and extent of any obstructive disease, and to detect any localized blockage, which might be amenable to surgical treatment.

Arteriography was not considered justifiable in the patient in view of the severe hypertensive heart disease.

Investigation of urinary tract obstruction

A number of techniques are available for investigating urinary tract obstruction (Table 3.22).

Table 3.22   Investigation of urinary tract obstruction

• Ultrasound
• Radio-hippuran–hippuran renography
• Intravenous pyelography
• Retrograde pyelography
• Cystoscopy
• Intravesical pressure measurements

Since the decision to carry out nephrectomy was made on the basis of the severity of the hydronephrosis and severe cortical atrophy seen in the ivp, no other investigations were considered necessary in the patient.

MANAGEMENT OF HYPERTENSION

The questions which the doctor has to decide when faced with a hypertensive patient, are shown in Table 3.23.

Table 3.23   Questions for the doctor in the hypertensive patient

• Does the patient really have high blood pressure?
• Is the hypertension primary or secondary
• If secondary, is there an operable cause
• renal   – renal artery stenosis
unilateral renal disease
• endocrine – pheochromocytoma
Conn's syndrome
Cushing's disease
• coarctation of the aorta
• If primary hypertension – whether to treat
how to treat

Does the patient have hypertension?

The answer to this question depends on the criteria used to define high blood pressure, which remain controversial.

This subject will be discussed in more detail under 'Natural History of Hypertension' (p. 101). However, for practical clinical reasons the limits of blood pressure widely accepted as being 'normal' are 140/90 for young subjects (up to 30 years of age) and 160/100 in older subjects.

The other important consideration is to establish that the patient does have *sustained* hypertension, and not an isolated raised blood pressure level initially due to anxiety. It is desirable, therefore, to record three blood pressure readings over a period of several weeks and base the management on the last measurement.

Labile hypertension

Lability of blood pressure – variation from reading to reading with occasional 'abnormal' levels – is most likely to be a manifestation of the considerable normal variability of blood pressure throughout the 24 hours. It is more prominent in the anxious individual.

There is no good evidence to date to suggest that this type of labile hypertension has any prognostic implication for the subsequent development of persistent hypertension.

A reasonable approach in these patients is to continue occasional, but infrequent, blood pressure checks provided it is judged that this will not lead to unjustifiable anxiety in susceptible individuals.

Secondary hypertension

The causes of secondary hypertension have already been shown in Figure 3.2. The value of the history and examination in detecting an underlying cause for the hypertension is shown in Table 3.24.

Specialist help will usually be necessary in the management of these patients.

Table 3.24 Value of history and examination in detecting secondary hypertension

• History	• Past	– Kidney disease
	• Present	– Urinary symptoms
		Symptoms of pheochromocytoma
	• Family	– 'Nephritis'
		Polycystic disease
• Examination	• Cushing's disease	
	• Enlargement of one kidney	– Hydronephrosis
	both kidneys	– Polycystic disease
	• Renal artery murmur	– Renal artery stenosis
	• Coarctation of aorta	– Absent femoral pulses
		Scapular pulsation
		Systolic murmur at back

Primary (essential) hypertension

The indications for treating essential hypertension are given in Table 3.25.

Table 3.25 Indications for treating essential hypertension

• Target organ damage	Heart	– ischaemia
		left ventricular failure
	Brain	– haemorrhagic stroke
	Kidneys	– renal failure
• Malignant hypertension	Severe hypertension	
	Grade 4 retinopathy	
	Uraemia	
• Blood pressure level	Diastolic > 110 mmHg	
	? Systolic	

The principal benefits of treating hypertension are prevention of death from left ventricular failure, cerebral haemorrhage and renal failure.

It has been clearly shown that antihypertensive treatment can achieve these aims in the more severe degrees of diastolic hypertension (>110 mmHg), but until recently there has been considerable doubt about the value of treating milder hypertension. Recent studies in Australia and the USA, however, have suggested that similar benefits result from treating mild hypertension (diastolic pressure 90–105 mmHg) with reduction in stroke, heart failure and myocardial infarction.

The management of mild hypertension will be discussed in more detail subsequently.

Systolic hypertension

The Framingham (USA) study has shown that the level of systolic pressure is as important prognostically as the diastolic pressure.

To date, however, there is very little evidence on the clinical benefits of treating systolic hypertension. Until adequate and acceptable evidence on its value is produced there is no justification for treating isolated systolic hypertension.

General measures in treating hypertension

The general measures which may be of value are shown in Table 3.26.

Table 3.26 General measures in treating hypertension

- Control of obesity
- Control of 'risk factors'
  - cigarette smoking
  - hyperlipidaemia
  - diabetes
  - contraceptive pill
- Improving physical activity
- Control of salt intake

Obesity

There is a direct correlation between obesity and blood pressure level. The potential benefits to the hypertensive patient of losing weight are shown in Table 3.27.

Table 3.27 Weight reduction in the hypertensive patient

- May reduce level of blood pressure
- Reduction of blood lipid levels
- Reduced tendency to diabetes
- Reduced risk of coronary artery disease
- Increased mobility and exercise potential

Compliance with a reducing diet is difficult and expensive. Constant encouragement to persist is necessary. In some cases, the motivation and support given by group dieting, e.g. Weight Watchers, is undoubtedly valuable, but again may involve considerable expense.

The important message to the patient is not that of a temporary diet, but of a permanent change in eating habits.

Control of risk factors

The association of hypertension with other major vascular risk factors, such as smoking and hypercholesterolaemia, greatly enhances the chance of a major cardiovascular or cerebrovascular catastrophe.

Smoking
Control of cigarette smoking reduces the risks. Giving up smoking is, however, very difficult for the heavy smoker. Some recommendations which may help have been discussed in Chapter 2.

Hyperlipidaemia
Although the relationship between hyperlipidaemia and coronary artery disease has been well-established in epidemiological studies, the clinical benefits of reducing blood lipid levels remain to be demonstrated. It would seem reasonable, however, to reduce blood cholesterol in the younger patient (arbitrarily, under 45 years of age) when there might be a theoretical chance of retarding development of more serious degrees of atherosclerosis.

Reduction of blood cholesterol levels should be attempted first with a low cholesterol diet.

Cholestyramine (Questran) may help if diet fails. Clofibrate should not be used except in severe hyperlipidaemia resistant to diet and cholestyramine, e.g. familial hypercholesterolaemia, since the side-effects are potentially hazardous (gallstones, possible increase in gastrointestinal cancer).

Diabetes
Although diabetics have accelerated atherosclerosis, it remains to be shown that control of the diabetes improves the vascular disease.

Contraceptive pill
The contraceptive pill increases the risk of stroke and myocardial infarction, especially in the older woman who smokes. If hypertension is also present, the risks are greatly increased.

Physical activity

The potential benefits of encouraging moderate physical activity in the hypertensive patient are indicated in Table 3.28.

Table 3.28 Potential benefits of exercise in the hypertensive patient

• Reduction of obesity
• Reduction of blood lipid levels
• Fall in systemic vascular resistance
• Possibly reduces risk of myocardial infarction

Isometric exercise – e.g. weight lifting, press-ups – should be avoided since it can increase blood pressure significantly during its performance.

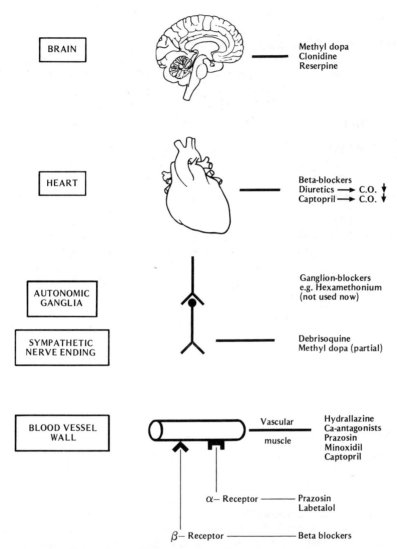

High blood pressure

BRAIN — Methyl dopa / Clonidine / Reserpine

HEART — Beta-blockers / Diuretics → C.O. ↓ / Captopril → C.O. ↓

AUTONOMIC GANGLIA — Ganglion-blockers e.g. Hexamethonium (not used now)

SYMPATHETIC NERVE ENDING — Debrisoquine / Methyl dopa (partial)

BLOOD VESSEL WALL — Vascular muscle — Hydrallazine / Ca-antagonists / Prazosin / Minoxidil / Captopril

α— Receptor — Prazosin / Labetalol

β— Receptor — Beta blockers

Figure 3.14 Site-related antihypertensive drugs

Salt intake

The relationship between salt intake and hypertension has been the subject of controversy for many years. The current view is that in some patients who may have a congenital defect in control of intracellular sodium levels, an increased salt intake can precipitate hypertension.

Since average salt intake in the United Kingdom is high (9–10 g/day) it would appear prudent for the hypertensive patient to reduce his or her daily intake by avoiding all added salt at the table. This will produce a more reasonable intake of 3–4 g/day.

Alcohol

Moderate alcohol consumption (less than 2 oz (6 cl) per day – one small whisky or 1 pint of beer) has no effect on blood pressure level.

Heavier drinking may increase the likelihood of hypertension and may also lead to alcoholic cardiomyopathy.

Coffee and tea

There is no evidence that moderate amounts of coffee or tea are harmful to hypertensive patients.

Specific treatment of hypertension

A wide variety of antihypertensive drugs are available which act at every level of the neurovascular pathways controlling blood pressure (Figure 3.14).

In view of the confusing plethora of drugs it is desirable for the doctor to become familiar with a few drugs acting at different sites in the neurovascular pathway. Table 3.29 indicates four of the basic hypotensive drugs which will suffice to control the majority of hypertensive patients.

Table 3.29   Basic hypotensive drugs

- Thiazide
- β-Blocker
- Peripheral vasodilator, e.g. hydrallazine
- Methyldopa

Thiazides

A thiazide diuretic may be used alone to control mild hypertension (diastolic pressure 90–105 mmHg) or in combination with other treatment for the more severe degrees of hypertension.

The mode of action is uncertain. Depletion of blood volume by the diuretic action is probably responsible for the initial hypotensive effect, but blood volume is soon restored. Subsequent control is probably by direct action on the peripheral vessels leading to reduced resistance by a mechanism as yet undefined.

Several thiazides in common use are shown in Table 3.30. The main side-effects are shown in Table 3.31.

Table 3.30   Thiazides in hypertension

	Dose
Hydrochlorothiazide (HydroSaluric)	25–100 mg once daily
Bendrofluazide (Aprinox)	2.5–5.0 mg once daily
Cyclopenthiazide (Navidrex)	0.25–0.5 mg once daily

Table 3.31 Side-effects of thiazides

• Hypokalaemia
• Hyperglycaemia
• Hyperuricaemia – gout
• Impotence

Supplementary potassium is usually unnecessary when thiazides are used to treat hypertension. When it is a problem, the most effective measure is to substitute a potassium-sparing diuretic for the thiazide (Table 3.32). If the hypotensive effect is attenuated too much, the potassium-retaining diuretic can be combined with the thiazide.

Table 3.32 Potassium-sparing diuretics

	Dose
Triamterene (Dytac)	150–250 mg daily (divided dose)
Amiloride (Midamor)	5–10 mg once daily
Spironolactone (Aldactone)	50–100 mg once daily

Although the two drugs should preferably be given singly, it is justifiable to use a combination product if compliance is a problem.

β-Receptor blockade

These drugs are frequently used as first-line single treatment for mild hypertension. They may also be used in combination with other drugs in treatment of more severe hypertension.

The mode of action remains controversial. The possible mechanisms are shown in Figure 3.15.

Pharmacologically, β-blockers can be distinguished by membrane-stabilizing activity, cardioselectivity and intrinsic sympathomimetic activity (Table 3.33). However, these pharmacological distinctions have little relevance to clinical control of blood pressure, and all the drugs are equally effective.

There are some circumstances when cardioselectivity is an advantage, as in hypertensive patients with bronchial asthma or intermittent claudication, since there is less tendency to exacerbate these associated conditions.

Among this profusion of drugs, it is desirable to become familiar with one non-selective membrane-stabilizing β-blocker, such as propranolol, and one cardioselective drug such as atenolol or metoprolol. Most patients will be managed very satisfactorily using just these two drugs.

The side-effects of β-blockers are shown in Table 3.34.

Where a β-blocker alone is insufficient to control the blood pressure adequately, it may be used with a thiazide. Although it is preferable to use the

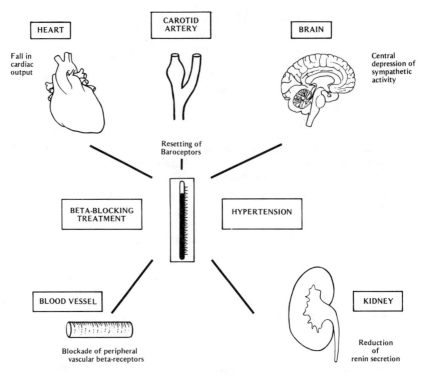

Figure 3.15   Possible mechanism of action of β-blockers

Table 3.33   Pharmacological distinctions between β-blocking drugs

	Membrane stabilizing activity	Cardioselectivity	Intrinsic sympathomimetic activity
Acebutolol	+	+	+
Atenolol	−	+	+
Labetalol	+	−	−
Metoprolol	+	+	−
Nadolol	+	−	−
Oxprenolol	+	−	+
Pindolol	+	−	+
Propranolol	+	−	−
Sotalol	+	−	−
Timolol	+	−	−

drugs separately, a combined preparation may be justifiable whenever compliance is a problem.

It is rarely justifiable, however, to initiate treatment of mild hypertension with a combined preparation of β-blockers and thiazides, since both drugs may not be necessary to control the blood pressure and the risk of side-effects is doubled.

Table 3.34   Side-effects of β-blocking drugs

- Bronchospasm
- Precipitation of latent heart failure
- Peripheral vascular insufficiency
     cold extremities
     intermittent claudication
- Fatigue – common
- Impotence
- Masking of hypoglycaemia in diabetics
- Nightmares and hallucinations – propranolol

Hydrallazine

This is an effective and safe drug for severe hypertension. The drug profile is shown in Table 3.35.

Table 3.35   Drug profile of hydrallazine

- Direct peripheral vasodilator
- Dose – 25 mg t.d.s. to 50 mg q.d.s
- Side-effects – postural hypotension – dizziness
                     throbbing headache
                     flushing
                     fluid retention –ankle swelling
                     syndrome like systemic lupus
                     erythematosus
- Use with a β-blocker to control reflex tachycardia

The development of a syndrome like systemic lupus erythematosus is a rare complication of hydrallazine treatment. It is dose-related and maximum dose should not exceed 200 mg/day.

The finding of antinuclear factor in the blood is a useful guide to the likely development of this syndrome. This test can therefore be used for regular screening purposes.

All direct peripheral vasodilators lead to reflex tachycardia. A β-blocker should, therefore, always be used in combination with this type of drug.

Methyldopa

This still remains a useful drug in patients with moderate to severe hypertension (diastolic pressure > 110 mgHg), especially when other drugs have failed. The drug profile is shown in Table 3.36.

Methyldopa is contraindicated in patients with depression.

Table 3.36   Drug profile of methyldopa

• Action	– partly central on brain partly on sympathetic nerve endings
• Dose	– 250 mg t.d.s. to 500 mg q.d.s.

• Side-effects	– drowsiness
	  depression
	  diarrhoea
	  fatigue
	  impotence
	  Parkinsonism – rare
	  liver damage – rare
	  haemolytic anaemia – rare

Summary of approach to the drug treatment of hypertension

The questions to be considered when treating hypertensive patients with specific drugs are:

- Who should treat? General practitioners or hospital specialist?
- Which patients should be treated?
- Which patients should not be treated?
- Which drugs should be used and in what order?
- What benefits are likely with treatment?

Who should treat the patient?

Most hypertensive patients can be treated quite satisfactorily at home by the general practitioner.

Specialist advice is desirable in the following circumstances:

- An operable cause of secondary hypertension is suspected (Table 3.37)

Table 3.37   Operable causes of secondary hypertension

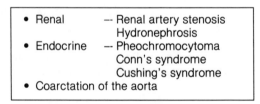

• Renal	— Renal artery stenosis Hydronephrosis

• Endocrine	— Pheochromocytoma
	  Conn's syndrome
	  Cushing's syndrome

• Coarctation of the aorta	

- The patient is resistant to treatment with all the standard drugs (Table 3.29)
- The patient has malignant hypertension – this is a medical emergency and immediate hospital admission should be sought

Which patients should be treated?

These are as follows:

- All adult patients below 65 years of age with a persistent diastolic pressure above 105 mmHg

- Patients with diastolic pressure of 90–105 mmHg if there are other adverse prognostic factors (Table 3.38).

Table 3.38 Adverse prognostic factors in patients with mild hypertension (diastolic pressure 90–105 mm Hg)

- Cardiac complications – angina
                        heart attack
                        left ventricular failure
- Previous haemorrhagic stroke
- Early impairment of renal function (raised blood urea)
- Bad family history of premature death from hypertension or its complications
- Other coronary risk factors – smoking
                        hypercholesterolaemia
                        diabetes

- Patients over 65 years of age with a diastolic pressure over 110 mmHg if they have left ventricular failure or a previous haemorrhagic stroke.

Which patients should not be treated

These are as follows:

- Those with labile hypertension where the diastolic pressure is inconsistently increased above 90 mmHg.
  The right course in these patients is periodic blood-pressure checks.

- A patient with sustained mild hypertension (diastolic pressure 90–105 mmHg) and no adverse prognostic features (Table 3.38).

- A patient with mild hypertension (diastolic pressure 90–105 mmHg) and obesity.
  The first line of treatment should be weight reduction.

- The elderly hypertensive patient in whom all attempts at reducing the blood pressure result in disabling postural hypotension.

Which antihypertensive drugs should be used?

Guidelines are as follows:

- The initial drug should be either a thiazide or a β-blocker.
  If asthma or claudication are also present, a thiazide should be chosen.

If diabetes or gout are present, a cardioselective β-blocker would be better.

A young male patient might also do better with a β-blocker than with a thiazide because of the greater risk of impotence with the thiazide.

- If either the thiazide or the β-blocker is ineffective alone in reducing the blood pressure, the two drugs can be combined

- If the combination is ineffective, a peripheral vasodilator such as hydrallazine should be tried, beginning with 25 mg t.d.s. and increasing to 50 mg q.d.s.

- If triple therapy with thiazide, β-blocker and peripheral vasodilator is still ineffective, methyldopa can be added, starting with 250 mg t.d.s. and increasing up to 500 mg q.d.s.

- If the patient's blood pressure is still unsatisfactory, hospital referral for specialist advice would be desirable

What benefits are likely with treatment?

These are as follows:

- Prolongation of life.

- Reduced chance of heart failure.

- Reduced chance of a haemorrhagic stroke.

- Reduced chance of hypertensive renal failure.

- A reduction in the incidence of myocardial infarction is also likely but this has not been shown as convincingly to date as the other benefits.

Special problems in the management of hypertension

Mild hypertension

This is arbitrarily defined as diastolic blood pressure of 90–105 mmHg.

Recent evidence, in the US Public Health Service Study, the US Hypertension Detection and Follow-up Study and the Australian National Blood Pressure Study, suggests that control of even mild hypertension may have long

Table 3.39 Guidelines in deciding treatment for the mild hypertensive

- Age – outcome worse in younger patients
- Sex – males have worse long term prognosis
- Family history of hypertension worsens prognosis
- Left ventricular hypertrophy (ECG) – worse prognosis
- Other 'risk' factors
    cigarette smoking
    hyperlipidaemia
    diabetes

term benefits in reduction of stroke and myocardial infarction. (These studies are critically reviewed in *The Lancet*, 16th January 1982, **1**, 149–156.) However, the decision to commit a young asymptomatic individual to lifelong hypotensive treatment, with the possibility of associated neurotic as well as drug-induced side-effect, is a very serious one and should not be undertaken lightly.

Guidelines which may help in making the decision are shown in Table 3.39.

β-Blockers and thiazides singly, or in combination, are the most useful drugs for long term treatment of mild hypertension.

Older patients with hypertension (>65 years)

The beneficial effects of treating asymptomatic and uncomplicated hypertension in older patients remain to be proved.

If heart failure or haemorrhagic stroke has occurred, blood pressure control is desirable.

Older patients are very prone to dizziness due to postural hypotension with most antihypertensive drugs. The diastolic pressure should therefore be reduced only to that level which avoids significant hypotensive symptoms, especially dizziness. A diastolic pressure of 110 mmHg is often the best level which can be comfortably tolerated.

Treatment should be simple to improve compliance, which is always a problem in older patients. Thiazides and β-blockers are probably the most useful drugs.

Peripheral vasodilators should be avoided because of the likelihood of postural hypotension.

Malignant hypertension

The diagnostic features of malignant hypertension are indicated in Figure 3.16.

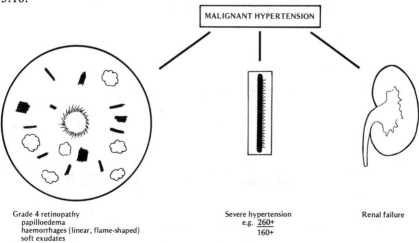

MALIGNANT HYPERTENSION

Grade 4 retinopathy
  papilloedema
  haemorrhages (linear, flame-shaped)
  soft exudates

Severe hypertension
e.g. 260+
      160+

Renal failure

Figure 3.16 Features of malignant hypertension

This is a medical emergency since cerebral haemorrhage, left ventricular failure and increasing renal failure are very likely. Prompt hospital admission is necessary.

The drugs used in treatment are shown in Table 3.40.

Table 3.40   Drugs for treating malignant hypertension

	Dose
Nitroprusside i.v.	0.5–8.0 µg/kg per min
Methyldopa i.v.	250–500 mg 4 hourly
Diazoxide i.v.	*small* boluses 100 mg
Labetalol oral	100–800 mg t.d.s.
i.v.	2 mg/min to maximum 200 mg

'Resistant' hypertension

A minority of severely hypertensive patients appears to remain resistant to a wide variety of hypotensive drugs. Some helpful points to managing these patients are suggested in Table 3.41.

Table 3.41   Approach to 'resistant' hypertension

- Check compliance – hospital admission often necessary
- Ensure maximal dose of drug has been tried
- Counteract fluid retention with effective diuretic
- Exclude antagonistic action of concomitant drug therapy
  - sympathomimetics
  - antidepressants
  - adrenal steroids
  - oestrogens
- Other hypotensive drugs which may not have been tried
  - calcium antagonists – nifedipine or verapamil
  - labetalol – combined α- and β-blocker
  - minoxidil – peripheral vasodilator
    (causes hirsuties in women)
  - captopril – angiotensin-converting-enzyme inhibitor
    (watch out for renal damage and bone marrow depression)

Choice of specific drugs for specific conditions

The hypotensive drug used may be decided by the type of hypertension being treated. Table 3.42 indicates some of these conditions.

Table 3.42 Hypotensive drugs 'tailored' to the condition treated

• Pregnancy	–	Methyldopa – safe for fetus
		Hydrallazine – safe for fetus
		(β-blockers interfere with uterine function)
• Heart failure	–	Diuretic
		Vasodilator
		(avoid β-blockers – cardiac depression)
• Diabetes	–	Avoid β-blockers – masks hypoglycaemia
		Avoid thiazide – aggravates diabetes
• Depression	–	Avoid methyldopa – more depression
		Avoid reserpine – more depression
• Renal failure	–	Hydrallazine – maintains renal blood flow
		Methyldopa – maintains renal blood flow
		β-Blockers – may control increased renin
		Captopril – neutralizes increased renin effect
		(Avoid K-sparing diuretics – hyperkalaemia)

Compliance with therapy

Since treatment of hypertension is usually lifelong, compliance is a major problem. Some guidelines to improve compliance are shown in Table 3.43.

Table 3.43 Improvement of compliance in hypertension

• Patient education	• hypertension and its complications
	• efficacy of treatment
• Simple drug regime	• as few drugs as possible
	• once, or at most, twice daily
	• avoid side-effects
• Maintain contact	• regular BP check at surgery
	• infrequent visits to surgery
	• use clinic nurse if available
	• follow-up missed visits

MANAGEMENT OF URINARY TRACT OBSTRUCTION

Possible causes of unilateral lower urinary obstruction producing the gross hydronephrosis in the patient are shown in Table 3.44.

Treatment has three aims (Table 3.45).

The nature of the obstructing lesion was uncertain in the patient. In view of the severe renal damage seen on the patient's intravenous pyelogram, more detailed urological investigation was not considered necessary since the decision was made to carry out nephrectomy.

At operation, a marked constriction was found at the vesico-ureteric junction. Histology of the constriction showed non-specific submucosal fibrosis without any significant inflammatory infiltration. The cause of the constriction remained unknown.

Table 3.44 Causes of unilateral lower urinary tract obstruction

- Congenital – uretero-vesical junction obstruction
- Tumour – intrinsic – carcinoma of bladder
  extrinsic – colonic carcinoma
  uterine carcinoma
  retroperitoneal glands
- Calculi
- Retroperitoneal fibrosis – methysergide (migraine)
  β-blockers

Table 3.45 Aims of treating urinary tract obstruction

- Relief of obstruction
  - catheterization
  - nephrostomy
  - pyelostomy
  - ureteric anastomosis
- Removal of the cause
- Control of infection

Disappointingly, nephrectomy did not result in improvement of the hypertension and continuation of medical treatment was necessary.

MANAGEMENT OF PERIPHERAL VASCULAR DISEASE

General measures

Cigarette smoking

Giving up smoking is the most important general measure in treating intermittent claudication, because of the close link between smoking and the development and progression of arteriosclerosis.

However, giving up cigarettes may be very difficult for many smokers. More specific practical advice on this subject is presented in Chapter 2.

Regular walking exercise

It has been suggested that regular exercise encourages the development of collateral vessels in the legs. The objective evidence to support this view remains to be established.

Buerger–Allen exercises

Raising and lowering the legs with dorsiflexion and plantar flexion of the feet when dependent, is also claimed to improve the blood supply to the legs. Supportive objective evidence is again lacking.

Symptomatic treatment

Peripheral vasodilators are used extensively for intermittent claudication but convincing evidence of efficacy remains to be presented.

If the drugs do lead to vasodilation it is likely that this occurs in the more healthy superficial vessels of the lower limbs which may divert blood away from the muscle vessels and so make the condition worse.

Drugs which are commonly used are shown in Table 3.46. They may be useful for their placebo effects provided they do not make the claudication worse.

Table 3.46   Drugs used in treating intermittent claudication

	Dose
Inositol nicotinate (Hexopal)	1.5–3.0 g daily
Thymoxamine (Opilon)	40 mg q.d.s.
Tolazoline (Priscol)	12.5–50 mg q.d.s.
Oxypentifyline (Trental)	100–200 mg t.d.s.

Surgical treatment

This is the only effective treatment in improving the blood supply to the lower limbs. The types of surgery available are shown in Table 3.47.

Table 3.47   Surgical treatment for intermittent claudication

- Lumbar sympathectomy – when reconstruction not possible
- Endarterectomy – for localized disease
- Insertion of prosthetic (Dacron) graft – for extensive disease
- Bypass graft – patient not well enough for major aorto-iliac reconstruction
- Percutaneous transluminal angioplasty – localized disease

The most promising approach with the least risk and inconvenience to the patient is *percutaneous transluminal angioplasty*. In this treatment the atherosclerotic obstruction is broken down by inflation of a balloon at the end of a catheter passed through the obstructed segment of artery.

NATURAL HISTORY OF HYPERTENSION

Because blood pressure is a continuous graded human characteristic it is impossible to define a specific upper limit beyond which 'hypertension' can be said to exist. Actuarial, insurance and clinical survey statistics have shown a steadily progressive increase in the major complications of hypertension (heart failure, stroke and renal failure) with increasing levels of both systolic and diastolic pressure.

'Normal' blood pressure is based on surveys of 'healthy' populations who have no clinically overt evidence of disease. On this basis it is generally accepted that 140/90 may be regarded as the upper limit of 'normal' blood pressure in young subjects (up to 30 years of age), and 160/100 in older subjects.

Incidence of hypertension

The incidence of hypertension in the United Kingdom is 10–15%. The incidence increases steadily with age. It is also more common in females, who tend to develop hypertension 10 years later than men.

Primary or secondary

Of patients presenting with hypertension, 90–95% have essential hypertension. The remaining 5–10% of cases are secondary to an underlying cause, the commonest cause being renal disease. Secondary hypertension is more likely in the younger patient.

Heredity

There is a familial incidence in essential hypertension. If both parents are hypertensive, half the offspring will be hypertensive; if only one parent is affected, the risk falls to 25%.

Presentation

Most patients with benign essential hypertension are asymptomatic. The only two convincing symptoms directly attributable to the high blood pressure are throbbing occipital morning headache and epistaxis. Other symptoms such as dizziness, 'pressure' headache, lack of energy, are due to anxiety and almost invariably develop *after* the patient has been told his blood pressure is high. More significantly, symptoms will occur when target organ damage is produced and will then relate to the heart, brain or kidneys.

Prognosis

The prognosis depends on a number of factors (Table 3.48).

Table 3.48 Prognostic factors in hypertension

• Age – outcome worse in younger patients
• Sex – outcome worse in males
• Height of systolic and diastolic pressure
• Target organ damage • Heart
• Brain
• Kidneys
• Positive family history of hypertension

The results of a 10 year survey of mortality in hypertensive patients in a typical family practice carried out by John Fry are shown in Figure 3.17. The overall mortality was 34%. The factors found by Dr Fry in this survey to increase the chances of dying are shown in Table 3.49.

Table 3.49   Factors increasing chances of dying in the hypertensive patients in Dr Fry's survey

- Male patient
- Young patient
- Family history of hypertension
- Increasing diastolic pressure

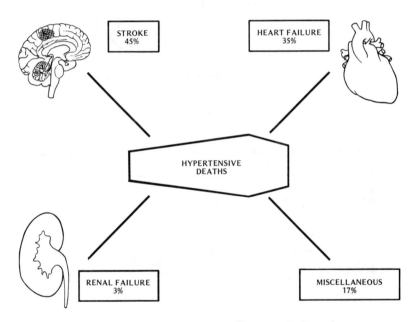

Figure 3.17   Survey of death in hypertensive patients in typical family practice (from John Fry)

The distribution of hypertension in the community is shown in Figure 3.18.

If patients are symptomatic on discovery of the hypertension, and the symptoms are directly attributable to the hypertension or to its complications, the prognosis is much worse, since half the patients will die within 5 years and three quarters will die within 10 years.

The prognosis in uncomplicated hypertension is good and the average duration of life is 20 years. With the onset of target organ damage, the prognosis will become poorer (Figure 3.19).

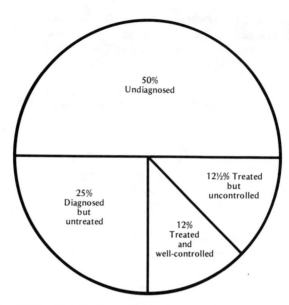

Figure 3.18   Distribution of hypertension in the community

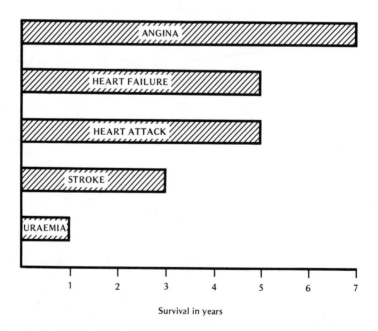

Survival in years

Figure 3.19   Prognosis in hypertension: average duration of life with target organ damage

The prognosis of hypertension will therefore depend very much on the extent of associated atherosclerosis since this is the basic cause of all target organ damage. The prognosis has been related to the fundal appearances which provides the simplest objective measure of arterial change (Table 3.50).

Table 3.50 Prognosis in hypertension related to fundal changes (5–10 year survival)

Retinopathy grade	Survival %
Retinopoathy grade	Survival (%)
1	80
2	45
3	15
4	5

The natural history of hypertension in the elderly is still unclear and the benefits of treatment are not yet established.

CAN WE MODIFY THE NATURAL HISTORY?

Since the aetiology of essential hypertension, which accounts for 90–95% of all hypertensive patients in practice, is unknown, there is no method of primary prevention.

In secondary hypertension, the most frequent cause is chronic pyelonephritis and this is potentially preventable.

All episodes of urinary tract infection in children should be treated promptly and effectively and arrangements made for adequate follow-up to ensure that all traces of infection have been eradicated. This will involve regular urine microscopy and bacteriology as well as clinical assessment.

When a young patient is prone to recurrent urinary tract infection it is advisable to investigate thoroughly to exclude any anatomical abnormality, such as an obstructive lesion, or functional abnormality, such as vesico-ureteric reflux, which may be responsible for the repeated infections and are remediable by operation.

In patients, especially children, who have recurrent urinary infection and no remediable underlying cause, a prolonged course of antibiotic treatment for a period of 6–12 months, changing the antibiotic each month, may help to minimize renal damage, and so reduce the chance of secondary hypertension.

Screening for hypertension

Since hypertension is so often asymptomatic, the only possible way of modifying the natural history is to detect it before target organ damage has occurred. This involves a screening programme.

The requirements for a worthwhile screening programme are shown in Table 3.51. Hypertension fulfils all these requirements.

Table 3.51 Requirements for a worthwhile screening programme

- Detection of a common disorder
- The condition is a hazard to health
- The condition is often asymptomatic
- Detection is easy
- The condition is amenable to treatment
- Treatment improves the prognosis

When screening surveys have been carried out, 5% of men and women between 35 and 64 years of age have been found to have diastolic pressures greater than 110 mmHg – a level clearly shown to benefit from treatment. Additionally 20–30% have diastolic levels of 90–109 mmHg which recent studies have also suggested will benefit.

Ninety per cent of patients in a family practice will have attended the surgery for one reason or another within a period of 5 years. The potential for detection of asymptomatic hypertension is therefore considerable.

USEFUL PRACTICAL POINTS

- Most hypertensive patients have essential hypertension. The most helpful pointer to this diagnosis is a positive family history.

- Secondary hypertension is more likely in the young. Renal disease is the most frequent underlying cause, and chronic pyelonephritis the commonest type of renal disease involved.

- Remember to look for femoral pulsation in the groin in hypertensive patients, especially young men, to exclude coarctation of the aorta.
  Remember also to listen over the abdomen for renal artery murmurs in hypertensive patients of all ages.

- Most hypertensive patients can be treated successfully with a thiazide, a β-blocker and a peripheral vasodilator such as hydrallazine.

- Avoid peripheral vasodilators in the elderly hypertensive because of postural hypotension.
  Be satisfied with less than perfect control of blood pressure in these patients to avoid incapacitating dizziness.

- Consider carefully before committing a young asymptomatic individual with mild hypertension to lifelong treatment. Assess associated adverse prognostic factors before making this decision.

4

Swelling of the legs

PRESENT HISTORY

A 42-year-old lady presented with a complaint of swelling of the legs.

Swelling of the legs

She had first developed swelling of the ankles about 1 year ago, but this only occurred in the evening, especially after she had been on her feet a long time.

Over the last few months, however, the swelling was becoming more persistent during the day and seemed to be slowly spreading up from the ankles to her legs.

She consulted her doctor about the legs and was told that they had a 'bad circulation' though she had never had any trouble with varicose veins or thrombosis in the veins of the legs. He gave her some 'water tablets' which helped to reduce the swelling at first but now seemed to be less effective. Her shoes always felt tight and uncomfortable and it interfered with her walking.

Chronic cough

Her other big problem was a chronic productive cough which had been present since she had a particularly bad attack of measles in childhood. She was told that she had 'damaged her lungs' and was prevented from joining in at games in school.

At first, the cough seemed troublesome only in the winter but it had gradually got worse so that for some time now she had cough and phlegm through most of the year. It would be especially bad first thing in the morning when she awoke, and she would usually bring up a lot of 'awful-looking phlegm'. She would feel better afterwards. On direct enquiry she admitted to noticing streaks of bright-red blood in the phlegm at times, especially when she had a recent 'chest cold'.

Although she was breathless if she tried to do too much, she did not think that she had become any more breathless than usual after the swelling of the legs had become bad.

Other relevant facts on direct enquiry

Alimentary system

Her *weight* had been increasing over the last month or two as indicated by her skirts getting tight.

Her *appetite* had been rather poor recently and she occasionally felt sick though rarely vomited. There was no previous history of indigestion.

Her *bowels* had been a bit loose over the last few months. She had not seen any blood or slime in the stools.

Urinary system

She had been passing *more urine* than normal recently but thought this was due to the 'water tablets'. She was starting to get up at night to pass urine which had never happened before. She denied any excessive thirst and had not noticed any discomfort, such as scalding, on passing urine and she had not had any pruritus vulvae.

Joints

Her joints had not been troublesome.

Central nervous system

She had not noticed any weakness of a limb or undue 'pins and needles'.

PAST HISTORY

Respiratory system

Her lungs had given her trouble since childhood. Apart from the chronic productive cough she had several attacks of *pleurisy* during the last few years. This usually affected the right side of her chest but she had one attack on the left. She had also been admitted to hospital about 3 years previously with 'pneumonia' and had to stay in for 6 weeks since there had been difficulty in controlling it.

Urinary system

She denied any previous kidney or bladder trouble.

FAMILY HISTORY

There was nothing relevant. In particular, there was no family history of lung trouble or bowel trouble with diarrhoea. There was no history of kidney disease.

PERSONAL HISTORY

She had three children. In spite of her chest trouble she had managed to cope quite well with the family. Recently, however, she was finding it more difficult to manage. She seemed to tire more easily and things seemed so much of an effort, especially as her legs 'felt heavy all the time'.

She smoked little, less than five cigarettes daily, and would only drink alcohol on special occasions.

DRUG HISTORY

Her only treatment was the 'water tablets'.

EXAMINATION

General

She was thin.
She was not breathless or cyanosed at rest but had a productive cough.
She had a sallow appearance though the conjunctivae, tongue and palms of the hand did not suggest anaemia.
Her eyes were rather *puffy*.
The fingers were clubbed.

Cardiovascular system

The neck veins were not visible, but pressure with the finger in the supra-clavicular area showed that the external jugular vein was capable of rapid distension. Pressure over the liver did not distend the neck veins.

There was marked pitting oedema of the feet, ankles and legs (Figure 4.1). The skin was pale, and there was no evidence of chronic venous insufficiency (Table 4.1).

Table 4.1   Signs of venous insufficiency in legs

• Varicose veins
• Blue or brown pigmentation
• Dilated superficial veins
• Skin ulcers
• Tenderness along line of veins

The pulse was normal. The radial and brachial arteries were not thickened. The blood pressure was 160/95. The apex beat was normal. There was a slight left parasternal lift but the pulmonary second sound was not palpable. There was a soft blowing midsystolic murmur localized to the apex. There was no triple rhythm and the pulmonary second sound was not increased.

109

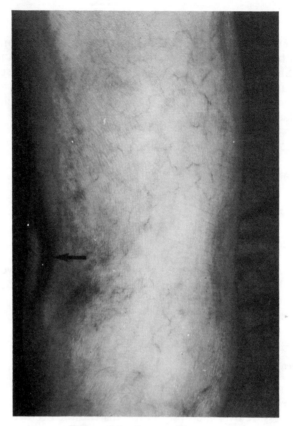

Figure 4.1   Leg oedema

Respiratory system

The lung findings are shown in Figure 4.2. Movement was reduced at both lung bases and all the signs were more marked at the right base than the left.

Abdomen

She had hepatosplenomegaly (Figure 4.3). The liver was palpable 5 cm below the costal margin and was firm, smooth and not tender. The splenic tip was felt 3 cm below the left costal margin. There were no dilated superficial veins and there was no ascites. There were no abdominal masses and the colon was not palpable or tender.

The kidneys were palpable. There was no renal angle tenderness.

Central nervous system

The fundi were normal. There was no abnormality in the central nervous system.

Swelling of the legs

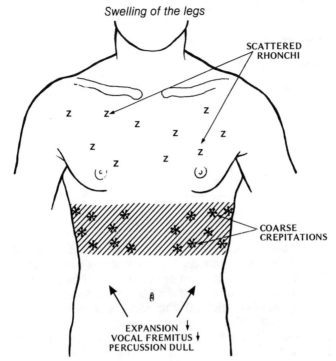

Figure 4.2   Physical signs in the lungs

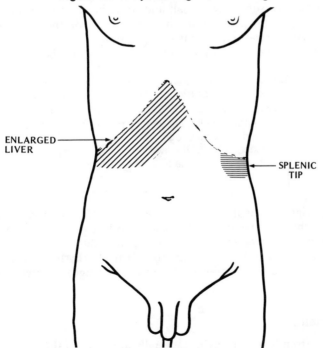

Figure 4.3   Abdominal findings in the patient

ANALYSIS OF THE HISTORY

Swelling of the legs

The main causes of leg oedema are shown in Table 4.2.

Table 4.2 Causes of oedema

- Heart failure
- Nephrotic syndrome
- Hepatic disease
- Local obstruction

Cardiac oedema

This is due to heart failure. If the left ventricle is affected the oedema collects in the lungs. If the right ventricle fails the oedema collects in the dependent area such as the legs (if ambulant) or the sacrum (if bed-ridden).

The mechanism of circulation of the tissue fluid is shown in simplified form in Figure 4.4. (This illustration takes no account of the hydrostatic pressure of the tissue fluid itself which is a minor factor.)

Accumulation of tissue fluid will occur if the hydrostatic pressure forcing salt and water out at the venous end of the capillary exceeds the osmotic pressure of the plasma proteins, as in *right ventricular failure*, or if the plasma protein osmotic pressure drawing salt and water back into the capillary falls below the hydrostatic pressure at the venous end of the capillary, as in *hypoproteinaemic states*, e.g. nephrotic syndrome.

The diagnostic criteria for right ventricular failure are shown in Table 4.3.

Table 4.3 Diagnostic criteria for right ventricular failure

- Increase in jugular venous pressure
- Oedema of the legs
- Congestion of the liver
- Triple rhythm due to 3rd heart sound
- Ascites may occur

Although right ventricular failure is by far the most likely cause of oedema in a patient with chronic lung disease, the lack of neck vein distension, the absence of hepatojugular reflux (which is an early sign of right ventricular failure), the lack of a protodiastolic (third heart sound) triple rhythm and the lack of tenderness over the enlarged liver, all indicate that right ventricular failure is not present.

Renal oedema

This results from loss of protein, especially albumin, in the urine leading to *hypoalbuminaemia* and reduced plasma osmotic pressure.

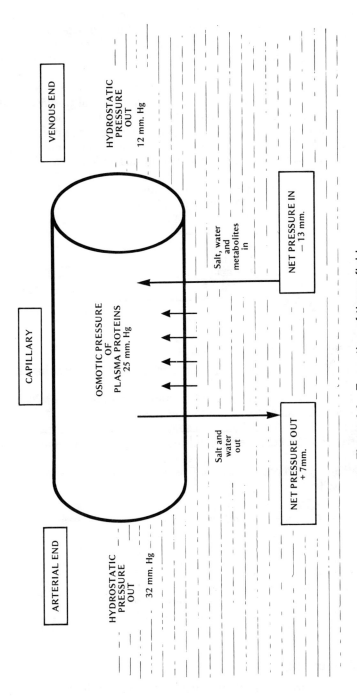

Figure 4.4 Formation of tissue fluid

The main feature distinguishing renal from cardiac oedema is that renal oedema is generalized and cardiac oedema gravitates to dependent parts.

The puffy eyes in this patient indicate periorbital oedema. Together with the absence of any other signs of right ventricular failure, *this points to oedema of renal origin.*

There is a less frequent type of renal oedema not due to albuminuria and hypoalbuminaemia. This is acute diffuse poststreptococcal *glomerulo-tubular nephritis* in which there is generalized oedema thought to be due to generalized capillary damage which increases the capillary's permeability to salt and water. The main clinical features of this condition are shown in Table 4.4.

There was no evidence of acute nephritis in this patient.

Table 4.4 Manifestations of acute diffuse glomerulo-tubular nephritis

• Generalized oedema
• Hypertension
• Haematuria
• Oliguria

Hepatic oedema

Oedema results from deficient production of albumin, leading again to hypoalbuminaemia.

An additional factor is an increased secretion of aldosterone which occurs in liver disease and leads to salt and water retention.

Ascites often occurs with hepatic oedema, probably because most cases are due to cirrhosis. The possible mechanisms causing ascites are shown in Table 4.5.

The patient had no past history of liver disease and no abdominal swelling to suggest ascites.

Table 4.5 Mechanisms of ascites in liver disease

• Hypoalbuminaemia
• Increase in aldosterone secretion
• Portal hypertension
• Renal impairment of salt and water excretion
• Increased levels of antidiuretic hormone (not metabolized in diseased liver)

Obstructive oedema

This may be due to venous obstruction or lymphatic obstruction. The main distinguishing feature is *pitting*, with venous but not lymphatic obstruction.

Additionally, the skin over lymphoedema is thickened with prominent hair follicles.

The causes of lymphatic obstruction are shown in Table 4.6.

The pitting of the patient's oedema excluded lymphatic obstruction and there was no evidence of venous insufficiency as shown in Table 4.1.

Table 4.6   Causes of lymphatic oedema

• Primary	• Congenital
	• Milroy's disease
• Secondary	• Recurrent lymphangitis
	• Neoplasia
	invasion
	lymph node compression
	• Filariasis in tropics

Chronic productive cough

Causes of a chronic cough with large amounts of purulent sputum are shown in Table 4.7.

The very long duration of the cough would exclude both lung abscess and bronchial carcinoma in this patient.

Table 4.7   Cough with profuse purulent sputum

- Bronchiectasis
- Lung abscess
- Necrotizing bronchial carcinoma

The features suggesting bronchiectasis in the patient are shown in Table 4.8.

Table 4.8   Features indicating bronchiectasis

- Initiated by measles in childhood
- Chronic history since first episode
- Worse on waking in morning
- Large amounts of offensive sputum
- Recurrent haemoptysis

Gastrointestinal symptoms

The patient had *anorexia*, *nausea* and occasional *diarrhoea*. There are many causes of this triad of symptoms (Table 4.9).

115

Table 4.9 Causes of the triad of anorexia, nausea and diarrhoea

• Gastrointestinal disease	• Gastritis
	• Gastric carcinoma
	• Hepatitis
	• Pancreatitis
	• Ulcerative colitis
	• Crohn's disease
	• Intestinal ischaemia
• Endocrine	• Addison's disease
	• Diabetes
	• Hyperparathyroidism
• Chronic renal failure	
• Malignancy anywhere	
• Drugs	• Digoxin
	• Alcohol

The absence of abdominal pain makes the diagnosis of inflammatory disease of the stomach, duodenum, hepatobiliary system and intestine unlikely.

The lack of weight loss suggests that there is no underlying malignancy, though the accumulation of oedema may counteract weight loss to some extent.

The absence of abdominal pain and blood in the stools is against the diagnosis of ulcerative colitis and Crohn's disease.

There was no profound fatigue, postural dizziness or pigmentation to suggest Addison's disease.

The lack of excessive thirst, weight loss and pruritus vulvae makes diabetes unlikely.

Hyperparathyroidism is excluded by the absence of muscle weakness, bone pain or deformity and drowsiness.

Since the oedema is considered of renal origin, *uraemia* is a possible cause of the anorexia, nausea and diarrhoea.

There is one other cause of the diarrhoea which is worth considering, and that is *amyloid disease* secondary to the bronchiectasis.

She had not been taking any drugs.

Polyuria and nocturia

The causes of polyuria are shown in Table 4.10.

Table 4.10 Causes of polyuria

• Diabetes mellitus
• Renal failure
• Diabetes insipidus
• Hyperparathyroidism
• Psychogenic

As already mentioned, diabetes mellitus is unlikely in the absence of poly-dipsia, loss of weight and pruritus vulvae.

In diabetes insipidus, the volume of urine passed is very great, up to 18 litres/day, and there is continuous thirst. This did not fit the patient's picture.

Hyperparathyroidism is unlikely for the reasons just discussed.

Psychogenic polyuria is associated with bizarre pictures of drinking and passing urine and is rarely evident at night, unlike this patient's nocturia. Evidence of an anxiety state was also lacking.

The most likely cause of the polyuria and nocturia in this patient is *renal failure*.

Past history

The past history of measles is significant.

Severe pulmonary infection can lead to bronchiolar blockage and pulmonary collapse, the necessary prerequisites for the development of bronchiectasis.

The mechanisms causing bronchiectasis are shown in Table 4.11.

Table 4.11   Mechanisms leading to bronchiectasis

• Congenital	• Cystic fibrosis
	• Bronchiectasis *per se*
	• Immotile cilia syndrome (Kartagener's syndrome)
• Bronchial obstruction	• Infection
	• Foreign body
	• Lymph node compression
• Necrotizing inflammation	• Tuberculosis
	• Staphylococcal pneumonia
	• Carcinoma

CONCLUSIONS FROM THE HISTORY

The main presenting problems were increasing swelling of the legs and chronic cough.

- The association of swelling round the eyes and peripheral oedema suggests a renal origin – *nephrotic syndrome.*

- The polyuria and nocturia support a renal origin for the oedema and suggest that renal failure is developing.

- The chronic cough with profuse offensive sputum, occasionally blood-stained, indicates *bronchiectasis*. This may well have been caused by the severe attack of measles in childhood.

- The association of bronchiectasis and renal disease may be explained by the development of *amyloid disease*.

   Support for amyloidosis is provided by the recent development of diarrhoea.

117

ANALYSIS OF THE EXAMINATION

Oedema

The combination of a pale puffy face and marked pitting leg oedema suggests *nephrotic syndrome*.

Right ventricular failure rarely produces facial oedema unless the heart failure is very severe. In these circumstances the skin would be cyanosed and not pale. The lack of cyanosis, raised jugular venous pressure, protodiastolic triple rhythm and tender liver excludes heart failure.

Cardiovascular findings

The left parasternal lift on palpation of the precordium indicates right ventricular hypertrophy secondary to the chronic lung disease. It is caused by pulmonary hypertension.

When pulmonary hypertension is severe, the pulmonary second sound is increased – not evident in this patient.

Respiratory system

The reduced basal chest expansion on both sides indicates bilateral basal disease.

The changes in mediastinal position, vocal fremitus and percussion note which accompany the common types of lung disease are shown in Table 4.12.

Table 4.12   Physical signs in lung disease

	Trachea	Vocal fremitus	Percussion
Fibrosis	←	↓	dull
Collapse	←	↓	dull
Effusion	→	↓	stony
Pneumothorax	→	↑	hyperresonant
Consolidation	↓	↑	dull
Cavitation	↓	↑	dull

Trachea: ← = towards side of pulmonary lesion;
→ = away from side of pulmonary lesion
Vocal fremitus: ↑ = increased; ↓ = reduced

From Table 4.12 it will be seen that the combination of a central mediastinum, reduced vocal fremitus and dull (but not stony dull) percussion note in the patient indicates either bilateral fibrosis or bilateral collapse. The presence of audible breath sounds excludes collapse, leaving *bilateral basal fibrosis* the likely diagnosis.

Coarse crepitations are produced by secretion within bronchi or cavities in the lungs. The crepitations heard at the patient's lung bases are due to bronchiectatic dilatation and pooling of secretions both in the bronchi and in adjacent cavitated lung lesions resulting from persistent infection round the diseased bronchi.

Abdominal findings

There was *hepatosplenomegaly*. The possible causes are shown in Table 4.13.

Table 4.13 Causes of hepato-splenomegaly

- Portal cirrhosis
- Blood dyscrasia, e.g. myeloma, leukaemia
- Reticulosis, e.g. Hodgkin's disease
- Sarcoidosis
- Amyloidosis

Portal cirrhosis

There was no past history of liver disease, she was not an alcoholic and there were no clinical signs of cirrhosis. (Figure 4.5).

Blood dyscrasia

The clinical features of leukaemia, myelomatosis and other proliferative disorders, such as polycythaemia vera, are shown in Table 4.14.

Table 4.14 Features of leukaemia, myelomatosis and other myeloproliferative disorders

• Marrow involvement	– anaemia leukopenia (infections) thrombocytopenia (bleeding)
• Bone lesions	– bone pain, e.g. backache pathological fractures
• Renal failure	

There was no evidence of anaemia, bleeding or bone problems in the patient.

Reticulosis

The clinical features of the main types of malignant lymphoma, including Hodgkin's disease, are shown in Table 4.15.

The patient did not fit the picture.

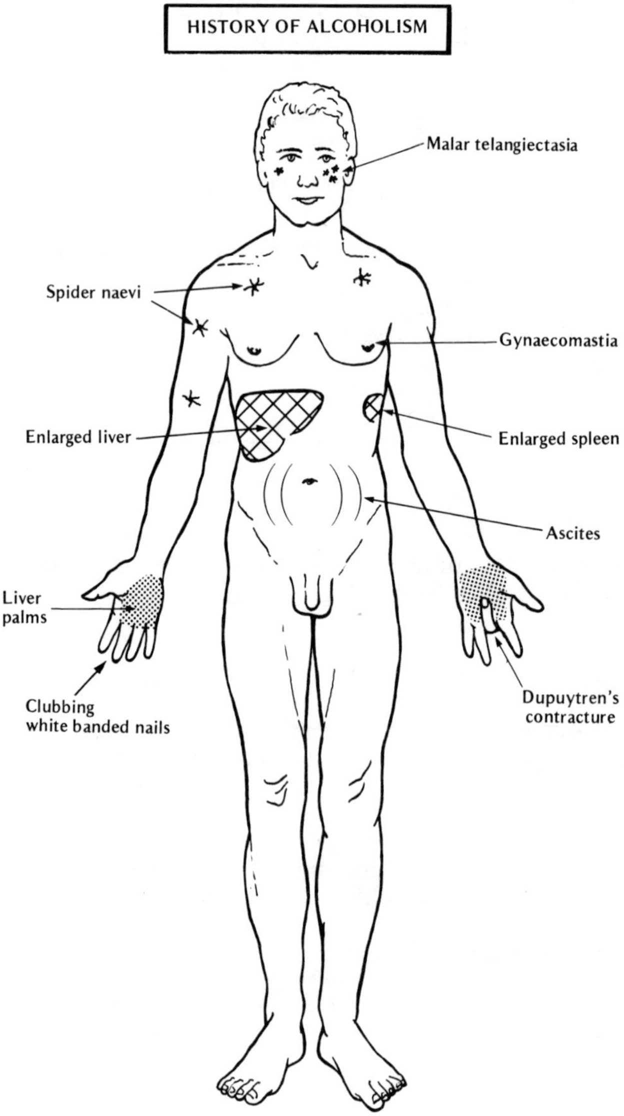

HISTORY OF ALCOHOLISM

Malar telangiectasia

Spider naevi

Gynaecomastia

Enlarged liver

Enlarged spleen

Ascites

Liver palms

Clubbing white banded nails

Dupuytren's contracture

Figure 4.5   Clinical signs of cirrhosis

Table 4.15   Features of reticulosis

- Hepatosplenomegaly
- Glandular enlargement
- Progressive anaemia
- Constitutional symptoms
    fever, weakness, weight loss
- Pruritus in 10% of patients

Sarcoidosis

The clinical features are shown in Figure 4.6. Apart from the pulmonary fibrosis, which tends to be diffuse and not basal in sarcoidosis, there was nothing else in the patient to suggest sarcoidosis as a cause of the hepatosplenomegaly.

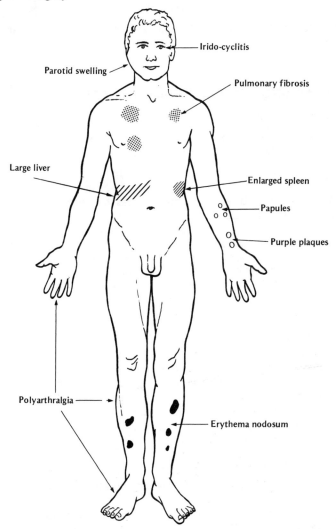

Figure 4.6   Clinical features of sarcoidosis

Amyloidosis

Secondary amyloidosis can follow chronic inflammatory and chronic suppurative disease. Bronchiectasis is a well-recognized cause of amyloidosis, and should be considered as a likely cause in this patient.

121

CONCLUSIONS FROM THE EXAMINATION

- The pale puffy face and leg oedema confirm nephrotic syndrome.

- The chest examination confirms bilateral basal bronchiectasis.

- The cardiovascular findings indicate pulmonary hypertension and right ventricular hypertrophy secondary to the chronic lung disease.

- The abdominal findings indicate hepatosplenomegaly, probably due to secondary amyloidosis.

INVESTIGATIONS FOR THE RENAL DISEASE

Urine examination

The nephrotic syndrome cannot be diagnosed without testing the urine.
The protein loss in the urine and the consequences are shown in Table 4.16.

Table 4.16   Clinical effects of protein loss in nephrotic syndrome

• Albumin	→	Oedema
• Thyroxine-binding globulin	→	Thyroid function unchanged
• Transferrin	→	Iron-deficiency anaemia
• Cholecalciferol-binding protein	→	Bone disease
• Anti-thrombin III	→	Venous thrombosis

The loss of albumin exceeds 3.5 g in 24 hours, the minimum loss required to cause generalized oedema.

The patient's albumin loss was measured on several occasions and ranged from 3 g to 8 g in 24 hours, thus confirming nephrotic syndrome.

One other relevant finding in the urine is the presence of *fatty casts* resulting from the secondary hyperlipidaemia commonly occurring in the nephrotic syndrome. None were present in the patient's urine.

Serum protein analysis

Oedema does not occur unless the serum albumin is reduced as a result of the albuminuria.

The serum albumin level in the patient on initial presentation was 29 g/l, the normal range being 35–50 g/l.

Renal function

Assessment of the degree of renal failure is made by measuring the *blood urea and creatinine* levels and the *serum electrolyte* levels.

The patient's results are shown in Table 4.17.

Table 4.17   Blood urea, creatinine and electrolyte levels in the patient

	Results	Normal range
Urea	13 mmol/l	(3.3–6.6)
Creatinine	400 μmol/l	(80–120)
Potassium	4.1 mmol/l	(3.5–5.0)
Sodium	128 mmol/l	(135–145)
CO_2	21 mm/l	(24–32)

The increase in the creatinine and urea levels indicates renal failure. The potassium is not yet elevated but should be carefully followed since a progressive increase in potassium level with advancing renal failure can cause serious cardiac dysrhythmia.

The low sodium level indicates a failure of sodium reabsorption by the defective kidney.

The low carbon dioxide level shows acidosis, which is another consequence of renal failure.

A more accurate assessment of the renal function is given by the *creatinine clearance test* which provides a measure of the glomerular filtration rate.

Intravenous pyelogram

Although not strictly necessary for the diagnosis of nephrotic syndrome, an i.v.p. may demonstrate large kidneys, as in this patient. Impaired excretion of dye indicates impairment of renal function.

INVESTIGATIONS FOR LUNG DISEASE

Chest X-ray

The patient's chest X-ray shows irregular basal shadowing with multiple cystic lesions (Figure 4.7).

It confirms the diagnosis of bilateral basal bronchiectasis.

Bronchography

Clinical examination and chest X-ray give all the information necessary to make the diagnosis of bronchiectasis.

Bronchography is only indicated if the bronchiectasis appears to be localized and surgical treatment is being considered. It is an unpleasant procedure for the patient with some risks.

Respiratory function tests

Detailed respiratory function testing is unhelpful.

The Wright Peak Flowmeter is adequate and will show whether there is small airway obstruction due to associated bronchitis.

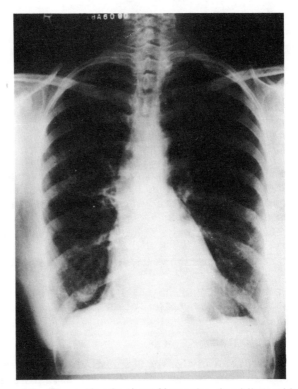

Figure 4.7 The patient's chest X-ray showing bilateral basal bronchiectasis

Electrocardiogram

The e.c.g. may be of prognostic help in detecting right ventricular strain which can lead to cor pulmonale.

INVESTIGATION FOR SECONDARY HYPERLIPIDAEMIA

Reduced plasma osmotic pressure stimulates hepatic lipoprotein synthesis, especially low-density lipoprotein and cholesterol. In the later stages the triglyceride level is also increased. The high-density lipoprotein usually remains normal.

Table 4.18 The patient's blood lipid results

	Results	Normal range
Cholesterol	9.2 mmol/l	(3.6–7.6)
High-density lipoprotein	1.2 mmol/l	(1.1–2.3)
Low-density lipoprotein	6.0 mmol/l	(2.6–5.1)
Triglyceride	1.8 mmol/l	(0.1–2.1)

The patient's results are shown in Table 4.18. As expected, the levels of cholesterol and low-density lipoprotein is increased; the levels of high-density lipoprotein and triglycerides are normal.

INVESTIGATION FOR AMYLOIDOSIS

Amyloidosis can only be diagnosed by biopsy and tissue staining with Congo Red. The sites for biopsy are shown in Figure 4.8.

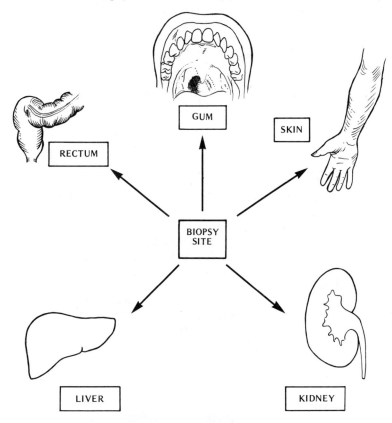

Figure 4.8   The sites for biopsy in suspected amyloidosis

The patient's rectal biopsy showed the typical pink staining of the amyloid with Congo Red, thus confirming the diagnosis.

MANAGEMENT OF NEPHROTIC SYNDROME

General Measures

Treatment of the causal condition

The nephrotic syndrome has a variety of causes (Table 4.19).

Table 4.19 Causes of nephrotic syndrome

• Infections	• Streptococcal
	• Hepatitis B
	• Syphilis
• Drugs	• Gold
	• Penicillamine
	• Tridione; mesantoin
	• Phenindione
	• Captopril
• Systemic disease	• Diabetes
	• Amyloidosis
	• Systemic lupus erythematosis
	• Polyarteritis nodosa
	• Sarcoidosis
	• Henoch–Schönlein purpura
	• Sjögren's syndrome
• Renal vein thrombosis	
• Neoplasia	
	• Hodgkin's disease
	• Carcinomatosis
	• Leukaemia

Where an underlying cause can be established it should be treated if possible.

Offending drugs should be withdrawn.

Diabetes should be controlled as strictly as possible.

Collagen disorders such as systemic lupus erythematosus and polyarteritis nodosa should be treated with steroids, which may also be of specific value for the renal disease.

The other conditions such as sarcoidosis, Henoch–Schönlein purpura and Sjögren's syndrome may also benefit from steroid treatment.

Renal vein thrombosis is treated by anticoagulants.

Neoplastic conditions might be treated with radiotherapy and/or cytotoxic drugs.

Malnutrition

Malnutrition follows the loss of protein in the urine and is often exacerbated by an associated anorexia.

Theoretically, a high-protein diet is desirable, but it is expensive. It has little permanent influence on maintaining the level of serum albumin.

Hypocalcaemia may occur as a result of loss of protein-binding cholecalciferol in the urine. Vitamin D supplements, such as calciferol tablets (10 000–50 000 units), would therefore also be of value.

Susceptibility to infection

Patients are unduly susceptible to infection because of a deficiency in circulating immunoglobulin, lost in the urine.

Prompt and effective antibiotic treatment is necessary for all infections. If renal failure is present the dose of acceptable antibiotics needs to be kept low, and some antibiotics should be avoided altogether because of the serious enhancement of their toxic effects (Table 4.20).

Table 4.20 Antibiotics to avoid in renal failure

- Neomycin
- Cephaloridine
- Chloramphenicol
- Nalidixic acid (Negram)
- Nitrofurantoin (Furadantin)
- Talampicillin
- Tetracyclines

Coagulation disorders

An increased tendency to venous thrombosis in the nephrotic syndrome occurs for the reasons shown in Table 4.21.

Table 4.21 Factors encouraging venous thrombosis in nephrotic syndrome

- Urinary loss of antithrombin III (heparin co-factor)
- Immobilization
- Vigorous diuresis
- Reduced plasma volume

This may lead to peripheral venous thrombosis or, not uncommonly, *renal vein thrombosis* – which will make the nephrotic syndrome worse.

The early detection and treatment of renal venous thrombosis is therefore important. Table 4.22 shows some helpful clinical diagnostic features. An intravenous pyelogram may show scalloping of the upper portions of the ureters caused by venous collaterals.

Table 4.22 Diagnostic features in renal vein thrombosis

- Sudden increase in albuminuria and oedema
- Pain in the loin
- Haematuria
- Pulmonary embolism

Conclusive diagnosis of renal vein thrombosis is by phlebography (Figure 4.9).

Heparin therapy is the treatment of choice.

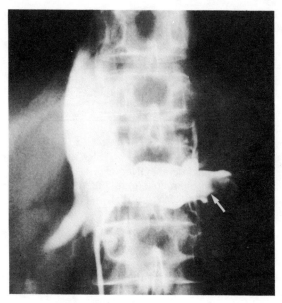

Figure 4.9 Phlebogram showing renal vein thrombosis

Hyperlipidaemia

The effect of the increase in low-density lipoprotein and cholesterol occurring in the nephrotic syndrome is to encourage atherosclerosis.

Clofibrate is currently considered hazardous because of its effect in encouraging gallstones and, in the long term, increasing mortality. Cholestyramine is unlikely to be well tolerated in the patient who already has uncomfortable gastrointestinal symptoms.

Since the clinical benefits of anti-lipidaemic therapy remain uncertain, specific drug therapy is not justified in this patient.

SYMPTOMATIC TREATMENT OF NEPHROTIC SYNDROME

Diuretics

Diuretics are the mainstay of treatment in the nephrotic syndrome. The diuretics that may be used are shown in Table 4.23. The better the renal function, the better the response to the diuretic.

Table 4.23 Diuretics used in the nephrotic syndrome

• Thiazides
• Frusemide
• Spironolactone

Thiazides are of value if renal function is good as indicated by a normal or minimally increased serum creatinine concentration. Hydrochlorothiazide 50–100 mg is an effective dose.

Frusemide, as a more-potent loop diuretic, is more effective than thiazides in the presence of renal impairment and the dose can be increased if necessary up to 500 mg–1 g daily.

Spironolactone is always worth trying in addition to a thiazide or loop diuretic, since secondary hyperaldosteronism is often present in the nephrotic syndrome. The dose is 100–200 mg daily.

When using diuretics it is important to watch out for adverse side-effects (Table 4.24). If spironolactone is used, especially if there is also some degree of renal failure, particular attention should be paid to the possibility of dangerous hyperkalaemia.

Table 4.24 Adverse effects of diuretics in the nephrotic syndrome

- Hypertension
- Hypokalaemia
- Oliguria
- Increase in renal failure

Dietary salt restriction

Salt intake should be reduced to no more than 3 g daily. This means allowing salt in the cooking but not added at the table.

Restricting salt will help eliminate oedema. However, caution is necessary if the patient is already salt-depleted because of renal failure, as indicated by a low serum sodium level (<130 mmol/l).

Correction of hypoalbuminaemia

Intravenous infusion of albumin is indicated in severe hypovolaemia and hypotension.

It is used in emergency situations only and is of transitory value only, as most of the infused albumin is soon lost in the urine.

It has no useful place in the routine management of nephrotic syndrome.

SPECIFIC TREATMENT OF NEPHROTIC SYNDROME

Over 80% of the patients with nephrotic syndrome have idiopathic glomerular lesions, and the specific management will depend on its pathological type (Table 4.25).

Steroids are of most value when the nephrotic syndrome is associated with minimal changes in the glomerulus. This minimal-change disease accounts for 80% of the cases in children but only 20% in adults.

The severity of the glomerular lesion can be decided by non-invasive and by invasive means (renal biopsy).

Table 4.25 Pathological types of glomerular disease causing nephrotic syndrome

- Minimal lesion (lipoid nephrosis)
- Membranous
- Membrano-proliferative
- Focal proliferative
    - Focal segmental glomerular sclerosis
    - Rapidly progressive glomerulo-nephritis

The non-invasive method is to determine the *selectivity* of protein loss in the urine. In minimal-change disease, only small molecular-weight protein is lost, such as albumin and transferrin. When the glomerulus is badly damaged all the plasma proteins are lost.

The initial steroid response in minimal-change nephrotic syndrome is good. Ninety per cent of children will respond initially, but the relapse rate is high and continued steroid administration may be necessary to maintain remission.

Regrettably, the rate of response to steroids in adults is poorer, about 60%.

The dose of prednisolone in both adults and children is 1 mg/kg body weight per day.

If the patient is going to respond, the response will usually be seen about the tenth day of treatment when urinary protein excretion decreases abruptly and a rapid diuresis occurs. Some useful guidelines in judging response to treatment are shown in Table 4.26.

Table 4.26 Guidelines in judging response to treatment in nephrotic syndrome

- Fall in body weight
- Reduction in oedema
- Fall in urinary protein excretion
- Increase in serum albumin level
- Fall in serum creatinine concentration

Other drugs used in treating nephrotic syndrome

Cyclophosphamide

This immunosuppressive drug is sometimes of value in prednisolone-resistant patients. The dose is 1.2–2.5 mg/kg body weight per day. The danger is marrow suppression.

Dipyridamole/warfarin combination

The addition of this combination to cyclophosphamide has sometimes been found effective in nephrotic syndrome due to diffuse membranous glomerulonephritis.

MANAGEMENT OF RENAL FAILURE IN NEPHROTIC SYNDROME

Nephrotic syndrome may lead to progressive renal failure, as in this patient.

Early intervention may prevent *secondary hyperparathyroidism*.

Phosphate-binding agents, such as aluminium hydroxide, and dietary phosphate restriction, will help to reduce the increased phosphate blood level which triggers off secondary hyperparathyroidism.

The *anaemia* of chronic renal failure may be helped with iron tablets and folic acid 1 mg/day.

With the onset of uraemic symptoms dietary *protein restriction* should be considered, though this will be complicated by the need to compensate for urinary protein loss.

MANAGEMENT OF AMYLOIDOSIS

Amyloidosis is a condition in which there is extracellular deposition of fibrous protein amyloid in various sites.

It is divided into primary and secondary types of amyloidosis. The sites affected are shown in Table 4.27. There is, however, a certain amount of overlap between the two types of the disease.

Table 4.27   Sites affected in amyloidosis

• Primary	• Tongue
	• Heart
	• Nerves
	• Gastrointestinal tract
	• Skin
• Secondary	• Liver
	• Spleen
	• Kidneys

Primary amyloidosis is often associated with myelomatosis. The causes of secondary amyloidosis are shown in Table 4.28.

The most frequent cause of secondary amyloidosis in the United Kingdom is chronic rheumatoid arthritis.

Table 4.28   Causes of secondary amyloidosis

• Chronic infection	• Bronchiectasis
	• Osteomyelitis
	• Tuberculosis
• Chronic inflammation	• Rheumatoid arthritis
	• Ankylosing spondylitis
• Heredo-familial e.g.	• Mediterranean fever
• Ageing	

General measures

There are no general measures which are relevant to the treatment of primary amyloidosis.

In secondary amyloidosis, the only measure likely to be of value is effective control of the underlying disorder which has led to the condition (Table 4.29).

Table 4.29 Treatment of the underlying disorder in secondary amyloidosis

• Chronic suppuration	– Antibiotics
	Surgery
• Chronic arthritis	– Non-steroidal anti-inflammatory drugs
	Steroids

Adequate control of the primary disease may sometimes halt the progress of the secondary amyloidosis.

Specific treatment

There is no specific therapy for any variety of amyloidosis.

However, because of the relationship between amyloidosis and myelomatosis and other plasma cell disorders, a combination of alkylating agent (melphalan) and prednisolone is sometimes tried with varying degrees of success.

Bone marrow depression may occur with melphalan, and occasional cases of leukaemia have been reported.

In the special case of amyloidosis secondary to familial Mediterranean fever, *colchicine* has been found of value.

MANAGEMENT OF BRONCHIECTASIS

General measures

Avoidance of irritants

Inflammation from any cause may exacerbate bronchiectasis. In practical terms, avoidance of this means adopting the measures recommended in Table 4.30.

Table 4.30 Avoidance of irritants in bronchiectasis

• Prohibition of smoking
• Avoid going out in fogs and smogs
• Avoid crowds in the 'flu' season
• Regular influenza vaccinations

Influenza vaccination gives some protection against influenza A and B. As the 'flu' virus strain frequently changes and new non A/non B strains occur, the standard vaccine may be ineffective.

Oxygen

This may be of value in severe exacerbations. It can be administered at home.

Specific treatment of bronchiectasis

Antibiotics

These form the mainstay of treatment.

An acute infection is likely to be due to *Haemophilus influenzae* or anaerobes, so prompt treatment with a broad-spectrum antibiotic, such as *ampicillin* or *amoxycillin*, is necessary.

Allergy to penicillin, or failure to respond within a few days as indicated by persistence of green or yellow sputum, warrants a change to a *tetracycline*, unless renal failure is present; in these circumstances *trimethoprim* should be used in reduced dose (100–200 mg daily).

If the sputum still remains infected, then sputum culture is necessary to decide the appropriate antibiotic to be given next.

Patients who have had repeated courses of antibiotics may have infections with resistant organisms, such as *Staphylococcus aureus* or *Pseudomonas aeruginosa*, so a penicillinase-resistant penicillin, a cephalosporin or an aminoglycoside, such as *gentamicin*, may be the drug of choice.

Postural drainage

This is of value in the prevention of infective episodes. The patient should be encouraged to carry it out at least twice, and preferably three times, each day, especially first thing in the morning and last thing at night.

The patient could lie head-down across the bed. A little gentle percussion over the lung bases by a co-operative spouse or relative is of added value.

Bronchodilators

These drugs may help if there is associated bronchitis with bronchospasm, which is a frequent occurrence in bronchiectatic patients. The choice of preparations is shown in Table 4.31.

Cough medicines

There is little scientific evidence that cough medicines increase expectoration, but they are widely used and may be of value as a placebo. There are many proprietary and non-proprietary preparations from which to choose.

Table 4.31 Bronchodilators

Oral	
• Aminophylline	100–300 mg as necessary
• Choline theophyllinate (Choledyl)	200 mg t.d.s.
• Theophylline (Nuelin)	60–200 mg t.d.s.
Aerosol	
• β-Receptor stimulants	salbutamol (Ventolin)
	terbutaline (Bricanyl)
	rimiterol (Pulmadil)
	fenoterol (Berotec)
• Anticholinergic	ipratropium (Atrovent)
• Sympathomimetic	orciprenaline (Alupent)

Surgery

Surgery is used less frequently now to treat bronchiectasis than it was 20–30 years ago. This is probably due to the effectiveness of modern antibiotics. Also most cases of bronchiectasis today seem to be diffuse rather than localized to one segment or lobe.

There are, however, some occasions when surgery is the preferred treatment (Table 4.32).

Table 4.32 Indications for surgery in bronchiectasis

• Localized bronchiectasis
• Persistent symptoms
• Uncontrollable haemoptysis
• Chronic fungal infection, e.g. aspergillosis

NATURAL HISTORY OF NEPHROTIC SYNDROME

The natural history of the nephrotic syndrome will depend very much on the pathological type of underlying glomerular disease (see Table 4.25).

Minimal-change disease

The long term prognosis for renal function is excellent, and a 10 year survival of at least 90% can be expected.

Diffuse membranous glomerulopathy

Spontaneous remission may occur commonly in children but in only 20% of adults.

The prognosis will depend on whether proteinuria persists. Where it does,

50% of the patients will die of intercurrent illness or develop renal failure within 10 years.

Membrano-proliferative glomerulonephritis

Spontaneous remissions are uncommon and the course is usually progressively downhill.

Over half the patients will develop renal failure or die within 10 years.

Focal sclerosis

There is no evidence that any form of treatment will prevent the relentless deterioration of this disease.

At least 50% will develop chronic renal failure or die within 10 years.

The prognosis is poorer if there is associated hypertension at the time of diagnosis.

There is a particularly bad type of focal glomerulonephritis in which the downhill course is rapidly progressive and death may occur within a few months. The distinctive pathological feature in the kidney is the *glomerular crescent*. The more extensive the crescents, the worse the prognosis. If 80% of the glomeruli are affected, death will usually occur within 6 months.

'Secondary' nephrotic syndrome

When the nephrotic syndrome is secondary to systemic disease, the prognosis will depend on this disease as well as on the degree of renal damage.

CAN WE MODIFY THE NATURAL HISTORY OF THE NEPHROTIC SYNDROME?

In practice, the underlying cause of the glomerulonephritis in most cases of nephrotic syndrome is unknown. Primary prevention is therefore not usually possible.

The only feasible preventive measure is the prompt and effective control of streptococcal infection, especially in young people.

Where the nephrotic syndrome is secondary to drugs or systemic disease, withdrawal of the offending drug and effective control of the systemic disease may induce a remission in the clinical manifestation of the nephrotic syndrome.

THE NATURAL HISTORY OF AMYLOIDOSIS

Generalized amyloidosis is a slowly progressive disease resulting in death within several years.

The prognosis will depend on the primary cause and the extent of involvement of the organs.

The prognosis in primary amyloidosis is very poor. In one extensive review the average survival was 15 months when there was no associated myeloma, and only 4 months when myeloma was also present.

The average survival in most large series is 1–4 years, though the occasional patient may live up to 10 years.

The causes of death are shown in Table 4.33

Table 4.33 Causes of death in amyloid disease

- Renal failure – commonest
- Cardiac arrhythmia
- Gastrointestinal haemorrhage
- Respiratory failure
- Intractable heart failure
- Intercurrent infection

CAN WE MODIFY THE NATURAL HISTORY OF AMYLOIDOSIS?

Secondary amyloidosis may improve with successful treatment of the underlying cause.

Otherwise, direct treatment of the amyloid has so far proved ineffective. Various drugs have been tried, including immunosuppressive drugs, but there is no convincing evidence of their efficacy. To the contrary, immunosuppressive drugs may actually encourage deposition of amyloid in various organs.

THE NATURAL HISTORY OF BRONCHIECTASIS

Prior to the introduction of antibiotics the prognosis of bronchiectasis was poor, as shown by a survey carried out in 1941 (Table 4.34).

Table 4.34 Prognosis in bronchiectasis in the pre-antibiotic era (1941)

- No. of patients surveyed — 789
- Period of survey — 2–14 years
- Overall mortality — 27.5%
- Average duration of symptoms to death — 5 years
- Average time from diagnosis to death — < 2 years

The main causes of death are shown in Table 4.35.

Table 4.35 Main causes of death in bronchiectasis

- Pneumonia
- Empyema
- Cerebral abscess
- Amyloidosis

With prompt control of infection by antibiotics most patients can now live an active and normal life though mortality is still high (Table 4.36).

Table 4.36 Survey of bronchiectasis (1981)

• No. of patients	116
• Period of survey (years)	14
• Mortality	20%
• No social disability	70%
• Satisfactory work record	70%
• Housebound	8%

A well-controlled patient with mild symptoms may have no decrease in life expectation at all.

Deterioration of the bronchiectasis is often associated with continued smoking.

Diffuse bronchiectasis with underlying mucoviscoidosis (fibrocystic disease) or immunological deficiency is associated with a very poor prognosis.

CAN WE MODIFY THE NATURAL HISTORY OF BRONCHIECTASIS

The most effective approach to bronchiectasis is preventive, since it commonly results from severe respiratory infection in childhood.

Prompt and intensive antibiotic treatment is essential. Additionally, adequate clinical and radiological follow-up should be continued through convalescence to confirm satisfactory and complete resolution of the infection. If there is evidence of collapse, *breathing exercises* and *postural drainage* should be carried out until the chest X-ray returns to normal.

These precautions are especially important after a severe attack of *measles* or *whooping cough*. Since these two conditions are among the worst 'offenders' in production of bronchiectasis, eradication by *vaccination* is an important preventive measure.

Where patients have hereditary disease, such as fibrocystic disease, which predisposes to bronchiectasis, *genetic counselling* may be helpful.

Prompt diagnosis and effective antibiotic treatment at all ages of all infections of the lower respiratory tract would help to prevent the development of bronchiectasis and its deterioration.

USEFUL PRACTICAL POINTS

- The two commonest causes of symmetrical leg oedema are heart failure and nephrotic syndrome. The clinical distinction between the two is that renal oedema is generalized (especially round the eyes) and cardiac oedema occurs in dependent areas only.

- The three essential features in nephrotic syndrome are oedema, albuminuria (>3.5 g in 24 h) and hypoalbuminaemia (<30 g/l).

137

- 75% of cases of nephrotic syndrome are due to primary glomerular disease and the remaining 25% are caused by systemic disorders.

- The mainstay of treatment of nephrotic syndrome is diuretics. Steroids are of value when glomerular involvement is minimal – this occurs in 80% of children but only 20% of adults.

- When a patient with longstanding inflammatory disease, such as rheumatoid arthritis, or chronic suppuration, such as bronchiectasis, develops nephrotic syndrome, amyloidosis should be considered.

- The best way of diagnosing amyloidosis is by biopsy of rectum, gums or other affected organ, and subsequent tissue staining with Congo Red.

5

Indigestion

PRESENT HISTORY

A 59-year-old ex-bus driver presented with a long history of indigestion becoming worse over the last few months.

Longstanding indigestion

He had a 20-year history of recurrent bouts of indigestion.

The pain occurred in the *epigastrium* and right *hypochondrium* and occasionally over the last year or so he had felt the pain in the *middle of his back*.

He described the pain as a dull *deep-seated aching pain*.

The pain occurred *between meals* and often when he was feeling *hungry*. It was *relieved by eating* and by *indigestion mixture*. Occasionally the pain would *wake him* in the middle of the night but would be relieved rapidly with indigestion mixture.

He would *vomit* sometimes with the pain but this was inconsistent. He had never seen any undigested food, blood or material resembling coffee grounds in the vomit.

The attacks of indigestion would usually last for 2 or 3 weeks at a time and then he would be free from indigestion for several months. He thought, however, that the attacks were getting more frequent and the pain-free intervals shorter.

There was no relationship between his epigastric pain and posture, e.g. lying in bed, bending.

Recent exacerbation of the indigestion

He had not been too concerned about his chronic indigestion because he could manage to control the pain with indigestion mixtures and it had not interfered with his work as a bus driver.

However, over the previous 3 months he found that the indigestion had become unresponsive to treatment and seemed to have changed its character.

The site of the pain had moved downwards to his periumbilical region. Instead of the usual dull gnawing ache the pain had become cramp-like and colicky.

The timing of the pain had also changed. Instead of occurring when he was hungry, often just before mealtimes, it was now troubling him about 15–30 minutes after he had eaten.

Finally, he was getting no relief either by eating more food or taking alkalis as he used to do.

He had now lost several days from work over the last few months because the pain had been really troublesome and he had found that strenuous work often made it worse.

Other relevant facts on direct enquiry

Alimentary system

Although he had not lost his *appetite*, he admitted that he was getting afraid to eat because of the severe pain.

He had noticed some *rumbling* in his abdomen recently which seemed to accompany the colicky pain.

He had developed some *diarrhoea* recently which he thought tended to occur whenever the colicky central abdominal pain was bad. He had no previous history of bowel disturbance.

He also admitted to occasional bright red *blood in his stools* but he had this for several years. He had not seen any blood in the loose motions accompanying the recent diarrhoea.

He had *lost* about a stone (6.5 kg) in *weight* over the last few months. He thought this was due to not eating because of the pain.

Cardiovascular system

He admitted to occasional attacks of tight *pain across his chest* with heaviness of the left arm. This occurred whenever he undertook any excessive physical effort, and had occurred several times at work.

He had the pain for about 2 years. It was infrequent, less than once a month on average, so he had never bothered to see his doctor about it.

Over the last few months he had noticed *aching in the front of both thighs* which seemed to come on whenever he was walking up a steep hill or climbing several flights of stairs. He didn't have to stop but had found that slowing his pace eased the pain.

He also admitted to aching in the calves on walking but this was not as consistent as the pain in the thighs.

Respiratory system

He had what he called a chronic 'smoker's cough'. He brought up grey or white sputum, often flecked with black spots, most mornings.

He was susceptible to 'winter bronchitis' when the sputum would become yellow or green.

Negative points

He denied any joint pains.
He had no skin rashes.
He was not prone to spontaneous bruising.
He had not seen any blood in his urine.
He had no paraesthesiae or limb weakness.

PAST HISTORY

He had a *heart attack* when he was 56 years of age.
   After discharge, from the hospital, he started to develop occasional chest pain on exertion.

FAMILY HISTORY

His father died of a heart attack when he was 52 years old.
His mother suffered with diabetes.

PERSONAL HISTORY

He had worked as a bus driver till he had his heart attack. He had then lost his Public Service Vehicle Driving Licence and had remained unemployed since.
   He was a *heavy smoker* – about 30 cigarettes a day – for most of his adult life. He had given up temporarily on medical advice after his heart attack but had restarted 18 months ago and was trying to smoke no more than 15 cigarettes a day.
   He drank 3 pints (1.7 litres) of beer twice or three times each week.

DRUG HISTORY

His only treatment was antacids, usually magnesium trisilicate mixture, but he would also use 'Rennies' tablets (chalk and light magnesium carbonate) when he thought it necessary.

EXAMINATION

The abnormal signs are shown in Figure 5.1.

General

The patient was thin – he looked as if he had lost weight.
He was not pale.
He had a well marked arcus senilis with xanthomatous deposits (Figure 5.2).
There was no butterfly rash on the face.
There were no enlarged lymph nodes in the neck and especially no left supraclavicular gland (Virchow's gland).
There was no finger clubbing or periungual erythema.

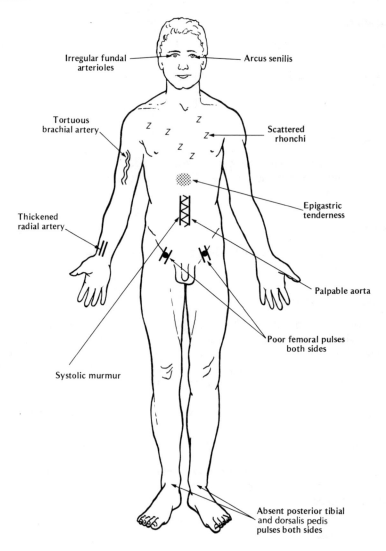

Irregular fundal arterioles

Arcus senilis

Tortuous brachial artery

Scattered rhonchi

Epigastric tenderness

Thickened radial artery

Palpable aorta

Poor femoral pulses both sides

Systolic murmur

Absent posterior tibial and dorsalis pedis pulses both sides

Figure 5.1 Abnormal physical signs

Cardiovascular system

The pulse rate was normal and regular.

The radial artery was thickened. The brachial artery was thickened and tortuous (locomotor brachial artery).

The blood pressure was 170/100 and equal in both arms.

The apex beat was normal.

The heart sounds were normal; there was no gallop; there were no murmurs.

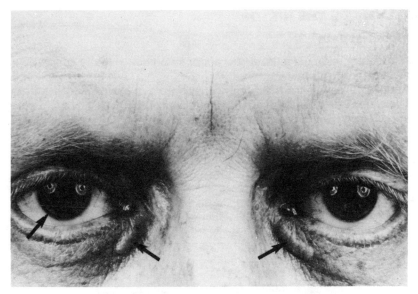

Figure 5.2 Arcus senilis with xanthelasma

Peripheral pulses

The femoral pulses were palpable but weak on both sides. Neither the posterior tibial nor the dorsalis pedis pulses was palpable in either foot.

Fundal arterioles

These were narrowed, irregular and tortuous on both sides. There was early arteriovenous nipping.

Respiratory system

The only abnormality was a few scattered high-pitched inspiratory rhonchi.

Abdomen

There was slight epigastric tenderness.
There was no abdominal distension or gastric 'succussion splash'.
No abdominal masses were felt.
The liver was not enlarged and the spleen was not palpable.
The abdominal aorta was easily felt but the pulsation was not considered to be expansile. There was a loud systolic murmur over the vessel.

Nervous system

No abnormality was found. There were no carotid or intracranial murmurs.

ANALYSIS OF THE HISTORY

Abdominal pain

The main presenting symptom was abdominal pain, initially epigastric and subsequently periumbilical.

Abdominal pain is the most frequent symptom of gastrointestinal disease.

There are three main types of abdominal pain (Table 5.1). The symptomatic features which help in deciding the cause of the abdominal pain are shown in Table 5.2.

Table 5.1   Types of abdominal pain

• Visceral	–	distension of organ muscle spasm in organ
• Peritoneal	–	inflammation of parietal peritoneum
• Referred	–	via common somatic and visceral afferent nervous pathway

Table 5.2 Helpful diagnostic features in abdominal pain

- Site
- Character
- Aggravating factors
- Relieving factors

Site of the pain

Visceral pain is deep-seated and vaguely localized according to the part of the gastrointestinal tract involved (Figure 5.3).

Peritoneal pain is usually felt over the affected organ though sometimes it may be referred, e.g. central diaphragmatic peritonitis may be referred to the tip of the shoulder.

Referred pain depends on the organ involved. Heart or lung pain may be felt in the upper abdomen while pain from the spine or nerve roots is referred to the appropriate abdominal dermatone.

The patient complained of pain at two different sites:

(1)   The *epigastric* pain is likely to be of gastroduodenal or biliary origin.
(2)   The *central abdominal* pain is probably due to involvement of the small intestine.

Character of the pain

Visceral pain is usually constant but may be colicky, as in renal colic but not gallstone colic which is usually constant. It is a deep-seated aching pain which in peptic ulcer is described typically as *gnawing*.

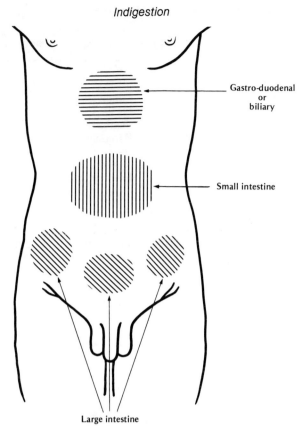

Figure 5.3 Sites of abdominal pain related to part of gastrointestinal tract involved

Peritoneal pain has a sharp superficial quality and is accompanied by marked local tenderness.

Referred pain may be stabbing, cutting or burning.

The patient described his epigastric pain as 'gnawing', which suggests peptic ulcer pain.

The periumbilical pain was colicky, which indicates spasm in the small intestine.

Aggravating factors

Relevant factors which may give some diagnostic help are shown in Table 5.3.

The relationship of the patient's epigastric pain to meals suggests peptic ulcer.

The occurrence of the pain before a meal, when the patient is hungry, rather than half an hour to 1 hour after eating, is more suggestive of duodenal ulcer than gastric ulcer, though this distinction is not always the case.

The patient's periumbilical pain is also related to meals, occurring about half an hour afterwards. The atypical site, however, makes it unlikely to be due to peptic ulcer.

Table 5.3 Diagnostic value of aggravating factors in abdominal pain

• Meals	– Peptic ulcer
• Aspirin and other anti-inflammatory drugs	– Peptic ulcer
• Bending or stooping	– Gastro-oesophageal regurgitation (hiatus hernia)
• Coughing, sneezing, movement	– Peritonitis
• Deep breathing	– Referred from lung disease
• Lying flat	– Pancreatitis
• Anxiety or stress	– Psychogenic pain

There is a condition designated *abdominal angina* which is due to atheroma of the mesenteric arteries. This pain occurs typically 15–30 min after eating.

The patient's pain may therefore be due to abdominal angina.

Relieving factors

The helpful diagnostic factors are shown in Table 5.4.

Table 5.4 Diagnostic value of relieving factors in abdominal pain

• Food	– Duodenal ulcer
• Alkalis	– Gastric or duodenal ulcer
• Bowel evacuation	– Colonic disease
• Sitting up	– Pancreatitis

The relief of the patient's epigastric pain by alkalis confirms peptic ulcer.

The beneficial effect of eating on the patient's pain suggests duodenal rather than gastric ulcer.

Alkalis and eating did not relieve the patient's periumbilical pain, which

Table 5.5 Differentation of gastric and duodenal ulcers

	Gastric ulcer	Duodenal ulcer
Relation to meals	1–2 h after	Just before
Effect of eating	Pain worse	Pain better
Vomiting	Common	Uncommon (unless pyloric stenosis)
Nocturnal pain	Rare	Frequent
Penetration to back	Rare	Common
Appetite	May be reduced	Usually normal
Weight loss	May occur (afraid to eat)	Rare
Malignant change	May occur	Extremely rare

confirms that it is not due to peptic ulcer. There were no other helpful relieving factors in relation to this pain.

The symptomatic differentiation between gastric and duodenal ulcer is shown in Table 5.5, though there is considerable overlap between the two conditions.

Flatulence

A complaint of 'flatulence' or 'wind' may imply various symptoms (Table 5.6).

Table 5.6 Types of flatulence

- Belching
- Passing flatus per rectum
- Abdominal distension
- Abdominal 'rumbling'

Belching is frequently due to swallowing air (aerophagy) which may result in several situations (Table 5.7). Rarely, belching is of organic origin due to pyloric obstruction caused either by peptic ulcer or carcinoma of the stomach.

Table 5.7 Situations leading to aerophagy

- Fear or anxiety
- Dry mouth
- Excessive salivation
- Eating in a hurry

Flatus per rectum is caused by excessive fermentation of food by intestinal bacteria with the production of carbon dioxide, methane, hydrogen and nitrogen.

It is most frequently due to eating food containing a substantial amount of non-digestible polysaccharides, such as beans, cabbage or broccoli. Flatus may also be due to organic disease when it is associated with malabsorption states.

Abdominal *distension* is due to excessive air in the bowel. It is caused either by aerophagy or by abnormal fermentation in the bowel.

Rumbling, or borborygmi, in the abdomen is usually of functional origin and due to excessive gut motility. It is a common manifestation of the *irritable bowel syndrome*, the features of which are shown in Table 5.8.

An abnormal increase in gut motility may occur in subacute intestinal obstruction. In these circumstances, other symptoms are common and occur with both small and large intestinal obstruction (Table 5.9).

147

Table 5.8   Irritable bowel syndrome

• Abdominal pain	– varying site constant or colicky
• Abdominal distension	
• Rumbling	
• Constipation	– pellet-like stools ribbon-like stools
• Morning diarrhoea	– loose or watery stools
• Anorexia and nausea	
• Associated symptoms of anxiety	

Table   5.9   Symptoms   in   intestinal obstruction

- • Colicky abdominal pain
- • Vomiting – may become faecal
- • Abdominal distension
- • Increasing constipation

The differentiation between obstruction of the small bowel and of the large bowel is shown in Table 5.10.

Table 5.10   Differentation between small and large bowel syndrome

	Large bowel	*Small bowel*
Onset	Slow	Fast
Site of pain	Lower abdomen	Periumbilical
Radiation	Flanks	–
Vomiting	Late	Early
Faecal vomiting	Rare	Sometimes
Constipation	Early	Late

Although the patient complained of abdominal rumbling, he had no other symptoms of irritable bowel syndrome, nor did he have any other symptoms to suggest intestinal obstruction.

Vascular insufficiency in the small intestine may act as the irritable stimulus causing the patient's borborygmi.

Diarrhoea

Acute diarrhoea

Acute diarrhoea is usually due to infection (Table 5.11).

A history of others suffering after eating the meal suggests food poisoning often due to staphylococci. Recent travel abroad may be relevant, especially with enteropathic *Escherichia coli.*

The length of the patient's history of diarrhoea excludes an acute infective cause of the type listed in Table 5.11.

Table 5.11 Infective causes of acute diarrhoea

- *Salmonella*
- *E. coli*
- Staphylococci
- *Shigella*
- Viruses

Chronic diarrhoea

The causes of subacute or chronic diarrhoea are shown in Table 5.12.

Table 5.12 Causes of chronic diarrhoea

- Ulcerative colitis
- Crohn's disease
- Carcinoma of the colon
- Diverticulitis
- Drugs
- Thyrotoxicosis
- Diabetes
- Mesenteric ischaemia
- Malabsorption states

Ulcerative colitis
Ulcerative colitis has distinctive features (Figure 5.4).

The patient's age, absence of severe constitutional symptoms, lack of bloody diarrhoea and absence of systemic involvement exclude this diagnosis.

Crohn's disease
The features are shown in Figure 5.5.

The lack of pain in the right iliac fossa and bloody diarrhoea, the absence of any perianal pain or abscesses and the absence of any symptoms of systemic involvement exclude this diagnosis.

Carcinoma of colon
Carcinoma of the ascending colon is usually associated with diarrhoea, while involvement of the descending colon usually produces increasing consti-

YOUNG PATIENT

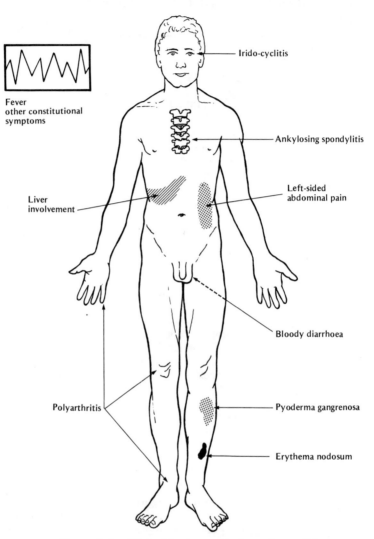

Fever
other constitutional
symptoms

Irido-cyclitis

Ankylosing spondylitis

Left-sided
abdominal pain

Liver
involvement

Bloody diarrhoea

Polyarthritis

Pyoderma gangrenosa

Erythema nodosum

Figure 5.4   Clinical features of ulcerative colitis

pation. Bleeding into the stools is frequent and anaemia is a common consequence.

There were no symptoms of anaemia in the patient (Table 5.13). However, it is not possible to exclude this diagnosis with certainty on the history alone – barium studies are necessary.

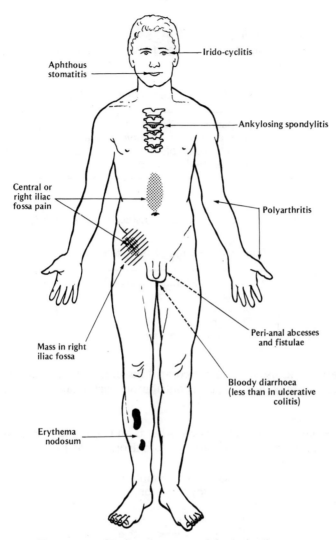

Figure 5.5   Clinical features of Crohn's disease

Table 5.13   Symptoms of Anaemia

- Weakness
- Breathlessness
- Palpitations
- Faintness
- Pallor
- Swelling of the feet

Diverticulitis

The features are shown in Table 5.14.

The absences of pain in the left iliac fossa and of urinary symptoms are against this diagnosis.

Table 5.14   Features of diverticulitis

- Colicky pain in left iliac fossa
- Constipation or constipation/diarrhoea
- Urinary symptoms often
- 'Acute abdomen' can occur

Drugs

The drugs which may cause diarrhoea are listed in Table 5.15.

Table 5.15   Drugs causing diarrhoea

- Magnesium-containing antacids
- Antibiotics
- Digitalis
- Guanethidine
- Excessive purgatives

The patient did use antacids to control his indigestion, often magnesium trisilicate. This may therefore be a contributory factor causing his diarrhoea.

Thyrotoxicosis

Diarrhoea may occur in thyrotoxicosis but is an uncommon symptom. There were no other symptoms to suggest thyrotoxicosis in the patient (Table 5.16).

Table 5.16   Symptoms of thyrotoxicosis

- Heat intolerance
- Excessive sweating
- Palpitations
- Tremors
- Irritability
- Increased appetite

Diabetes

Diarrhoea may occur in diabetes as a result of autonomic neuropathy affecting the bowel. It usually occurs at night.

The patient had no thirst or polyuria to suggest diabetes. There was no postural faintness which is the other important manifestation of autonomic neuropathy.

There is therefore nothing to suggest that the patient has diabetes.

Mesenteric ischaemia

Chronic small intestinal ischaemia is due to obstruction of the superior mesenteric artery by atherosclerosis (Figure 5.6).

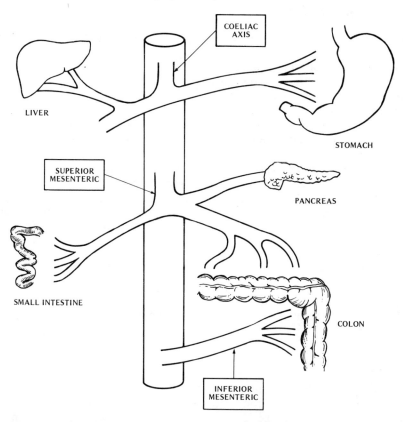

Figure 5.6   Anatomy of the mesenteric arteries

The typical symptoms of this condition are postprandial colicky periumbilical pain, 15–30 minutes after eating, associated with diarrhoea.

The pattern of the patient's symptoms fits this picture very well, making it likely that he does have intestinal ischaemia due to superior mesenteric artery obstruction.

Involvement of the inferior mesenteric artery leads to ischaemic colitis which has an acute onset with severe left-sided abdominal pain and bloody diarrhoea. Gangrene of the bowel occurs in 10–15% of these patients.

There were no symptoms to suggest ischaemic involvement of the colon in the patient.

Malabsorption states

Malabsorption in the bowel leads to pale bulky offensive stools which float and are difficult to flush away.

The absence of such stools in the patient excludes the diagnosis of malabsorption.

Blood in the stools

The patient complained of passing bright-red blood in the stools over several years.

This indicates bleeding from the rectum or the descending colon. Bleeding from more proximal sites in the gastrointestinal tract is likely to produce *dark stools*, and not bright-red blood in the stools, because of the breakdown of the haemoglobin during passage through the bowel.

The most frequent cause of bright-red blood in the stools is *bleeding piles*, and this was confirmed by the patient who knew he had suffered with piles for several years.

More serious disease affecting the descending colon, such as ulcerative colitis or carcinoma, can also lead to frank blood in the stools. Colitis has already been excluded by the absence of other typical features (see Figure 5.4). Carcinoma can only be excluded satisfactorily by a barium enema examination.

Chest pain

The attacks of chest pain on exertion over the previous 3 years clearly indicate *angina*.

The significance of this symptom is in indicating the presence of athero-sclerotic disease.

Leg pain

The pain in the thighs, coming on with walking and relieved by resting, indicates intermittent claudication. The site of the pain helps to localize the level of atherosclerotic/thrombotic obstruction of the abdominal aorta and its branches (Figure 5.7).

The pain in both of the patient's thighs points to vascular obstruction in the lower part of the abdominal aorta. Sometimes with this type of obstruction pain occurs in the buttocks.

An interesting and rare additional manifestation of terminal aortic occlusion is *impotence* due to an impaired blood supply to the penis preventing adequate erection (*Leriche's syndrome*).

A frequent site of atherosclerotic obstruction in the lower limbs is the femoral artery either in its superficial or its deep branches. This produces the classical calf pain on walking.

Chronic cough

The chronic cough with production of daily grey or white sputum indicates non-infected chronic bronchitis. Superadded acute infection turns the sputum green or yellow.

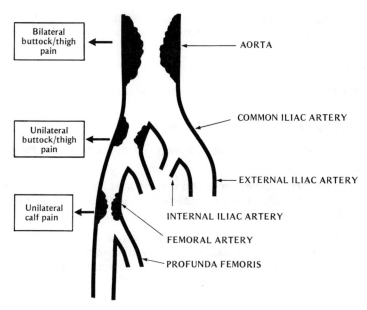

Figure 5.7 Sites of vascular obstruction in intermittent claudication

The main causal factor was the patient's cigarette smoking.

PAST HISTORY

The heart attack indicates the presence of coronary atherosclerosis and fits into the pattern of generalized atherosclerosis suggested by the history.

FAMILY HISTORY

His father's heart attack at the relatively early age of 52 years suggests the likelihood of a genetic predisposition to atherosclerosis in the patient.

The mother's diabetes reinforces this genetic susceptibility since the association between diabetes and arterial disease is well recognized.

PERSONAL HISTORY

Bus Driving

The development of ischaemic heart disease in the patient precludes the holding of a licence to drive a public service vehicle or a heavy goods vehicle. A bus driver who has had a heart attack is no longer legally entitled to continue his bus driving. The reason is obvious, since the risk of a recurrence of a heart attack within a period of 5 years is ten times that of the healthy individual of the same age.

Personal car driving is quite acceptable and legal provided the patient is not subject to angina during driving. The patient should wait 3 months after a heart attack before resuming car driving.

Smoking

This is the major cause of the patient's arterial disease

CONCLUSIONS FROM THE HISTORY

- The long history of indigestion suggests a peptic ulcer, most likely duodenal.

- The recent periumbilical pain and diarrhoea is likely to be due to small intestinal ischaemia caused by atherosclerosis of the superior mesenteric artery.

- The patient has generalized arteriosclerosis manifesting itself in ischaemic heart disease due to involvement of the coronary arteries, intermittent claudication due to involvement of the terminal aorta and/or iliac arteries, and mesenteric ischaemia (Table 5.17).

Table 5.17   Atherosclerotic pattern of the history

• Heart attack	– coronary atherosclerosis
• Angina	– coronary atherosclerosis
• Claudication	– aorto-iliac atherosclerosis
• Central abdominal pain	– mesenteric atherosclerosis

ANALYSIS OF THE EXAMINATION

Arcus senilis

This indicates premature arteriosclerosis.

Alimentary system

The only abnormality was epigastric tenderness. This is often present with an active peptic ulcer.

There was no evidence of gastric carcinoma (Figure 5.8). This should always be considered when the typical symptoms of peptic ulcer change as in this patient (Table 5.18).

Cardiovascular system

There are a number of abnormal findings (Table 5.19). All these findings indicate extensive peripheral arterial disease.

Table 5.18   Change in patient's symptoms

- Altered site of pain
- Altered relationship to eating
- Failure to respond to alkalis
- Change in nature of the pain
- Development of diarrhoea with the pain

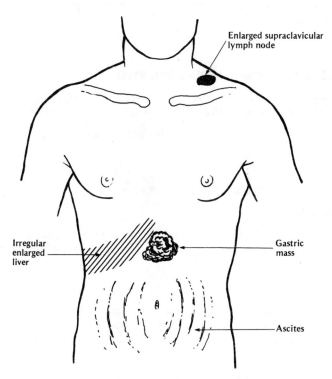

Figure 5.8   Signs of carcinoma of stomach

Table 5.19   Abnormal cardiovascular findings in the patient

- Tortuous fundal arteries
- Thickened radial artery
- Locomotor brachial artery
- Systolic bruit over abdominal aorta
- Reduced femoral pulses
- Absent foot pulses

The systolic murmur over the abdominal aorta indicates obstructive disease which is very likely to be associated with similar disease affecting the mesenteric arteries. This leads to intestinal ischaemia.

Involvement of the abdominal aorta would also impair the blood supply to the gluteal muscles and the lower limbs, thus producing claudication affecting the patient's thighs.

Respiratory system

The only finding was scattered rhonchi over both lungs. This is due to the patient's chronic bronchitis.

CONCLUSIONS FROM THE EXAMINATION

- The vascular findings indicate extensive arterial disease affecting the abdominal aorta and all the peripheral arteries to the limbs.

- The abdominal findings suggest active peptic ulceration.

INVESTIGATION OF PEPTIC ULCER

Barium meal

The simplest and most useful test in the diagnosis of peptic ulcer is a barium meal examination. The advantages and disadvantages of the barium meal are shown in Table 5.20.

Table 5.20   Advantages and disadvantages of barium meal examination in the diagnosis of peptic ulcer

• Advantages	–	Simple
		Inexpensive
		Widely available
• Disadvantages	–	May miss the ulcer (10–30%)
		Poor differentiation between benign and malignant gastric ulcer

A benign *gastric ulcer* may show as a niche of barium in the wall of the stomach or as a more substantial ulcer often on the lesser curve (Figure 5.9).

A *gastric carcinoma* is usually shown as an extensive filling defect (Figure 5.10).

A *duodenal ulcer* shows as a deformity of the duodenal cap, as in this patient (Figure 5.11). An ulcer crater may be seen superimposed on the deformity but this is difficult to detect.

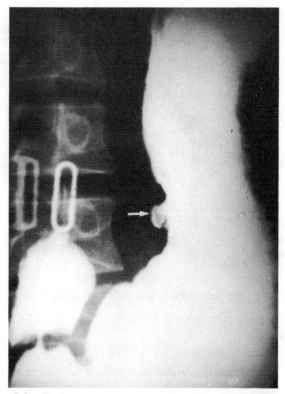

Figure 5.9 Barium meal examination showing gastric ulcer

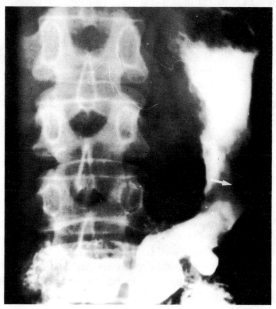

Figure 5.10 Barium meal examination showing carcinoma of the stomach

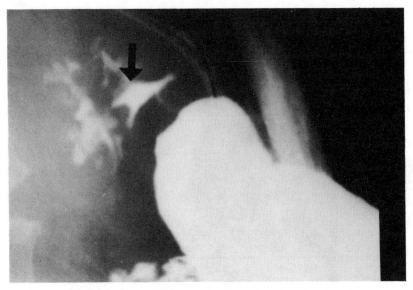

Figure 5.11 Barium meal examination showing duodenal ulcer

Endoscopy

This is a valuable investigation in both the diagnosis and management of peptic ulcer. The advantages and disadvantages are shown in Table 5.21.

Table 5.21 Advantages and disadvantages of gastroscopy

• Advantages	– Accurate
	Reliable
	Distinguishes between benign and malignant lesions
	Biopsy can be taken
	Can assess healing of ulcer
	Can control bleeding (diathermy, laser)
• Disadvantages	– Not readily available
	Uncomfortable for patient
	Complications can occur:
	perforation of oesophagus
	bursting of recent perforation
	bursting of recently healed ulcer

The indications for gastroscopy in preference to barium meal examination are shown in Table 5.22.

The two investigations may well complement each other and enhance diagnostic accuracy. Endoscopy would show active ulceration in 50% of dyspeptic patients with non-specific changes in the barium meal and in 30% of patients in whom the barium meal is entirely normal.

160

Table 5.22   Indications for gastroscopy

- To exclude malignancy
- Equivocal or normal barium meal
- To assess response to treatment
- Failure to respond to conventional treatment
- To detect cause of bleeding
- Previous stomach operation (barium meal difficult to interpret)

Gastroscopy was not considered necessary in the patient since the barium meal showed clearly the presence of duodenal ulceration.

Gastric acidity studies

This has no place in the routine management of peptic ulcer.

INVESTIGATION OF MESENTERIC ISCHAEMIA

The only investigation of value is aortography and selective angiography of the mesenteric vessels.

INVESTIGATIONS OF PERIPHERAL VASCULAR DISEASE

Angiography is the definitive investigation here also. It is required for the following two reasons:

(1)   Detection of peripheral arterial disease.
(2)   Localization of any blockage with a view to the feasibility of surgical treatment.

Figure 5.12 shows the patient's arteriogram with extensive atherosclerotic obstruction affecting the aorta and iliac arteries.

INVESTIGATION OF ISCHAEMIC HEART DISEASE

The patient's ischaemic heart disease has manifested as a previous heart attack and current angina.

Electrocardiogram

This is a necessary test in the diagnosis of myocardial infarction but is of limited value in angina.

The diagnosis of angina is based primarily on the history. The resting e.c.g. is often normal unless a previous heart attack has occurred. An exercise e.c.g. is of more value in diagnosing cardiac ischaemia under stress. A positive test will confirm ischaemia but a negative test will not exclude it.

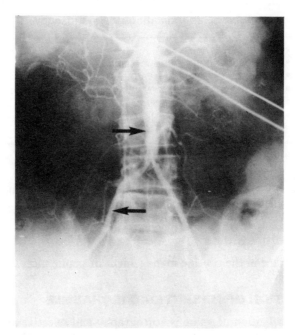

Figure 5.12   Arteriogram showing obstruction of the abdominal aorta and iliac arteries

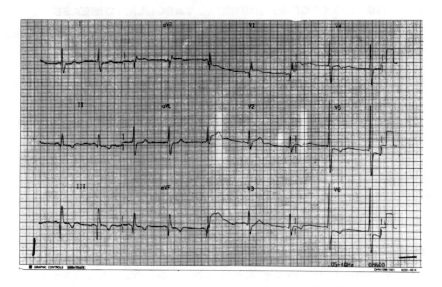

Figure 5.13   Electrocardiogram showing old inferior infarction

The patient's e.c.g. is shown in Figure 5.13. There is a stabilized inferior infarction with deep Q waves in leads III and aVF but no S–T elevation to indicate recent ischaemia.

Chest X-ray

This is of no value in the diagnosis of angina.

It may be of prognostic value in showing cardiac enlargement, which is of adverse significance.

The patient's chest X-ray was normal.

Blood lipids

This test is of very little value in this patient since there is no evidence that lowering a raised blood cholesterol at the age of 59 years is of any therapeutic value.

MANAGEMENT OF PEPTIC ULCER

The aims of treatment of peptic ulcer are shown in Table 5.23.

Table 5.23 Aims of treatment of peptic ulcer

- Relief of symptoms
- Healing of the ulcer
- Prevention of recurrence
- Prevention of complications

Medical treatment can relieve pain and heal the ulcer, but is unlikely to prevent a recurrence of the ulcer or the development of complications. Treatment is based on four approaches (Table 5.24).

Table 5.24 Approach to treatment of peptic ulcer

- General measures
- Symptomatic measures
- Specific medical treatment
- Surgical treatment

General measures in treating peptic ulcer

The general measures which may be of value are shown in Table 5.25.

Table 5.25 General measures in treating peptic ulcers

- Bed-rest
- Stopping smoking
- Diet
  - Frequent small meals
  - Avoidance of fried foods
  - Avoidance of spices
- Avoid gastric irritant drugs
  - Aspirin
  - Non-steroidal anti-inflammatory drugs
  - Steroids
- Sedation

Bed-rest

This is an effective measure for control of ulcer pain and healing of the ulcer.

It can be undertaken at home under the care of the family doctor but is probably more effective in hospital because of the detachment from domestic and business worries.

The risks of bed-rest (Table 5.26) should be balanced against the benefits of healing the ulcer quickly. It may well be that all that is required is a break from the strain of work while remaining fully ambulant.

Table 5.26 Risks of bed-rest in treatment of peptic ulcer

- Deep vein thrombosis
- Lung infection
- Urinary retention and infection

Smoking

Stopping smoking can accelerate the healing of a gastric ulcer but is less effective in duodenal ulcer.

Diet

Dietary modification is of very little value in the healing of peptic ulcer and a normal diet is probably best.

However, it is sensible to avoid any food which is known to provoke the indigestion, such as fried food or spices. It is also advisable to take small frequent meals for their acid-neutralizing effect, which is unfortunately very transient.

Drugs

It is important to avoid drugs listed in Table 5.25 since they irritate the stomach mucosa and exacerbate the ulcer pain or cause bleeding from the ulcer.

Sedation

Patients with chronic painful peptic ulcer are often tense and anxious.

A short course of a tranquillizer, such as diazepam (Valium) 2–5 mg t.d.s., may be of value if the anxiety is a major problem.

Symptomatic treatment of peptic ulcer

Although the role of gastric hydrochloric acid in the development of peptic ulcer has not been defined, there is a close link between the production of ulcer pain and the level of gastric acidity. Control of the pain can be achieved by neutralization of gastric acid with alkali mixtures (antacids).

There are many antacids available. They can be divided into two groups according to their solubility in water (Table 5.27).

Table 5.27　Antacids used in treating peptic ulcer

• Water-soluble	• Sodium bicarbonate
	• Calcium carbonate
• Water-insoluble	• Aluminium – hydroxide
	phosphate
	glycinate
	• Magnesium – carbonate
	hydroxide
	trisilicate

Water-soluble antacids

Although the water-soluble antacids are very effective at increasing gastric pH and controlling ulcer pain, they are easily absorbed into the systemic circulation and may cause *alkalosis*. This is especially likely to occur if there is associated pyloric stenosis with vomiting.

The main adverse effects of prolonged alkalis are shown in Table 5.28.

Table 5.28　Adverse effects of alkalis

• Renal impairment		
• Mental changes	–	apathy
	–	personality change
	–	delirium
	–	stupor
• Tetany		

Water-insoluble antacids

Aluminium hydroxide and *magnesium trisilicate* are two of the most widely-used simple antacids and are usually very effective at relieving pain.

Doses of 15–30 ml of the mixture, or 250–500 mg of the tablets, are used between meals and at bedtime. The mixtures are generally more effective than the tablets at relieving pain. Additional doses, even at hourly intervals, can be taken as necessary to control the pain.

There are many compound proprietary preparations available for the relief of ulcer pain (Table 5.29), but they are more expensive than the simple remedies and there is no evidence that they are any more effective than the simple non-proprietary preparations.

Table 5.29   Some compound proprietary drugs used in peptic ulcer

Name	Form	Content	Dose	Price level*
Actal	tablets	Alexitol	1–2 chewed or sucked	A
	suspension	Alexitol	5–10 ml	C
Asilone	tablets	Al. hydroxide	1–2 chewed or sucked	C
	gel	Al. hydroxide	5–10 ml	C
	suspension	Mag. oxide	5–10 ml	C
Gaviscon	tablets	Sodium bicarb. Al. hydroxide	1–2 tablets chewed	C
	granules	Mag. trisilicate	1 sachet	D
	liquid	Sod. bicarbonate	10–20 ml	C
Gelusil	tablets	Al. hydroxide	1–2 chewed or sucked	B
	suspension	Mag. trisilicate	5–20 ml	B
Polycrol	tablets	Al. hydroxide Mag. carbonate Mag. hydroxide	1–2 chewed	B
	gel	Al. hydroxide Mag. hydroxide	5–10 ml	C

* Scale from A = cheapest to D = most expensive

Table 5.30 lists some side-effects of antacids.

Table 5.30   Side-effects of antacids

• Aluminium hydroxide	– Constipation
• Magnesium trisilicate	– Diarrhoea
• Sodium bicarbonate	– Alkalosis
• Calcium carbonate	– Alkalosis
	Hypercalcaemia
	Constipation
	Rebound hypersecretion of acid

There is no evidence that use of any of these antacids in their standard doses promotes healing of peptic ulcer.

Anticholinergic drugs

These drugs inhibit vagal production of gastric acid. They are rarely used now because of their limited effectiveness in standard dose and their side-effects. The preparations most used are shown in Table 5.31.

Table 5.31 Anticholinergic drugs used in peptic ulcer

• Pro-banthine		– 15 mg t.d.s.
		30 mg at night
• Kolanticon	gel	– 10–20 ml every 4 h
	tablets	– 5–10 mg every 4 h
• Nacton		– 2–4 mg every 6 h

The common side-effects are shown in Table 5.32.

Table 5.32 Side-effects of anticholinergic drugs

- Glaucoma – especially the elderly
- Difficulty with visual accommodation
- Dry mouth
- Urinary retention
- Constipation

Specific treatment of peptic ulcer

The treatments which have been shown to heal peptic ulcer are shown in Table 5.33.

Table 5.33 Treatments which heal peptic ulcer

- H_2-receptor antagonists
  cimetidine (Tagamet)
  ranitidine (Zantac)
- Carbenoxolone
- High-dose antacids
- Colloidal bismuthate

H_2-receptor antagonists

Cimetidine and ranitidine are very effective agents in reducing gastric acid production and healing peptic ulcer. Fifty per cent of gastric and duodenal ulcers can be expected to heal within 3 weeks and 90% within 6 weeks.

The dose required is shown in Table 5.34. The side-effects are shown in Table 5.35.

Table 5.34   Dose of cimetidine and ranitidine in treating peptic ulcer

• Cimetidine	–	200 mg t.d.s. and 400 mg at night for 4–6 weeks
		400 mg at night for maintenance
• Ranitidine	–	150 mg b.d. for 4–6 weeks
		150 mg daily for maintenance

Table 5.35   Side-effects of cimetidine

• Gynaecomastia	
• Diarrhoea	
• Dizziness	
• Rashes	
• Mental confusion	
• Blood dyscrasia	– leukopenia
	thrombocytopenia
• Interference with other drugs	– warfarin
	phenytoin

The problem with cimetidine, and probably with ranitidine also, is that pro-longed maintenance treatment is required since there is a high rate of relapse when treatment is stopped. It may be that treatment will need to be continued indefinitely but the hazards of prolonged treatment are unknown, especially the risk of gastric carcinoma.

The current view is that cimetidine, and probably ranitidine also, should be continued in a nocturnal maintenance dose of 400 mg for at least 1 year and then stopped. If there is a recurrence of the ulcer, one further course of treat-ment can be tried. If there is a second relapse on stopping treatment, alter-native measures, especially surgery, should be considered. Some physicians will continue intermittent short courses of cimetidine for recurrences over a longer time before recourse to surgery.

Prolonged maintenance treatment beyond a year should be confined to patients over 60 years old who are unfit for surgery.

Carbenoxolone (Biogastrone)

This is a liquorice derivative which can promote healing of peptic ulcer. It is more effective in gastric ulcer than duodenal ulcer.

The dose is 50–100 mg three times daily after meals for 4–6 weeks.

The main problem with carbenoxolone is the frequent side-effects (Table 5.36).

Table 5.36   Side-effects of carbenoxolone

• Salt retention	–	oedema
		hypertension
		heart failure
• Hypokalaemia	–	muscle weakness

The drug is contraindicated in elderly patients because of its liability to sodium retention and the precipitation of heart failure. The most useful indication of sodium retention with carbenoxolone is increasing weight.

Deglycyrrhizinized liquorice (*Caved (-S)*) is claimed to be free of the side-effects of carbenoxolone but is of doubtful efficacy. *Duogastrone* is a slower-release preparation of carbenoxolone in capsule form for treatment of duodenal ulcer.

Carbenoxolone is rarely used now since the introduction of the H_2-receptor blockers.

High-dose antacids

Very large doses of antacids such as 200–300 ml of aluminium hydroxide daily in divided doses can lead to healing of duodenal ulcer, but may be difficult for the patient to take and therefore unacceptable.

Colloidal bismuthate (De-Nol)

This drug has been shown to produce ulcer healing comparable to the H_2-receptor blockers, 80–90% in 4–6 weeks. It is claimed that healing is longer-lasting but this remains to be convincingly shown.

The dose is 5 ml (120 mg) four times daily for 4–6 weeks. Long term treatment should be avoided because of the risk of bismuth toxicity.

INDICATIONS FOR SURGERY IN PEPTIC ULCER

The indications for surgery are shown in Table 5.37. The operations available are shown in Table 5.38.

Table 5.37   Indications for surgery in peptic ulcer

• Failed medical treatment
• Complications
Uncontrollable bleeding
Perforation
Stenosis – pyloric
'hour-glass'
• Suspicion of malignancy in gastric ulcer
• Unacceptable disruption of work and/or leisure
• Recurrent ulcer following previous surgery

Table 5.38   Available operations
for peptic ulcer

- Vagotomy and pyloroplasty
- Partial gastrectomy
- Gastro-enterostomy

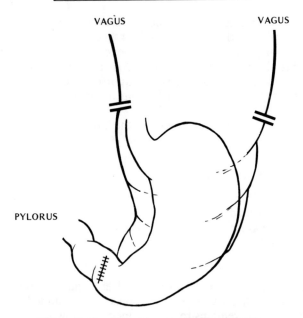

Figure 5.14   Vagotomy and pyloroplasty

The most popular operation is vagotomy and pyloroplasty (Figure 5.14).
The side-effects of surgery are shown in Table 5.39.

Table 5.39   Side-effects of surgery for peptic
ulcer

• Mechanical	• Vomiting
	• Dumping
	• Diarrhoea
• Nutritional	• Iron deficiency anaemia
	• B_{12} deficiency
	• Osteomalacia
	• Osteoporosis

COMPLICATIONS OF PEPTIC ULCER

There are three main complications of peptic ulcer. These are shown in Table
5.40 with their management.

Table 5.40 Complications of peptic ulcer and their management

• Bleeding	–	Blood transfusion
		H_2-receptor antagonists
		Surgery
• Perforation	–	Surgery
• Stenosis	–	Correct dehydration
		Restore electrolytes
		Aspirate stomach
		Surgery

MANAGEMENT OF CHRONIC INTESTINAL ISCHAEMIA

The only definitive treatment is surgical removal of any localized obstruction in the mesenteric artery, or a bypass graft (Figure 5.15).

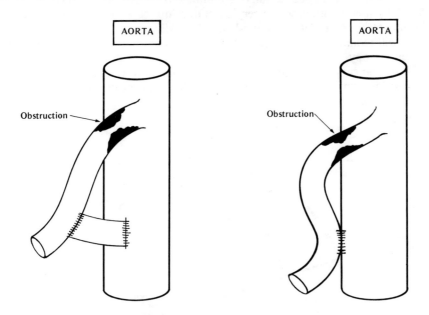

Figure 5.15 Bypass grafts for mesenteric ischaemia

NATURAL HISTORY OF PEPTIC ULCER

Prevalence of peptic ulcer

Precise figures are difficult to obtain because only a small number of patients with peptic ulcer are admitted to hospital to be included in surveys. In addition, accurate diagnosis requires radiology and/or endoscopy, and only a minority of patients in general practice will undergo these investigations. With these reservations, the prevalence of peptic ulcer in the Western world has been assessed at 12% for the male population and 9% for females. Duodenal ulcer is more common than gastric ulcer in the ratio of 4:1 in adults. Males predominate in both conditions.

The frequency of duodenal ulcer has been increasing in the West over the past 30 years. The reason for this is unknown.

Incidence

The incidence of peptic ulcer in the West is 2.5/1000 per year. The peak incidence of gastric ulcer is in the fifth decade, 10 years later than duodenal ulcer.

Prognosis

The outcome of gastric ulcer differs from that of duodenal ulcer.

Duodenal ulcer is a condition of spontaneous remissions and relapses while 50% of patients with gastric ulcer do not develop recurrence. Within a year of healing 60% of patients with duodenal ulcer will have a relapse and a further 25% will remain asymptomatic but show evidence of recurrence of ulceration on endoscopy.

A 20 year survey of the prognosis of duodenal ulcer was carried out by John Fry in his family practice (Figure 5.16). He found gastric ulcer followed a similar course.

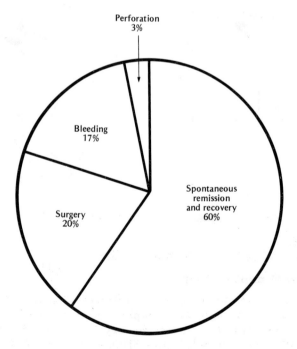

Figure 5.16 Prognosis of duodenal ulcer (from survey by John Fry)

Operation

Over 5–10 years, one in two patients with gastric ulcer and one in five patients with duodenal ulcer come to operation.

Mortality

The overall mortality in gastric and duodenal ulcer is 5/100000 per year. Death from gastric ulcer usually exceeds that from duodenal ulcer. Death from peptic ulcer is more likely in older patients.

CAN WE MODIFY THE NATURAL HISTORY OF PEPTIC ULCER?

The aetiological factors which have been suggested in gastric and duodenal ulcer are shown in Table 5.41. Very few of these possible factors are capable of modification.

Table 5.41   Aetiological factors in gastric and duodenal ulcers

	Gastric ulcer	*Duodenal ulcer*
Heredity	Marked (3 × general population)	Marked (3 × general population)
Smoking	Marked	Slight
Drugs	Aspirin Other anti-inflammatory	Nil
Hormones	Little effect	Oestrogens protect
Stress	Probably no effect	May exacerbate
Social class	Commoner in poor	Commoner in poor
Blood group	Commoner in 0	Commoner in 0
Gastric acidity	Normal	Increased
Duodeno-gastric reflux	Common	Uncommon
Associated disease	None	Coronary disease Chronic bronchitis Cirrhosis Hyperparathyroidism

Smoking

The effect of smoking in the development and cause of gastric ulcer is more significant than in duodenal ulcer.

There are two possible mechanisms of exacerbation:
(1) Nicotine decreases pancreatic bicarbonate secretion and so impairs neutralization of acid in the duodenum
(2) Nicotine relaxes the pyloric sphincter and so encourages duodeno-gastric reflux

Psychological stress

This is always being invoked as a factor in the development of peptic ulcer.

There is, however, no good objective evidence to support this view.

External stress is very difficult to quantify, and even if quantification were possible, the more important factor is the way that the particular individual responds to the stress. Response will depend very much on his or her personality and this cannot be easily changed.

Drugs

Regular use of aspirin and other anti-inflammatory drugs such as those frequently used in treating arthritis should be avoided as far as possible.

NATURAL HISTORY OF INTESTINAL ISCHAEMIA

Acute intestinal ischaemia

The four main causes of acute ischaemia of the small bowel are shown in Table 5.42.

Table 5.42 Causes of acute ischaemia of the small bowel

- Embolism in superior mesenteric artery:
    Rheumatic heart disease
    Atrial fibrillation from any cause
- Thrombosis following atheroma
- Low-flow non-occlusive states:
    Fall in cardiac output
    Digoxin → splanchnic vasoconstriction
    Haemoconcentration
    Disseminated intravascular coagulation
- Thrombosis of superior mesenteric vein

Acute intestinal ischaemia leads to infarction of the bowel with shock, peritonitis and paralytic ileus.

Laparatomy and surgery are urgently required but the outcome is poor. Survival after acute intestinal infarction is shown in Table 5.43.

Table 5.43 Survival in acute intestinal infarction

- Embolism superior mesenteric artery   – 25%
- Thrombosis superior mesenteric artery   – 20%
- Thrombosis superior mesenteric vein   – 5%

Chronic intestinal ischaemia

A clear picture of the natural history of this condition is not yet available since it is a difficult diagnosis to make and frequently a diagnosis of exclusion only.

However, the main risk in chronic intestinal ischaemia is that thrombosis will occur in the atherosclerotic vessel and precipitate acute infarction with its associated poor prognosis.

Even after surgery, the prognosis is likely to be poor, since the intestinal ischaemia is just one manifestation of a more widely spread atherosclerosis.

CAN WE MODIFY THE NATURAL HISTORY OF INTESTINAL ISCHAEMIA?

Acute ischaemia

Modification of the natural history of acute intestinal ischaemia consists mainly in prevention of emboli by long term anticoagulation treatment in atrial fibrillation and rheumatic heart disease.

Chronic ischaemia

The aetiology of this condition is that of atherosclerosis itself. The main factors involved in the development of atherosclerosis are shown in Table 5.44.

Table 5.44 Aetiological factors in atherosclerosis

• Cigarette smoking
• Hypertension
• Hypercholesterolaemia
• Diabetes
• Obesity

Smoking

This is the most important factor. Stopping smoking has been shown to be of value in all forms of occlusive arterial disease.

Hypertension

Control of hypertension will retard the development of atherosclerosis. It is likely that control of systolic pressure is as important as diastolic pressure. However, the evidence of clinical benefit of controlling systolic pressure is as yet lacking.

Hypercholesterolaemia

Control of a high blood cholesterol is likely to be of value in younger patients only.

Diabetes

Control of diabetes has yet to be shown to be of value in preventing or retarding its atherosclerotic complications.

Obesity

The risk of obesity is mainly because of the associated hypertension, hyperlipidaemia and carbohydrate intolerance. Objective evidence of the value of weight reduction in retarding atherosclerosis remains to be presented.

USEFUL PRACTICAL POINTS

- Postprandial colicky central abdominal pain with diarrhoea and weight loss is very suggestive of superior mesenteric artery obstruction.

  This condition is almost invariably associated with other symptoms and signs of generalized arteriosclerosis.

- The relationship of pain to meals, and the occurrence of nocturnal pain, is not a reliable guide in distinguishing gastric and duodenal ulcer.

- A change in the established pattern of indigestion in gastric ulcer should always suggest the possibility of malignancy.

- Cimetidine and ranitidine are currently the most effective drugs available for healing both gastric and duodenal ulcer.

  Long term maintenance therapy is likely to be necessary because of the frequent relapse on stopping the drug, but the hazards of such therapy remain to be evaluated.

- There is no evidence that any type of medical treatment currently available for peptic ulcer will prevent relapses or reduce complications such as bleeding or perforation.

- The chronic use of the water-soluble antacids (sodium bicarbonate, calcium carbonate) in the symptomatic treatment of peptic ulcer should be avoided, because of the risk of alkalosis.

6

Diarrhoea

PRESENT HISTORY

A young lady of 25 years first presented with an 18 month history of increasing diarrhoea.

Diarrhoea and abdominal pain

The diarrhoea had started about 18 months ago. It consisted of periodic episodes of diarrhoea lasting for a week or two but gradually getting more frequent and more severe.

At present bowel actions were occurring nine or ten times daily and were often associated with *colicky lower abdominal pain*.

Nature of the stools

The stools were loose and watery and, over the last month or so, she had noticed *blood and slime*. She had an earlier episode of blood in the stool a year previously and her general practitioner had diagnosed 'piles' and given her some ointment. The bleeding had settled over a week or so though she continued to have mild diarrhoea, about two or three times daily.

Since then her bowels periodically became worse over periods of 2 or 3 weeks at a time, but she had managed to cope until about 1 month before presentation, when she became a lot worse with more diarrhoea, colicky pain, blood and slime in the motions, weakness, loss of appetite and loss of weight.

Relevant negative points on direct enquiry

She denied any *joint* trouble.
She denied any *back* trouble.
She had not had any *eye* problems.
She had not noticed any *skin* problems.
She had never had any *perianal* trouble, especially abscess.

177

PAST HISTORY

There was nothing relevant.

FAMILY HISTORY

Her sister, aged 35 years, had suffered with bowel trouble for a number of years, and her mother had some trouble with her spine but the patient did not know the details.

PERSONAL HISTORY

She had two small children, aged 2 and 4 years, and was having difficulty coping owing to the periodic flare-ups of her diarrhoea. This was also leading to problems with her husband who liked to go out and socialize but was prevented from doing so by her bowel trouble.

She did not smoke.

She did not drink alcohol.

DRUG HISTORY

Her present treatment comprised:

salazopyrin 0.5 g q.d.s.
codeine phosphate 30 mg t.d.s.
ferrous sulphate 300 mg t.d.s.

She had never taken the contraceptive pill.

EXAMINATION

General

She was mildly pyrexial, 38.5 °C, pale, weepy and depressed. She was mildly dehydrated with a dry skin and tongue. There was no evidence of glossitis or aphthous ulceration in the mouth. There was early finger clubbing. There were no skin lesions, joint abnormality or eye problems.

Abdomen

The physical signs are shown in Figure 6.1.

The abdomen was distended but there was definite tenderness over the left side and the descending colon was palpable and tender. There was no rebound tenderness. The liver was not palpable. Bowel sounds were normal.

Rectal examination showed external anal tags and marked tenderness inside the rectum; soft faeces were felt and some blood-streaking was seen when the gloved finger was withdrawn.

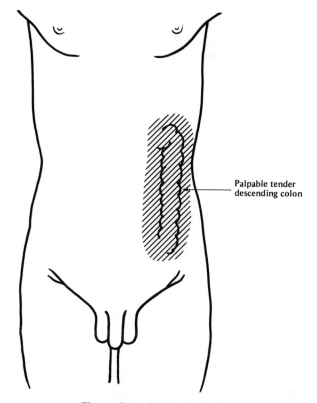

Palpable tender
descending colon

Figure 6.1   Abdominal signs

Cardiovascular system

The pulse was 110/min and regular.
The blood pressure was 130/85.
The heart sounds were normal with no murmurs.

Respiratory system

No abnormality was found.

Central nervous system

No abnormality was found.

INVESTIGATION

Proctoscopy

This was attempted but impossible because of pain and spasm in the anal
sphincter.

Sigmoidoscopy

Sigmoidoscopy was carried out under a general anaesthetic, and this showed a red congested granular mucosa which bled easily – this was thought to be the typical appearance of *ulcerative colitis*.

Rectal biopsy

Rectal biopsy from the recto-sigmoid junction showed surface epithelial destruction, mucosal congestion and haemorrhage, heavy mucosal infiltration with inflammatory cells, infection in the submucosa and some crypt abscesses – this picture was also considered highly suggestive of ulcerative colitis.

Barium enema

A barium enema examination was requested to determine the extent of the colitis, but when it was attempted in the X-ray department, the patient was reported to have 'collapsed' and so the examination was not carried out.

TREATMENT

Intravenous fluid replacement was not considered necessary, nor was blood transfusion indicated since her haemoglobin was only mildly reduced to 10.8 g/dl. She was given large doses of prednisolone orally, 60 mg a day reducing slowly over the succeeding 2 weeks, together with local hydrocortisone enemas twice daily. Antibiotics were not considered necessary.

On this regime, she improved rapidly and the diarrhoea was controlled and the stools became normal within 8 days. She was discharged on sulphasalazine (Salazopyrin) 0.5 g four times daily. A barium enema examination was booked for her as an outpatient.

PROGRESS

Review in 6 months showed that she had remained well, with no recurrence of the diarrhoea. She had become *pregnant* and so the *barium enema examination had been cancelled*. The subsequent pregnancy was uneventful, and after she had her baby she failed to reattend the medical clinic.

She was referred back to the clinic 2 years after her first admission with a severe recurrence of diarrhoea, blood and mucus in the stool and colicky abdominal pain over the previous 2 months. Three weeks earlier she had developed some *pain and swelling in her right knee* and 10 days earlier had noticed some *painful red lumps* over her shins.

She was readmitted to hospital and given a further course of high-dose prednisolone and hydrocortisone enemas and responded favourably within a week. In addition to controlling her diarrhoea, there was improvement in her right knee and the lumps on her legs became less painful and smaller. She was discharged to continue Salazopyrin, codeine phosphate tablets for symptomatic control of diarrhoea and iron tablets.

Her subsequent progress out of hospital was not so satisfactory since her bowel actions remained at 3–4 daily and the stools tended to be loose, though blood-streaking was infrequent. A further acute flare-up occurred 8 months later, necessitating readmission to hospital. Attempts were made to persuade her to undergo sigmoidoscopy and barium enema examination but she adamantly refused both investigations. She was treated once more with a high-dose prednisolone regime and local steroid enemas with some initial improvement, but insisted on early discharge because of problems at home with the three children. She was advised to continue prednisolone at home 10 mg twice daily as well as Salazopyrin, codeine phosphate and iron.

Review at the clinic showed that her condition was not settling down but she was unwilling to come back into hospital for further intensive treatment. Local steroid enemas were tried nightly at home with limited success. Six months later she was readmitted to hospital as an emergency with bowel actions up to 18 times daily, blood and mucus continually in the stools and considerable loss of weight.

On this occasion, she agreed to have a barium enema examination. This was reported as showing *extensive changes of ulcerative colitis* from the rectum to the hepatic flexure of the colon (Figure 6.2).

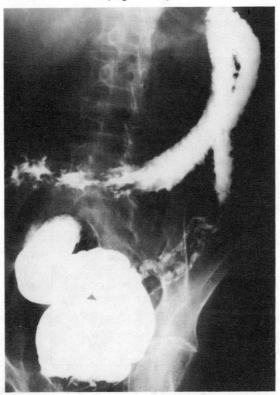

Figure 6.2   Barium enema showing changes of ulcerative colitis from rectum to hepatic flexure

In view of the frequent severe recurrences of the disease and the extensive involvement of the colon, a *panproctocolectomy* was carried out.

Histology showed the features of florid *Crohn's disease* affecting the whole of the colon; the terminal ileum was completely normal.

ANALYSIS OF THE HISTORY

Diarrhoea

Acute diarrhoea is usually due to *infection*: the common infecting organisms are shown in Table 6.1. Diagnostic clues may be obtained from the history but will usually require confirmation in the laboratory. If other individuals have been affected after eating together, *'food poisoning'* often due to staphylococcal infection is the likely cause. Recent travel abroad suggests *'Traveller's diarrhoea'* caused by enteropathic *E. coli*. *Pseudomembranous colitis* is a serious condition caused by the toxins of *C. difficile* and often follows a course of antibiotics; diagnosis is made by sigmoidoscopy and stool examination for the toxins of *C. difficile*.

Table 6.1   Causes of acute diarrhoea

• Infections	• *Salmonella*
	• *E. Coli*
	• Staphylococci
	• *Shigella*
	• Amoebiasis
	• *Campylobacter*
• Toxaemia	• Pseudomembranous colitis (*C. difficile*)

In this patient, the diarrhoea is clearly *chronic diarrhoea*: the common causes are shown in Table 6.2.

Table 6.2   Common causes of chronic diarrhoea

• Ulcerative colitis
• Crohn's disease
• Carcinoma of colon
• Diverticulitis
• Irritable colon syndrome
• Malabsorption states
• Ischaemic colitis
• Drugs
• Thyrotoxicosis
• Diabetes

The length of the history would exclude carcinoma of the colon. Diverticulitis does not usually cause severe constitutional disturbance with rectal bleeding and the same applies to irritable bowel syndrome. Malabsorption leads to bulky offensive stools without bleeding, and multiple deficiency states, and is therefore excluded in this patient. Ischaemic colitis with infarction of the colon occurs usually in young women taking the contraceptive pill and produces lower abdominal pain, fever and rectal bleeding; the length of the history and the systemic complications are against this diagnosis. The patient had not taken any drugs such as purgatives, digoxin or magnesium-containing antacids which might cause diarrhoea. There was no clinical evidence of diabetes (with autonomic neuropathy causing diarrhoea) or thyrotoxicosis.

The clinical course in this patient over $3\frac{1}{2}$ years with recurrent episodes of severe diarrhoea with blood and mucus in the stools indicates that the likely diagnosis is either *ulcerative colitis* or *Crohn's disease*, and this patient's case clearly shows the great difficulty in differentiating between the two conditions on clinical grounds alone. Some of the points which may help are shown in Table 6.3.

Table 6.3 Clinical points in differentiating between ulcerative colitis and Crohn's disease

	Colitis	*Crohn's disease*
Abdominal pain	Lower abdomen left iliac fossa	Central abdomen right iliac fossa
Diarrhoea	Severe	Moderate
Rectal bleeding	Frequent and severe	Infrequent and mild
Abdominal tenderness	Common	Sometimes
Abdominal mass	Not present	Very common
Perianal disease	Rare	Common
Fistulae	Very rare	Common
Malabsorption	Not present	Common
Mouth ulcers	Not present	Common

This patient has had frequent episodes of severe diarrhoea with profuse rectal bleeding – this favours the diagnosis of ulcerative colitis.

Abdominal pain

Abdominal pain is common in both ulcerative colitis and Crohn's disease. It is usually colicky, precedes bowel action and is relieved by defaecation.

The localization of the pain in this patient to the lower abdomen suggests a colonic origin and therefore ulcerative colitis.

In Crohn's disease the frequent involvement of the ileum leads to small intestinal pain which is periumbilical. Another important feature about the pain in Crohn's disease is that it often occurs soon after eating; this relationship was not evident in this patient.

Constitutional symptoms

Constitutional symptoms such as fever, anorexia and weight loss are more common as chronic manifestations in Crohn's disease. During exacerbations of ulcerative colitis, however, constitutional symptoms may be marked.

During the course of the patient's illness she has had frequent and severe exacerbations with prominent constitutional disturbances, and therefore this is a less helpful differentiating point in this patient.

Painful knee joint

The patient had a swollen painful right knee joint.

Joint problems occur in 10–20% of patients with ulcerative colitis and Crohn's disease (Table 6.4). Peripheral arthritis is often mono-articular and frequently affects the knee joint, as in the patient. Arthritis is more common with extensive bowel disease and reflects its activity, again exemplified by the patient, whose arthritis developed during an acute exacerbation of the disease.

Table 6.4   Arthritis associated with ulcerative colitis and Crohn's disease

	Ulcerative colitis (%)	Crohn's disease (%)
Ankylosing spondylitis	6	6
Sacro-iliitis	20	18
Peripheral arthritis	10	16

Red painful lumps on the legs

This indicates *erythema nodosum* which may occur in both conditions and is also related to the activity of the disease. It is often associated with arthritis. Both the arthritis and erythema nodosum are thought to be due to the deposition of immune complexes in the affected tissue leading to an inflammatory reaction.

There are other systemic manifestations of ulcerative colitis and Crohn's disease, and these are shown in Table 6.5.

Family history

This is very relevant in the present case. Her sister suffered with bowel trouble and her mother with back trouble.

There is a definite familial incidence of 10%–17% in patients with ulcerative colitis and Crohn's disease. The commonest pattern is an affected sibling, as in this case. Where a family history is present, the disease tends to begin earlier in life.

Her mother's back trouble could have been ankylosing spondylitis, since this too occurs more frequently in relatives of patients with ulcerative colitis or Crohn's disease.

Personal history

The patient was under considerable stress in looking after her children and in her relationship with her husband.

Table 6.5 Systemic manifestations of ulcerative colitis and Crohn's disease

Related to activity of the disease
- Aphthous ulceration in the mouth
- Skin lesions
  - erythema nodosum
  - pyoderma gangrenosum
- Acute arthritis
- Eye involvement
  - conjunctivitis
  - episcleritis
  - uveitis

Unrelated to disease activity
- Skeletal
  - sacro-iliitis
  - ankylosing spondylitis
- Biliary
  - pericholangitis
  - primary sclerosing cholangitis
  - carcinoma of the bile duct
  - gallstones
- Hepatocellular
  - chronic active hepatitis
  - cirrhosis
- Thrombo-embolic due to thrombocythaemia and increase in clotting factors
- Kidney stones, especially after ileostomy

The role of psychological factors in the initiation and development of ulcerative colitis and Crohn's disease remains controversial. Significant emotional stresses are often related to the onset and exacerbations of the disease. However, it is very difficult, especially in a young person, to distinguish the severe psychological effects of this type of chronic disabling disease from the psychological state of the patient before the disease started. Additionally, psychotherapy has been disappointing in treating the disease. It is likely that psychological factors are more important in the exacerbations of the disease rather than its onset.

CONCLUSIONS FROM THE HISTORY

- The initial presentation in a young lady of constitutional symptoms, chronic diarrhoea and bloody stools containing mucus, suggests either *ulcerative colitis* or *Crohn's disease.*

- She subsequently developed arthralgia and erythema nodosum which support the above differential diagnosis and indicate the auto-immune nature of the condition.

- In the family history, her sister's bowel trouble, and her mother's back trouble, which could be ankylosing spondylitis, lend further support to the diagnosis of auto-immune bowel disease in the patient, manifesting as either ulcerative colitis or Crohn's disease.

- The patient's lower abdominal pain, rather than periumbilical pain or pain in the right iliac fossa, and the absence of any perianal symptoms, are more in favour of *ulcerative colitis* than Crohn's disease.

- The patient was under considerable stress in her domestic life but it is not possible to be definite as to whether this is a cause or a consequence of her disease.

ANALYSIS OF THE EXAMINATION

Constitutional findings

The initial presentation in this patient was not with a severe exacerbation of the disease and so constitutional disturbance was limited. She did have slight pyrexia and mild dehydration. With the later more severe exacerbation just prior to operation, she was profoundly ill with marked fever, dehydration, weakness, cachexia and hypotension.

Anaemia

She was pale due to anaemia. The common type of anaemia in ulcerative colitis is due to iron deficiency characterized by a *microcytic hypochromic* blood picture: this is caused by *chronic blood loss*. It may be detected clinically by koilonychia (Figure 6.3).

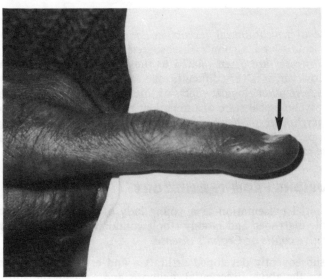

Figure 6.3   Koilonychia

In Crohn's disease there may be an alternative cause for the anaemia, *vitamin B_{12} deficiency* due to defective absorption from a diseased terminal ileum, and in this case the anaemia is *macrocytic*.

Apart from glossitis due to iron deficiency anaemia or macrocytic anaemia, another mouth abnormality sometimes seen in Crohn's disease is aphthous ulceration. There was no glossitis in the patient, and koilonychia was not possible because of the finger clubbing.

Finger clubbing

This occurs in both conditions and is related to disease activity (Figure 6.4).

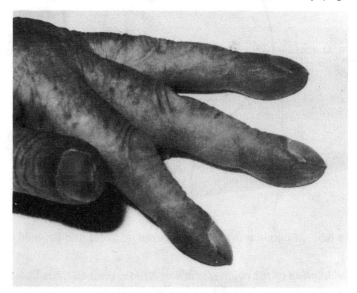

Figure 6.4 Clubbing

Abdominal findings

The left-sided abdominal tenderness and palpable tender descending colon suggest an active descending colitis, and therefore favour ulcerative colitis. In Crohn's disease, tenderness is more likely to be central or in the right iliac fossa, and often accompanied by a mass in this region due to frequent involvement of the terminal ileum and caecum (Figure 6.5).

When the colon is affected by Crohn's disease, 50% of the patients develop *perianal and perirectal disease*. This is indicated by a bluish-red discolouration of the perianal skin, a painful perianal abscess discharging pus or by a perianal fistula.

The absence of these findings in the patient in the presence of definite clinical signs of an active inflammation of the descending colon was against a clinical diagnosis of Crohn's disease.

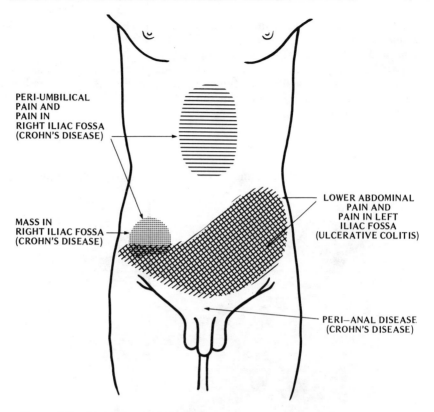

PERI-UMBILICAL
PAIN AND
PAIN IN
RIGHT ILIAC FOSSA
(CROHN'S DISEASE)

MASS IN
RIGHT ILIAC FOSSA
(CROHN'S DISEASE)

LOWER ABDOMINAL
PAIN AND
PAIN IN LEFT
ILIAC FOSSA
(ULCERATIVE COLITIS)

PERI–ANAL DISEASE
(CROHN'S DISEASE)

Figure 6.5   Abdominal findings in ulcerative colitis and Crohn's disease

Toxic dilatation of the colon (toxic megacolon) is much more likely to occur in ulcerative colitis than in Crohn's disease. In this condition the patient becomes seriously ill with severe constitutional symptoms, severe abdominal pain, a distended tender abdomen, rebound tenderness and absent bowel sounds. The colon is distended, bacterial growth flourishes, peritonitis is frequent and mortality is high, 20–30%. Colectomy is usually necessary.

The factors which may precipitate this condition are shown in Table 6.6.

The other local complications which may occur are shown in Table 6.7 and Figure 6.6.

Table 6.6   Factors precipitating toxic megacolon

- Spontaneous
- Barium enema examination
- Excessive potassium depletion
- Anticholinergic drugs
- Excessive use of narcotics

188

Table 6.7 Local complications in ulcerative colitis and Crohn's disease

	Colitis	*Crohn's disease*
Acute dilatation	Common	Uncommon
Perforation	Common	Uncommon
Massive haemorrhage	Common	Uncommon
Benign stricture	Uncommon	Common
Obstruction	Uncommon	Common
Fistulae	Uncommon	Common
Perianal disease	Uncommon	Common
Carcinoma		
colon	Common	Uncommon
small bowel	Never	Sometimes

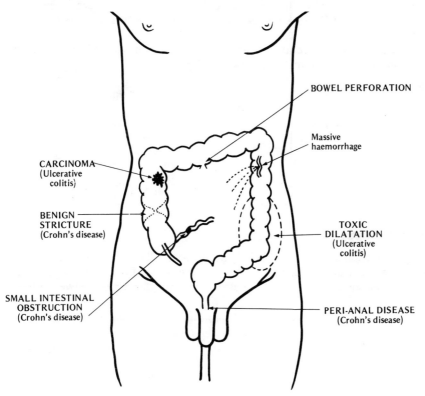

Figure 6.6 Abdominal complications of ulcerative colitis and Crohn's disease

CONCLUSIONS FROM THE EXAMINATION

The general findings were:

- pyrexia

- anaemia
- finger clubbing

These signs are common in both ulcerative colitis and Crohn's disease. The abdominal findings were:

- left-sided abdominal tenderness
- palpable tender descending colon

These positive signs together with the absence of perianal disease are in favour of ulcerative colitis rather than Crohn's disease.

INVESTIGATIONS

Procto-sigmoidoscopy

This is of more value in ulcerative colitis, where the rectum is invariably involved, than in Crohn's disease where less than half the patients have rectal disease.

The findings in ulcerative colitis are detailed in Table 6.8. In Crohn's disease, there may be mild non-specific hyperaemia.

Table 6.8 Proto-sigmoidoscopic findings in ulcerative colitis

• Mild	Hyperaemia and oedema
• Moderate	Red granular mucosa
	Contact bleeding
• Severe	Ulcerated mucosa
	Spontaneous bleeding

Rectal biopsy

Although rectal biopsy is not strictly necessary to diagnose ulcerative colitis if there are a typical clinical picture and positive sigmoidoscopic appearances, it is a very important test in the sometimes difficult distinction between ulcera-

Table 6.9 Histological differentiation between ulcerative colitis and Crohn's disease

	Colitis	*Crohn's disease*
• Distribution	Mucosal	Transmural
• Cells	Plasma cells	Plasma cells
	Polymorphs	Lymphocytes
	Eosinophils	Macrophages
• Glands	Mucin depletion	Not affected
	Gland destruction	
	Crypt abscesses	
• Additional	None	Aphthous ulcers
		Granulomas

190

tive colitis and Crohn's disease (Table 6.9). It may also be helpful in detecting carcinoma and in excluding pseudomembranous colitis.

The patient's rectal biopsy showed predominant mucosal involvement with crypt abscesses and so favoured ulcerative colitis.

Barium studies

Barium studies are essential in the diagnosis of both ulcerative colitis and Crohn's disease to determine the extent and the severity of the disease.

Ulcerative colitis

A barium enema is necessary in ulcerative colitis to examine the colon. The changes which may be seen are shown in Table 6.10.

Figure 6.7 shows the typical changes of extensive ulcerative colitis on barium enema with uniform constriction, shortening and loss of haustral pattern.

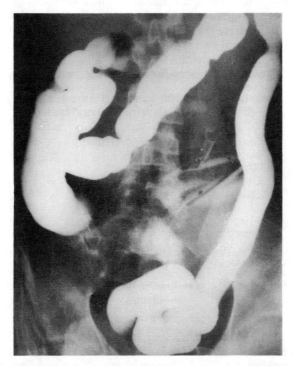

Figure 6.7 Barium enema showing extensive ulcerative colitis

The precautions which must be kept in mind before embarking on a barium enema examination in ulcerative colitis are shown in Table 6.11.

Table 6.10   Barium enema changes
in ulcerative colitis

Shallow ulceration
Loss of haustral pattern
Uniform constriction and shortening
Pseudopolyps

Table 6.11   Precautions for barium enema in
ulcerative colitis

Radiologist fully aware of the diagnosis
Preparatory emptying of the bowel best avoided
Barium should be run in at low pressure

Crohn's disease

In this condition, it is the small intestine which needs to be visualized by barium. This can be achieved either by a barium meal and follow-through examination, or, better, by a small intestinal 'enema' in which duodenal intubation is carried out and the small intestine then 'flushed' through with barium.

The changes which may be seen in Crohn's disease are shown in Table 6.12.

Table 6.12   Small intestinal changes on
barium examination in Crohn's disease

Terminal ileum narrow and irregular
Segmental involvement
'Cobblestone' appearance
Deep transverse linear fissures
Strictures
Sinuses
Fistulae

Figure 6.8 shows involvement of the terminal ileum with stenosis due to Crohn's disease.

Table 6.13   Radiological differentiation between ulcerative colitis and Crohn's
disease

	Ulcerative colitis	*Crohn's disease*
Rectal involvement	Invariable	Less frequent (50%)
Mucosal appearance	Shallow ulcers	Deep linear ulcers 'Cobblestones'
Pattern of involvement	Continuous	Segmental
Sinuses/fistulae	Rare	Common
Strictures	Rare	Common

Some factors which help in the radiological differentiation of ulcerative colitis and Crohn's disease are shown in Table 6.13.

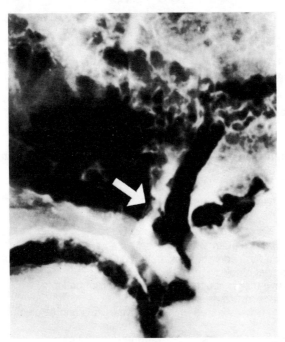

Figure 6.8 Barium study in Crohn's disease showing involvement of the terminal ileum resulting in constriction

Colonoscopy

The whole of the colon can be examined with a fibreoptic colonoscope. It has no place in the routine diagnosis of ulcerative colitis but may be helpful when doubt exists about Crohn's disease, and also when multiple biopsies are necessary to exclude carcinomatous change in longstanding ulcerative colitis.

Blood count

A blood count may be helpful in several ways (Table 6.14).

Table 6.14 Blood count in ulcerative colitis and Crohn's disease

• Polymorph leucocytosis	– active disease
• Low haemoglobin	– anaemia
• Blood film	– microyctic hypochromic anaemia
	macrocytic anaemia
• ESR	– activity of disease
	progress of disease with treatment

The blood count varied at different times in the patient, in showing iron deficiency anaemia and an increased white count and high ESR during exacerbations.

MANAGEMENT

The treatment of ulcerative colitis and Crohn's disease is similar in many respects and will involve general measures and specific treatment.

General measures

Diet

A good well-balanced non-irritant diet is necessary. The requirements are indicated in Table 6.15.

Table 6.15   Dietary requirements in ulcerative colitis and Crohn's disease

• Adequate calories, protein, vitamins and minerals
• Reduce fibre content in exacerbation of diarrhoea (less fruit and vegetables)
• Remove milk products in lactose-intolerant patients
• If malabsorption present –   reduce fat
extra vitamin D and calcium
extra folate
• If severely ill   – parenteral nutrition

Anaemia

The causes of the anaemia are shown in Table 6.16.

The commonest anaemia is iron deficiency due to *chronic blood loss*. This will produce a microcytic hypochromic picture on blood film. Oral iron is suitable for treatment if tolerated, otherwise intramuscular iron is indicated.

Vitamin B_{12} deficiency occurs in Crohn's disease when the terminal ileum, where B_{12} is normally absorbed, is affected. This will produce a macrocytic blood picture. Treatment is with vitamin B_{12} injections.

The causes of *folate deficiency* are shown in Table 6.17. The anaemia produced is macrocytic. Treatment is with folic acid tablets.

Table 6.16   Causes of anaemia in ulcerative colitis and Crohn's disease

• Blood loss
• Deficiency of vitamin B_{12}
• Deficiency of folate
• Chronic disease

Table 6.17   Causes of folate deficiency in Crohn's disease

> • Inadequate dietary intake (fresh fruit, leafy vegetables)
> • Inadequate absorption (duodenojejunal disease)
> • Sulphasalazine (Salazopyrin) therapy)

Antidiarrhoeal drugs

These drugs reduce intestinal motility and may result in symptomatic improvement of the diarrhoea. Some of the useful preparations are shown in Table 6.18.

Anticholinergic drugs such as atropine preparations are sometimes used to control painful abdominal cramps. They are best avoided as they may precipitate toxic megacolon.

Table 6.18   Antidiarrhoeal drugs

• Codeine phosphate tabs	30–60 mg t.d.s.
• Diphenoxylate (Lomotil)	10 mg initially
	5 mg every 6 hours
• Loperamide (Imodium)	4 mg initially
	2 mg up to 8 times daily

Rapport of patient with the doctor

In a chronic, relapsing, demoralizing condition often unresponsive to treatment, good rapport between the patient and the doctor is of considerable importance. Unrealistic expectation of response to therapy, e.g. a total cure, may easily impair this relationship. The doctor and the patient together should define attainable goals for the treatment, related primarily to improving the patient's quality of life.

The difficulties in the relationship between the doctor and the patient and his relatives may be prevented by early education of the patient and his family about the disease, and they should be given a realistic assessment of what can and cannot be expected with modern treatment.

In patients who are already deeply concerned over their chronic symptoms and poor physical health, undue emphasis on psychological factors may not be helpful.

Specific treatment

The treatment of ulcerative colitis and Crohn's disease with specific drugs will depend on several factors (Table 6.19).

The assessment of the severity of the disease is shown in Table 6.20.

In a *mild attack* bowel movements are usually from 6–8/day and there are few constitutional disturbances. The mild attack may be treated at home by the general practitioner.

A *severe attack* produces severe constitutional manifestations and a much greater frequency of bowel action. Treatment should always be carried out in hospital.

Table 6.19 Factors determining treatment in ulcerative colitis and Crohn's disease

- Location of disease
- Extent of involvement of bowel
- Activity of disease
- Duration of disease

Table 6.20 Assessment of severity of disease

• Clinical	• Number of bowel movements
	• Constitutional effects
	fever
	abdominal pain
	abdominal tenderness
	loss of weight
• Investigations	• Procto-sigmoidoscopy
	• Hb level
	• ESR
	• Level of serum albumin
• Systemic manifestations	• Arthritis
	• Erythema nodosum
	• Pyoderma gangrenosum
	• Eye complications

Mild attack

The treatment is shown in Table 6.21.

Local steroid treatment daily over 2–3 weeks will not lead to sufficient absorption to cause adrenal suppression.

Sulphasalazine is split by bacteria in the small intestine and colon into sulphapyridine, which is largely responsible for the side-effects (Table 6.22),

Table 6.21 Treatment of a mild attack

- Sulphasalazine (Salazopyrin) 1 g q.d.s. initially
                                    0.5 g q.d.s. for maintenance

- Local steroid preparations
  - hydrocortisone
    - suppository (25 mg%)
    - colifoam (10%)
    - enema (10%)
  - prednisolone
    - suppository (5 mg)
    - enema (20 mg)

and 5-aminosalicylic acid, which is the active component in colitis or ileitis and probably achieves its anti-inflammatory effect by inhibition of inflammation-producing prostaglandins.

Table 6.22   Side-effects of sulphasalazine

- Headache
- Gastrointestinal upset
- Arthralgia
- Rashes
- Blood dyscrasia • haemolysis
              • leukopenia
              • agranulocytosis

Severe attack

This should be regarded as a medical emergency and the patient admitted to hospital. The treatment is shown in Table 6.23. The use of potent broad-spectrum antibiotics is still controversial but should probably be tried in a severely ill patient going downhill and unsuitable for operative treatment.

Table 6.23   Treatment of a severe attack

- Replace plasma volume by i.v. saline or plasma
- Blood transfusion if severe anaemia
- Parenteral nutrition (hyperalimentation)
- Prednisolone i.v. 60–80 mg daily
- Hydrocortisone enemas 100 mg twice daily
- ?Broad spectrum antibotics

The patient should be reassessed frequently. If the response is not satisfactory within 24–48 hours, surgery should be considered. During this period *perforation of the bowel* should be suspected if there is a rising pulse rate and falling blood pressure – pain may be masked by the high dose of steroids. Another serious complication is *toxic dilatation of the colon*, which has been discussed earlier.

If the patient responds to treatment within 48 hours, the dose of intravenous prednisolone can be replaced by oral prednisolone and the dose progressively

Table 6.24   Common side-effects
of steroids

- Weight gain
- Fluid retention → oedema
- Hypertension
- Diabetes
- Hypokalaemia
- Mental disturbance

reduced to 20 mg/day which should be continued for 6–8 weeks. While the patient is on steroid treatment, possible side-effects should be remembered (Table 6.24).

Oral feeding replaces intravenous fluids, first liquid food then solids.

Sulphasalazine is introduced in a dose of 1 g every 6 hours initially, reducing to 2 g/day for maintenance treatment. This drug is of limited value in controlling disease activity but is useful in preventing relapses.

Other drugs used in management

Azathioprine (Imuran)

Immunosuppressive treatment with azathioprine is based on the assumption that ulcerative colitis and Crohn's disease may have an auto-immune basis. The drug is not effective in controlling an acute exacerbation but may be of some value in preventing relapses. It may produce bone marrow depression leading to pancytopenia.

Sodium cromoglycate (Nalcrom)

This drug prevents release of chemical factors from mast cells which mediate allergic reactions. It is of limited value in preventing relapses in ulcerative colitis and Crohn's disease. It may be useful when patients cannot take sulphasalazine.

Indications for surgery

The indications are shown in Table 6.25.

Table 6.25 Indications for surgery

• Severe unresponsive attack
• Toxic dilatation of the colon
• Perforation of the bowel
• Massive haemorrhage from the bowel
• Benign stricture causing obstruction
• Abscesses and fistulae (Crohn's disease)
• Extensive chronic unresponsive symptomatic disease
• Carcinoma of the colon
• Precarcinomatous change on colonoscopy
• Longstanding (> 10 years) pancolitis

NATURAL HISTORY OF ULCERATIVE COLITIS AND CROHN'S DISEASE

Ulcerative colitis

Prevalence and incidence

The prevalence of the disease is 40–80 per 100 000 of the population. The annual incidence is 3–6/100 000 population.

198

Age and sex

Females are more commonly affected than males. There is a bimodal age distribution – 15-20 years and 55-60 years. There is no evidence of a higher socio-economic or educational status of patients.

Prognosis

Figure 6.9 shows the prognosis after the first attack. The prognosis is therefore good in 87% of patients, who will be able to lead a reasonably full and active life during their periods of remission, though with each recurrence both morbidity and mortality may be progressively increased.

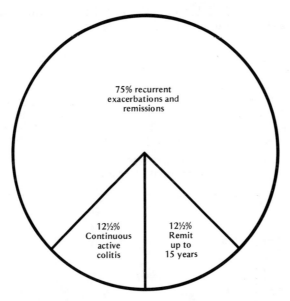

75% recurrent exacerbations and remissions

12½% Continuous active colitis

12½% Remit up to 15 years

Figure 6.9   Prognosis of ulcerative colitis

Mortality

The 5 year mortality in patients with moderate or severe disease ranges between 5% and 15% and will depend very much on the extent of the disease –

Table 6.26   Causes of death in ulcerative colitis

• Acute	• massive haemorrhage
	• toxic megacolon
	• systemic infection
	• pulmonary embolism
• Late	• carcinoma of colon

local proctitis will do well but pancolitis will lead to the highest death rate. The mortality also increases with age. The main causes of death are shown in Table 6.26.

Surgery

Between 20% and 25% of patients will require colectomy at some time, but once the first postoperative year has passed the prognosis is similar to the general population.

Systemic complications

The incidence is shown in Table 6.27. The peripheral arthritis and skin and eye involvement are related to activity of the disease.

Table 6.27 Incidence of systemic complications in ulcerative colitis

• Skin and eyes		3–10%
• Arthritis	• peripheral	10%
	• sacro-iliitis	20%
	• ankylosing spondylitis	2–10%
• Hepato-biliary	• clinical disease	1–3%
	• abnormal liver function tests	50–90%

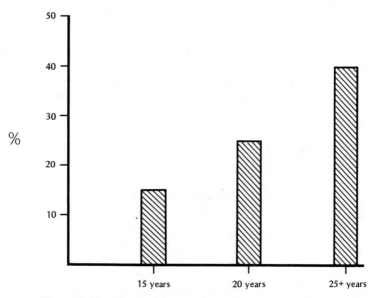

Figure 6.10   The incidence of carcinoma in pancolitis

Carcinoma of the colon

The development of carcinoma of colon depends on the extent and duration of the disease, and also a family history of colonic carcinoma. The overall incidence is 3–5%.

With pancolitis of at least 10 years' duration, the incidence of carcinoma is 10–20 times that in the general population. The risk increases progressively with the duration of the disease (Figure 6.10).

Crohn's disease

Prevalence and incidence

The prevalence is 20–40/100000 of the population. The annual incidence is 1/100000.

Age and sex

There is no sex difference. There is a similar bimodal age distribution to ulcerative colitis – 15–20 years and 55–60 years.

Mortality

The overall mortality is 5–18% and also depends on extent of bowel involvement.

Surgery

The majority of patients come to surgery in view of the unsatisfactory response to medical treatment. The indications for surgery are shown in Table 6.28.

Table 6.28   Indication for surgery in Crohn's disease

- Intestinal obstruction
- Massive haemorrhage
- Fistulae, especially to bladder
- Chronic unresponsive symptomatic patient
- Carcinoma of small intestine

Table 6.29   Prognosis after resection in Crohn's disease

• Recurrent symptoms	25% at 5 years
	50% at 10 years
• Further resection	15% at 5 years
	25% at 10 years
• Mortality	7% at 5 years
	12% at 10 years

The prognosis after operation is not as favourable as in ulcerative colitis (Table 6.29).

CAN WE MODIFY THE NATURAL HISTORY?

The aetiology of both ulcerative colitis and Crohn's disease remains unknown. Some possible mechanisms have been suggested (Table 6.30).

Table 6.30 Possible mechanisms in the aetiology of ulcerative colitis and Crohn's disease

- Transmissible infective agent ?virus ?bacterial
- Immunological disturbance
- Heredity
- Psychosomatic disturbance
- Impairment of blood supply
- Neurogenic – disturbed motility pattern
- Environmental – factor in food or drugs

Since the basic cause has not been established it is not possible to suggest any basic approach to delay the onset or limit the extent of the disease.

On the other hand, the introduction of corticosteroids, as well as the improvement in supportive techniques such as total intravenous feeding, has improved the short term prognosis in both conditions. The result is a remission rate of 85% in an acute severe attack. Steroid treatment is unlikely to influence the long term prognosis and, unlike sulphasalazine, has little value in preventing relapses.

The earlier detection of carcinoma may improve the long term prognosis. Since the risk of carcinoma is greatest in pancolitis of at least 10 years' duration, there is a case for regular colonoscopy and biopsy. Unfortunately, the lesion may occur in several different sites at the same time.

Because of the frequent multicentric origin of carcinoma and the difficulty in adequate examination of every possible precarcinomatous site, prophylactic pan-proctocolectomy is often advised in patients with longstanding pancolitis.

USEFUL PRACTICAL POINTS

- It may be difficult to differentiate Crohn's disease from ulcerative colitis. The most helpful clinical points are infrequent rectal bleeding, a right-sided abdominal mass, perianal disease and evidence of malabsorption.

- Crohn's disease responds less well long term to medical treatment than ulcerative colitis. Most patients with Crohn's disease come to surgery at some time.

- The postoperative surgical prognosis in ulcerative colitis is very good, unlike Crohn's disease where there is a steadily increasing postoperative recurrence rate, necessitating further surgery.

- A mild attack of ulcerative colitis can be treated at home with sulphasalazine and local steroid enemas or suppositories. A severe attack requires hospital treatment with intravenous fluids and intravenous steroids.

- Carcinoma of the colon is a serious risk in pancolitis of at least 10 years' duration and the incidence increases progressively with time.

7

Jaundice

PRESENT HISTORY

A 43-year-old woman presented with a 2 month history of jaundice and itching of the skin. More recently, she had developed swelling of the feet and distension of the abdomen.

Jaundice

Her husband had noticed that her skin had been getting yellow for about 2 months. Although she thought that some days she looked less yellow than other days, overall she was getting progressively more yellow over the 2 months since it started.

Pruritus

Her skin had begun to itch, over the previous month. It tended to be worse in bed and was begining to keep her awake.

Abdominal swelling

She had noticed that her abdomen was swelling over the previous 4 weeks. There was no significant abdominal pain apart from the general discomfort of a big abdomen which was producing difficulty getting her dresses on.

At the same time as her abdomen was swelling, she had also developed *swelling in her feet* and this was steadily getting more marked.

Other relevant factors on direct enquiry

Stools

The stools were getting very *pale* and now looked 'like putty'. She had not noticed the stools floating in the pan and they flushed away quite easily. She had not really looked for or noticed any change in the colour of her urine.

She had not had diarrhoea.

Appetite

Over the same period of 8 weeks she had been *off her food* and seemed to get more tired than usual doing her housework.

Flatulence

She had suffered from occasional *flatulent dyspepsia* for a number of years, especially after fatty foods. She had never had any severe attacks of upper abdominal pain.

Weight

She had *lost about 7 lb* (3 kg) in the past few months.

PAST HISTORY

Jaundice

She had a previous attack of jaundice about 8 years earlier. She had been told that this was probably due to a drug she had been taking 'for her nerves'.

High blood pressure

She had been found to have high blood pressure 3 years earlier and had been taking methyldopa since then.

Arthritis

Over the last year or so she had been having some pain and swelling in the finger joints, wrist joints and knees. She had been taking indomethacin for the pain with considerable relief. She did not think it made her flatulence worse.

There was no past history of pleurisy, skin rashes, thyroid trouble, kidney disease or thrombophlebitis.

She had not had a recent operation requiring general anaesthesia.

FAMILY HISTORY

The only relevant fact was that one of her sisters had suffered from *chronic bowel trouble* with diarrhoea for many years.

There was no history of liver trouble in any member of the family.

PERSONAL HISTORY

She had always been a *very moderate drinker* – only an occasional glass of sherry on a social occasion.

She smoked about 10 cigarettes daily for the past 20 years or so.

DRUG HISTORY

She was taking *methyldopa* (Aldomet) and *cyclopenthiazide* (Navidrex) for her hypertension.

She had experienced 'trouble with her nerves' for some years. Her original tablets had been stopped when she developed jaundice, but over the last few years she had been taking regular *diazepam* (Valium).

She had also been taking *indomethacin* (Indocid) for control of her painful joints.

She was *not* on the oral *contraceptive pill*.

EXAMINATION

The abnormal signs are shown in Figure 7.1.

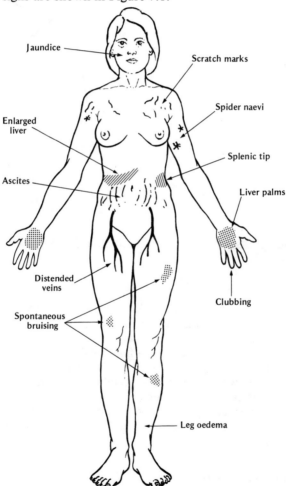

Figure 7.1 Clinical signs in the patient

General

She was deeply *jaundiced* with *scratch marks* over the chest and arms.

There were several *bruises* on her legs for which she could not account.

She did not look cachetic. There was no arcus senilis or xanthelasma. There were no enlarged lymph nodes in the neck.

Palpation of the breasts was normal.

She had *palmar erythema* and mild *clubbing* of the fingers.

There were several *spider naevi* over her upper arms and cheeks (Figure 7.2).

There was no evidence of any permanent arthritis changes in the hands, wrists or knees and no tenderness or swelling at the time of the examination.

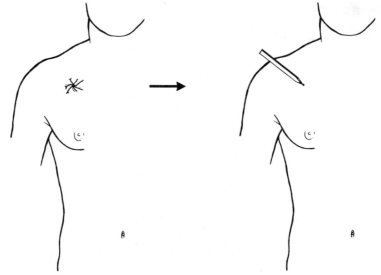

Figure 7.2   Spider naevus on chest obliterated by pencil pressure

Abdomen

This was *distended*, more in the flanks than in the centre. The umbilicus was everted. There were some *dilated veins* along the lateral sides of the abdomen, the direction of venous flow being upwards.

Shifting dullness was present but a fluid thrill was not obtained.

The *liver was enlarged* 3 cm below the right costal margin. The surface was firm and smooth with no obvious nodularity. There was no tenderness. Palpation of the liver was accompanied by a distinct sensation of *dipping* through fluid before coming onto the surface of the liver.

The *tip of the spleen* could also be felt below the left costal margin.

The gallbladder was not palpable.

Cardiovascular system

The pulse was normal. The arterial wall was not thickened.

The blood pressure was 180/105.

The apex beat was normal.

There was no abnormality of heart sounds, no triple rhythm and no murmurs.

Respiratory system

The lungs were normal.

Nervous system

The mental state was clear.

There were no tremors.

There were no pyramidal signs.

The fundi showed slight arteriolar irregularity but no arteriovenous nipping and no retinal abnormality.

ANALYSIS OF THE HISTORY

Jaundice

The major problem is the progressive jaundice.

The metabolic pathways of the bile are shown in Figure 7.3.

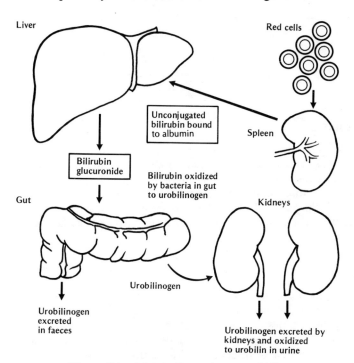

Figure 7.3   Metabolic pathways of bile

The three main types of jaundice, and their associated clinical features, are shown in Table 7.1.

Table 7.1 The types of jaundice and their clinical features

	Haemolytic	*Hepatocellular*	*Obstructive*
Jaundice	mild	mild to moderate	severe
Symptoms	nil (except in crisis)	malaise, anorexia, distaste for smoking	pruritus
Urine	dark	normal or dark	dark
Stools	dark	normal or pale	pale

The colour of the stool is the simplest indication of obstructive jaundice, and in this patient was 'putty coloured', typical of obstruction.

Urine colour is more difficult for the patient to evaluate and so is less helpful.

Causes of jaundice encountered in clinical practice are shown in Table 7.2.

Table 7.2 Common causes of jaundice

- Gallstones
- Hepatitis – acute
              chronic
- Cirrhosis
- Carcinoma of pancreas
- Drugs
- Alcohol
- Haemolytic – hereditary
                acquired

Gallstones

These are a frequent cause of obstructive jaundice.

There may be a history of flatulent dyspepsia, as in this patient. Attacks of constant or colicky pain in the right hypochondrium occur. A family history of gallbladder disease may be present.

Although the patient has flatulent dyspepsia, the absence of attacks of pain, together with the absence of a family history, makes gallstones an unlikely diagnosis.

Hepatitis

Hepatitis may be caused by three types of virus (Table 7.3).

It usually causes a hepatocellular type of jaundice though obstruction due to intrahepatic cholestasis may sometimes occur.

In *acute hepatitis* there may be a recent contact with a jaundiced patient (hepatitis A) or with an injection or blood transfusion (hepatitis B).

In hepatitis A infection there is usually a prodromal symptomatic period

(Table 7.4). This is followed by a hepatocellular type of jaundice with dark urine, normal stools (if no obstructive element) and upper abdominal discomfort.

Table 7.3 Types of viral hepatitis

- Hepatitis A
- Hepatitis B
- Hepatitis non-A non-B

Table 7.4 Prodromata in hepatitis A

- Malaise
- Fever
- Sore throat
- Anorexia
- Nausea
- Loss of taste for smoking

In addition to similar gastrointestinal symptoms in hepatitis B, skin rashes and arthralgia may occur.

The absence of any prodromata, the prolonged duration of the jaundice and its obstructive nature make the diagnosis of acute viral hepatitis untenable.

Chronic hepatitis may cause obstructive jaundice, and may also be associated with extra-hepatic manifestations, so it remains a possible diagnosis. It will be discussed in more detail subsequently.

Carcinoma of the pancreas

The clinical features of carcinoma of the pancreas are shown in Table 7.5.

The patient does have some suspicious features – anorexia, loss of weight, progressive obstructive jaundice – but has no abdominal pain or thrombophlebitis.

Pancreatic carcinoma remains a possibility.

Table 7.5 Clinical features of carcinoma of pancreas

- Usually males
- Anorexia and weight loss
- Penetrating upper abdominal pain
- Steadily progressive obstructive jaundice
- Thrombophlebitis common

Drugs

Some of the more commonly used drugs which may cause liver toxicity are shown in Table 7.6.

Most of these drugs cause a hepatocellular type of jaundice, but there are several which produce cholestatic (obstructive) jaundice (Table 7.7).

The patient has been taking diazepam (Valium) for several years and this may be a relevant factor in causing her jaundice.

There is one other important association between drugs and liver disease – some may be implicated in the development of chronic active hepatitis (Table 7.8).

Table 7.6   Common hepatotoxic drugs

• Psychotropic	– monoamine oxidase inhibitors, e.g. Nardil
	tricyclic antidepressants, e.g. Tofranil
	phenothiazines, e.g. Largactil
	benzodiazepines, e.g. Valium
• Anti-inflammatory	– phenylbutazone (Butazolidine)
	indomethacin (Indocid)
	penicillamine (Distamine)
	gold (Myocrisin)
• Antihypertensives	– methyldopa (Aldomet)
	hydrallazine (Apresoline)
• Antidiabetic	– chlorpropamide (Diabinese)
	tolbutamide (Rastinon)
• Anticonvulsant	– phenytoin (Epanutin)
• Antispasmodic	– dantrolene (Dantrium)
• Antibiotic	– sulphonamides, e.g. Kelfizine
	nitrofurantoin (Furadantin)
	antituberculous drugs, e.g. isoniazid

**Table 7.7   Drugs causing chol-
estatic jaundice**

- Tricyclic antidepressants
- Phenothiazines
- Benzodiazepines
- Gold salts
- Chlorpropamide
- Tolbutamide
- Oral contraceptives

**Table 7.8   Drugs associated with chronic active
hepatitis**

- Isoniazid – tuberculosis
- Nitrofurantoin (Furadantin) – urinary infection
- Dantrolene (Dantrium) – muscle relaxant
- Methyldopa (Aldomet) – hypertension

The patient has been on methyldopa (Aldomet) for several years for her hypertension. This may therefore be another hepatotoxic factor leading to the jaundice.

Methyldopa (Aldomet) may also cause haemolytic anaemia and so contribute to the jaundice in another way.

Alcoholism

Alcohol is the usual cause of *cirrhosis* in the United Kingdom.

The degree of jaundice in alcoholic cirrhosis is usually mild and cholestasis is minimal.

The absence of an alcohol history excludes this diagnosis in the patient.

Haemolytic jaundice

Haemolytic anaemia may be due to intrinsic defects of the red cell or to extrinsic factors (Table 7.9).

Unconjugated bilirubin, produced by haemolysis, is not excreted by the kidney so that the urine is free of bilirubin. The jaundice is usually mild, and there are few symptoms unless a haemolytic crisis occurs (Table 7.10).

Table 7.9 Causes of haemolytic anaemia

• Intrinsic defects	• Congenital spherocytosis
	• Congenital ellipsocytosis
	• Thalassaemia
	• Sickle cell disease
• Extrinsic factors	• Auto-immune
	• Drugs
	methyldopa
	quinine
	quinidine
	• Cold haemoglobinuria
	• Hypersplenism (any cause)
	• Mismatched blood transfusion

Table 7.10 Clinical features in a haemolytic crisis

• Increasing lassitude
• Muscle cramps
• Backache
• Raynaud's phenomenon
• Mottling of the skin

Although the patient is being treated with methyldopa (Aldomet), which may cause a haemolytic anaemia, the obstructive type of jaundice and the absence of symptoms and signs of anaemia make this diagnosis unlikely.

213

Abdominal swelling

The causes of abdominal swelling are shown in Table 7.11.

Table 7.11 Common causes of
abdominal swelling

- Fat
- Flatus
- Faeces
- Fetus
- Fluid

Fat

The rapid onset of the swelling over 4 weeks makes fat very unlikely.

Flatus

Flatus is associated with intermittent swelling, especially after meals, and abdominal rumbling with belching or passing flatus from the rectum.

The constancy of the abdominal swelling and the absence of other manifestations of excessive bowel activity exclude this diagnosis.

Faeces

Abdominal swelling due to faeces is a result of some measure of intestinal obstruction. In these circumstances other symptoms occur, such as abdominal pain, vomiting and absence of stool and flatus.

None of these symptoms occurred in this patient.

Fetus

There was no possibility of pregnancy, since she had an early menopause at the age of 40 years.

Fluid

The most likely cause of the abdominal swelling is *ascites*.

Swelling of the legs

The causes of swelling of the legs are shown in Figure 7.4.

Right ventricular failure

There was no past history of heart disease, no dyspnoea to indicate left ventricular failure – which when longstanding, is a common cause of right ventri-

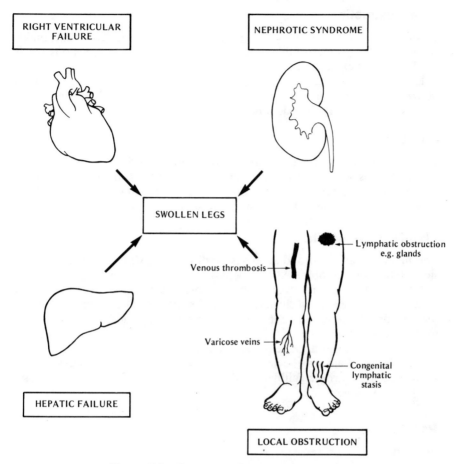

RIGHT VENTRICULAR FAILURE

NEPHROTIC SYNDROME

SWOLLEN LEGS

Lymphatic obstruction e.g. glands

Venous thrombosis

Varicose veins

Congenital lymphatic stasis

HEPATIC FAILURE

LOCAL OBSTRUCTION

Figure 7.4   Causes of swelling of the legs

cular failure – and there was no history of chronic lung disease, perhaps the commonest of all causes of right ventricular failure.

Nephrotic syndrome

There was no past history of kidney disease, and there were no current urinary or uraemic symptoms and no swelling around the eyes, so common in renal oedema.

Nephrotic syndrome is therefore very unlikely.

Hepatic failure

The history indicates liver disease. The combination of leg swelling with ascites strongly suggests a *hypoproteinaemic state* in this patient due to hepatic failure to synthesize proteins, especially albumin.

Local obstruction

The absence of a past history of leg vein thrombosis or varicose veins makes *venous insufficiency* an unlikely cause of the leg oedema. A venous origin would also not explain the ascites.

The rapidity of onset of the leg swelling is very much against *lymphatic obstruction* which is usually chronic, unless the obstruction is extrinsic from rapidly developing lymphadenopathy.

Pruritus

The systemic causes of pruritus are shown in Figure 7.5.

The obvious cause of pruritus in this patient is the *obstructive jaundice*.

The mechanism responsible for the pruritus is the retention of bile salts in the circulation and their deposition in the skin.

Flatulent dyspepsia

This manifests as postprandial epigastric discomfort with a feeling of distension. Relief is often obtained by belching.

Although the condition often has no organic basis, it does appear on occasions to be related to chronic gallbladder disease. The probable reason is the disordered digestion of fat resulting from the gallbladder disease leading to fatty food intolerance.

A number of cases are due to excessive air swallowing.

A cholecystogram may be necessary to decide whether flatulent dyspepsia is associated with chronic gallbladder disease, and it therefore remains a possibility in this patient.

Past history

Jaundice

The previous attack of jaundice was attributed to *drug toxicity*. If so, it is unlikely to be relevant to the present liver disorder.

If the drug had produced hepatocellular jaundice, the effects would have improved rapidly on withdrawal of the drug.

If the drug had been one of these associated with the development of chronic active hepatitis, the established disease would have become manifest within 1–2 years of exposure.

It is possible that the jaundice was not caused by drug toxicity but by an attack of *acute viral hepatitis*. If this was a hepatitis A infection, it would have little relevance to her present condition, since type A hepatitis very rarely progresses to chronic hepatitis. However, both type B hepatitis and non-A non-B hepatitis can cause chronic hepatitis and this may therefore be a significant possibility in the patient's past history.

Hypertension

The only relevance of this condition is the treatment with the potentially

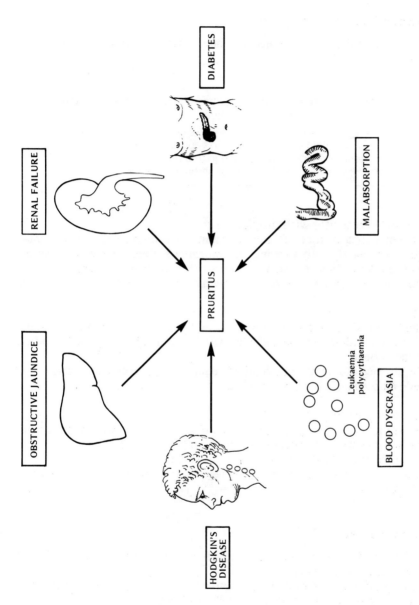

Figure 7.5   Systemic causes of pruritus

hepatotoxic methyldopa which is associated with the development of chronic active hepatitis.

Polyarthralgia

There are several possible connections between polyarthralgia and jaundice. (Table 7.12).

Table 7.12 Relationships between polyarthralgia and jaundice

• Rheumatoid arthritis leading to hepatic amyloidosis • Hepatotoxicity of drugs used in treatment • Extrahepatic manifestation of chronic hepatitis

Rheumatoid arthritis with amyloidosis
The absence of a history of gradual symmetrical involvement of the small joints of the hands with swelling and morning stiffness makes rheumatoid arthritis unlikely. There is also no evidence of amyloidosis of the gut which is a common manifestation of secondary amyloidosis and would cause diarrhoea.

Drugs
She had been taking *indomethacin* (Indocid) to control the painful joints, but this is a drug leading to hepatocellular jaundice and not obstructive jaundice, as in the patient.

The absence of any recent operation requiring a general anaesthetic would exclude *halothane*, a hepatotoxic agent.

Chronic hepatitis
There are a variety of extra-hepatic manifestations associated with chronic active hepatitis and arthralgia is one of them (Figure 7.6).

The patient's arthralgia may fit into this category.

There were no symptoms to suggest any of the other systemic manifestations.

Family history

The sister with a chronic bowel problem may be relevant, since this may represent *ulcerative colitis*.

Relatives of patients with chronic active hepatitis may have disorders considered to be of auto-immune type, such as ulcerative colitis.

Personal history

The smoking and minimal drinking are irrelevant.

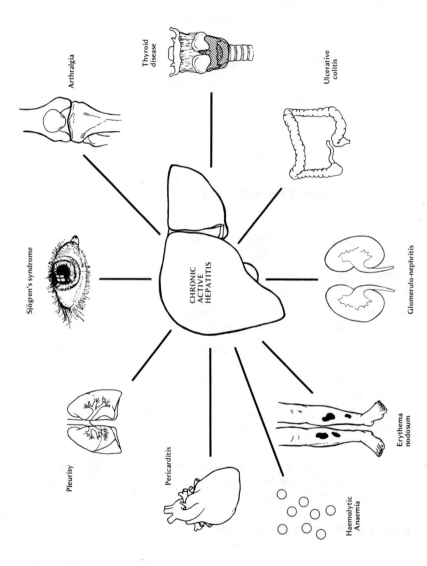

Figure 7.6 Extrahepatic complications of chronic active hepatitis

Drug history

The patient is taking three potentially hepatotoxic drugs (Table 7.13).

The *indomethacin* (Indocid) is likely to be irrelevant since this produces a hepatocellular and not obstructive jaundice.

Diazepam (Valium) can produce a cholestatic type of jaundice and so may be relevant here.

Methyldopa (Aldomet) is also highly relevant since this may lead to a chronic active hepatitis.

Table 7.13 Hepatotoxic drugs taken by the patient

• Methyldopa
• Indomethacin
• Diazepam

CONCLUSIONS FROM THE HISTORY

These are as follows.

- The putty-coloured stools indicate that the patient's jaundice is obstructive. The pruritis supports this view.

- The abdominal swelling associated with the jaundice suggests the possibility of ascites due to cirrhosis.

- The polyarthralgia may be an extrahepatic manifestation of the auto-immune type of chronic active hepatitis.

- The liver disease may be related to treatment with two potentially hepatotoxic drugs:
  Diazepam (Valium) – cholestatic jaundice
  Methyldopa (Aldomet).

- The ulcerative colitis in the patient's sister may be relevant if the patient has chronic active hepatitis, since both conditions have an auto-immune basis.

- Another possible cause of chronic active hepatitis in the patient may be the previous attack of jaundice, since this may have been due to hepatitis B infection which can progress to chronic active hepatitis.

ANALYSIS OF THE EXAMINATION

General

Useful negative points

The absence of a cachectic appearance and obvious excessive weight loss is against malignant liver involvement.

Similarly, the absence of enlarged neck glands excludes secondary deposits from an abdominal carcinoma, and also excludes reticulosis.

The absence of xanthelasma is against a diagnosis of primary biliary cirrhosis. The absence of any lumps in the breasts excludes carcinoma of the breast with hepatic mestastases.

Jaundice

The deep jaundice and the scratch marks on the skin indicate *obstructive jaundice.*

Bruising

Spontaneous bruising in a jaundiced patient indicates *hypoprothrombinaemia* due to impaired synthesis in a damaged liver.

Signs of cirrhosis

The signs of cirrhosis in the patient are shown in Figure 7.7.

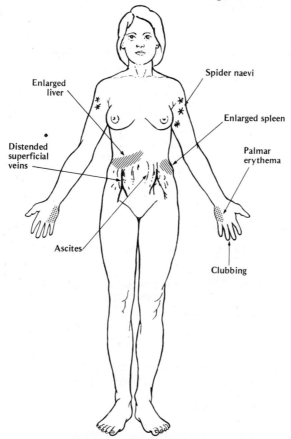

Figure 7.7   Signs of cirrhosis in the patient

Abdominal swelling

The typical signs of ascites are shown in Table 7.14. The patient showed all these features except the fluid thrill.

The absence of the fluid thrill is probably related to the quantity of abdominal fluid. Two litres are required to produce distension in the flanks with shifting dullness, but considerably more is necessary to allow a fluid thrill to be felt.

Causes of ascites and their differentiation are shown in Table 7.15.

The signs in this patient suggest *cirrhosis* as the cause of the ascites.

Table 7.14   Typical signs of ascites

- Abdominal distension especially in flanks
- Everted umbilicus
- Fluid thrill
- Shifting dullness
- Dipping (ballottement)

Table 7.15   Common causes of ascites and their differentiation

	Fever	Liver size	Skin lesions	Other
Cirrhosis	usual	variable	present	–
Ca metastases	often	large, nodular	rare	signs of primary Ca
Right ventricular failure	rare	large, smooth, tender	none	J.V.P. ↑
Constrictive pericarditis	rare	large, not tender	none	J.V.P. ↑

Hepatosplenomegaly

The common causes of hepatosplenomegaly are noted in Table 7.16.

Table 7.16   Common causes of hepato-splenomegaly

- Infection — Glandular fever
  Leptospirosis
- Cirrhosis
- Blood diseases — Chronic leukaemia
  Myelofibrosis
- Reticulosis
- Amyloidosis
- Sarcoidosis
- (Tropical diseases, e.g. Kala Azar)

Infection

There were no features to suggest either glandular fever (Table 7.17) or lepto-spirosis (Table 7.18).

Table 7.17 Clinical features of glandular fever

- Fever
- Sore throat
- Enlarged glands
- Skin rash

Table 7.18 Clinical features of lepto-spirosis

- Fever
- Conjunctivitis
- Muscle pains
- Canal swimming or sewer worker

Blood disease

The clinical features associated with blood diseases are shown in Table 7.19. Apart from spontaneous bruising, none of these features was present in the patient.

Table 7.19 Clinical features of blood diseases associated with hepatosplenomegaly

- Anaemia
- Bone pain (especially backpain)
- Bleeding
- Pathological fractures
- Uraemia
- Massive splenomegaly in myelofibrosis

Reticulosis

Reticulosis is usually associated with enlargement of the lymph glands. No lymphadenopathy was found in the patient.

Amyloidosis

The causes of amyloidosis are shown in Table 7.20. The organs involved in primary and secondary amyloidosis are shown in Table 7.21, but there is a certain amount of overlap of organ involvement in the two types of amyloidosis.

There was no evidence of an underlying cause of secondary amyloidosis.

Nor was there any evidence of involvement by amyloidosis of the heart, lungs, skin, joints, nervous system or gastrointestinal tract.

Table 7.20 Causes of amyloidosis

• Primary	– often with myelomatosis
• Secondary	• chronic suppuration
	Bronchiectasis
	Osteomyelitis
	Empyema
	• chronic inflammation
	Rheumatoid arthritis
	Ankylosing spondylitis
• Ageing	– old age

Table 7.21 Organ involvement in amyloidosis

• Primary	• Heart
	• Lungs
	• Skin
	• Joints
	• Nervous system
• Secondary	• Gastrointestinal tract
	• Liver
	• Kidney

Sarcoidosis

The wide variety of lesions in sarcoidosis apart from hepatosplenomegaly are shown in Table 7.22.

Table 7.22 Features of sarcoidosis

• Lungs	Hilar lymphadenopathy
	Infiltration
• Eyes	Conjunctivitis
	Uveitis
	Sjögren's syndrome
• Nervous system	Meningitis
	Space-occupying lesion
	Diabetes insipidus
• Joints	Polyarthralgia
• Skin	Erythema nodosum
	Plaques
	Lupus pernio
• Heart	Myocarditis
• Other	Hypercalcaemia
	Renal calculi

There was no evidence of involvement of the lungs, eyes, nervous system, skin or heart, which makes sarcoidosis an unlikely diagnosis.

A definitive differentiation can be made with a Kveim test.

Cirrhosis

The clinical features which suggest cirrhosis as the likely cause of the hepato-splenomegaly in the patient are summarized in Table 7.23.

Table 7.23 Clinical features establishing cirr-hosis as the cause of the patient's hepato-splenomegaly

• Portal hypertension	– Ascites Collateral veins
• Hepatic failure	– Liver palms Spider naevi

Nervous system

Hepatic encephalopathy is a serious complication of severe liver disease. The features are shown in Table 7.24.

There was no evidence of encephalopathy in the patient.

Table 7.24 Features of hepatic encephalopathy

- Foetor hepaticus
- Flapping tremor
- Drowsiness
- Confusion
- Slurred speech
- Ataxia
- Spastic paraparesis

Cardiovascular system

The only abnormality was the moderate degree of hypertension, associated with mild arteriosclerotic changes in the fundi.

There was no evidence of any adverse effects of hypertension on the heart (Table 7.25).

Table 7.25 Clinical signs of adverse effects of hyper-tension on the heart

- Apex displaced to the left
- Sustained heaving left ventricular apex
- Presystolic triple rhythm ('atrial' gallop)
- Loud P2 indicating pulmonary hypertension
- Crepitations at lung bases indicating congestion

CONCLUSIONS FROM THE EXAMINATION

- The deep jaundice and scratch marks confirm obstructive jaundice.
- She has evidence of cirrhosis of the liver.
- The abdominal swelling is confirmed as ascites.
- The spontaneous bruises indicate severe liver dysfunction.
- There was no evidence of the serious complication of cirrhosis – hepatic encephalopathy.
- The only other significant condition on examination is uncontrolled moderate hypertension.

INVESTIGATIONS

Urine examination

Urine examination for bile pigments is helpful in distinguishing the three types of jaundice (Table 7.26).

The patient's urine showed an increase in bilirubin and urobilinogen, indicating hepatocellular jaundice without complete obstruction.

Table 7.26   Urinary bile pigments in the different types of jaundice

	Haemolytic	*Hepatocellular*	*Obstructive*
Bilirubin	Absent	Increased	Increased
Urobilinogen	Increased	Increased	Absent

Liver function tests

These tests are essential in any jaundiced patient.

The help given by the different parameters is shown in Table 7.27.

The differentiation between the different types of jaundice is shown in Table 7.28.

The patient's results are shown in Table 7.29. This indicates clearly the picture of *obstructive jaundice with associated hepatocellular damage*.

When doubt still remains regarding intrahepatic or extrahepatic obstruction, a *'steroid whitewash'* test may help. Prednisolone is given in a dose of 30 mg daily for 5 days and the effect on the level of serum bilirubin determined.

Table 7.27   Value of different liver function tests

• Bilirubin	Degree of jaundice
• Alkaline phosphatase	Degree of obstruction (cholestasis)
• Transaminases	Amount of liver cell damage
• Albumin level	Hepatic synthesis

A drop of at least 40% will indicate intrahepatic cholestasis, while no significant fall occurs in extrahepatic obstruction.

Table 7.28 Differentiation between the types of jaundice by liver function tests

	Haemolytic	Hepatocellular	Cholestatic
Bilirubin	Increase (unconjugated)	Increase	Marked increase
Alkaline phosphatase	Normal	Slight increase	Marked increase
Transaminase	Normal	Marked increase	Slight increase
Albumin	Normal	Reduced	Normal

Table 7.29 Patient's liver function tests

		Normal range
Bilirubin	46 mol/l	(5–17)
Alkaline phosphatase	685 iu/l	(102–289)
Gamma-GT	119 iu/l	(6–42)
Albumin	28 g/l	(35–50)

Serum autoantibodies

The serological abnormalities which occur in chronic active hepatitis are shown in Table 7.30.

Some of these antibodies are also found in other types of liver disease, and the relative incidence is shown in Table 7.31.

Table 7.30 Incidence of serum autoantibodies in chronic active hepatitis

• Increase in immunoglobulins	– 50–70%
• Smooth muscle antibodies	– 40–80%
• Antinuclear antibodies	– 20–50%
• Antimitochondrial antibodies	– 10–20%
• LE cells	– 10–20%
• Antigastric	
• Antithyroid	– <5%
• Antiadrenal	

Table 7.31 Relative incidence of same serum autoantibodies in liver diseases

	Antinuclear	Smooth muscle	Mitochondrial
Chronic active hepatitis	55	65	25
Primary biliary cirrhosis	30	50	90
Alcoholic cirrhosis	5	0	0
Obstruction of common bile duct	0	0	3

Since primary biliary cirrhosis is an important differential diagnosis in chronic hepatitis, some helpful features are shown in Table 7.32. The most important differentiating method is by liver biopsy and this will be discussed subsequently.

The patient's serum autoantibody result is shown in Table 7.33. Antinuclear and smooth muscle antibodies are present, but no antimitochondrial antibodies – a strong factor against the diagnosis of primary biliary cirrhosis.

The patient's immunoglobulins are all increased, especially IgG, a typical result in *chronic active hepatitis.*

Table 7.32 Differentiation between primary biliary cirrhosis and chronic active hepatitis

	Primary biliary cirrhosis	Chronic active hepatitis
Pruritus	Frequent	Variable
Xanthelasma	Common	None
Serum cholesterol	Increased	Normal
Alkaline phosphatase	Marked increase	Variable
Serum antibodies	Mitochondrial high	Mitochondrial low

Table 7.33 Patient's serum auto-antibodies

Antinuclear	– 100
Smooth muscle	– 20
Mitochondrial	– 0
Rheumatoid factor	– Positive
IgG	– 19.2 g/l (high)
IgA	– 5.2 g/l (high)
IgM	– 3.2 g/l (high)

Virus studies

Chronic active hepatitis may be associated with the hepatitis virus. This relationship is predominantly with type B hepatitis virus, but occasionally with non-A non-B virus. Type A virus is only extremely rarely involved.

The detection of previous infection with hepatitis B is usually done by assessing the presence of its surface antigen in the blood (HB_sAg). It is more commonly found in the older male with chronic active hepatitis (HB_sAg-positive) where symptoms are slight and extrahepatic manifestations rare.

The young female with chronic active hepatitis, severe symptoms and extrahepatic involvement is usually HB_sAg-negative.

Hepatitis B surface antigen was *not found* in this patient. Additionally, no antibodies were found to the core antigen of the hepatitis B virus, which confirms the lack of involvement of the hepatitis B virus in the present case.

Table 7.34 summarizes the important differences between HB_sAg positive and negative chronic active hepatitis.

Table 7.34 Comparison of HB_sAg-positive and negative chronic active hepatitis

	HB_sAg-negative	HB_sAg-positive
Sex	Female	Male
Age	15–25	Over 50
	Menopause	
Extrahepatic manifestations	Frequent	Rare
Smooth muscle antibodies	High titre	Low titre
LE cells	15%	None
Response to steroids	Good	Uncertain

Liver biopsy

This is the definitive test in the diagnosis of liver disease.

Chronic active hepatitis

The typical features of chronic active hepatitis are shown in Figure 7.8.

The patient's liver biopsy showed all the features of Figure 7.8, which confirms the diagnosis of chronic active hepatitis.

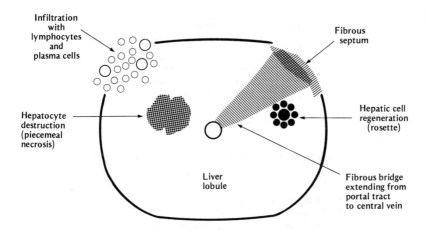

Figure 7.8 Histology of chronic active hepatitis

229

Chronic persistent hepatitis

It is important to distinguish chronic persistent hepatitis from chronic active hepatitis, since the clinical features may be similar but the prognosis is very much better in chronic persistent hepatitis. The distinction is made on the basis of the liver biopsy (Table 7.35).

Table 7.35   Histological differentiation between chronic active and persistent hepatitis

	Active hepatitis	*Persistent hepatitis*
Piecemeal necrosis	frequent	rare
Site involved	portal → lobule	portal only
Lobular structure	abnormal	normal
Fibrosis	common	slight
Bridging	common	rare
Regeneration	common	rare
Progression to cirrhosis	common	rare

Primary biliary cirrhosis

Another important differential diagnosis is primary biliary cirrhosis. The histological features are shown in Table 7.36. The most distinctive feature is the presence of periductal granulomata.

There is one other condition which should be considered if the liver biopsy shows changes of chronic active hepatitis in a patient under 30 years old – Wilson's disease. This is an inherited defect of copper metabolism. The diagnostic features are shown in Table 7.37.

Table 7.36   Histological features
of primary biliary cirrhosis

- Periductal granulomata
- Proliferation of bile ducts
- Piecemeal necrosis
- Fibrosis

Table 7.37   Diagnostic features of Wilson's disease

- Family history of liver disease
- Hepatosplenomegaly
- Neurological disturbances
- Kayser–Fleischer rings in eyes (slit-lamp)
- Increased urinary copper excretion
- Increased serum ceruloplasmin concentration

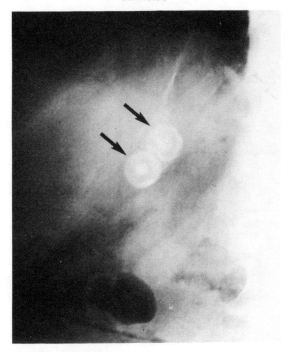

Figure 7.9   Plain X-ray of the abdomen showing radio-opaque gallstones

Plain X-ray of the abdomen

This may be of value in a patient with jaundice by showing radio-opaque gall-stones (Figure 7.9). The patient's X-ray was normal.

Barium meal

This is a helpful investigation in two ways: (1) it may show *oesophageal varices* associated with cirrhosis (Figure 7.10) and (2) it is also of diagnostic value in detecting *pancreatic carcinoma*, when the duodenal loop may be widened.

The patient's barium meal examination was normal.

Cholecystography

Although this investigation is of value in showing gallstones and gallbladder contraction, the X-ray pictures obtained are very poor once jaundice has become established. It was not carried out in this patient.

Transhepatic percutaneous cholangiography

In this investigation, radio-opaque dye is injected directly into the liver through a needle inserted into the liver through the chest wall. It is of value in

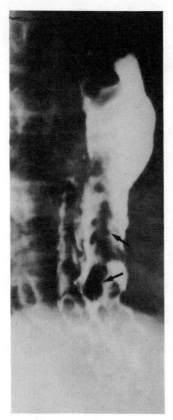

Figure 7.10   Barium meal showing oesophageal varices

showing a dilated biliary tree in cholestatic jaundice and sometimes defining the site of the obstruction.

In this patient, the investigation confirmed some *biliary dilatation* but showed no site of obstruction.

MANAGEMENT

General measures

The only general measure of value in any form of chronic liver disease is complete abstinence from alcohol.

Symptomatic treatment

Pruritus often responds to cholestyramine (Questran) 4 g four times daily. The mechanism of its action is to bind the bile salts in the gut and so prevent absorption into the circulation.

Bleeding

Bleeding in liver disease may be due to several factors (Table 7.38).

Improvement of prothrombin and factor VIII synthesis, due either to liver cell damage or to failure of absorption of vitamin K in obstructive jaundice, can be corrected by vitamin K administration. Vitamin K can be given either intravenously, 2.5–20 mg for a haemorrhagic crisis, or 10–20 mg by mouth daily for long term prophylaxis.

The treatment available for control of bleeding from oesophageal varices is shown in Table 7.39.

Table 7.38   Bleeding in liver disease

- Defective synthesis of prothrombin and Factor VIII
- Impaired absorption of vitamin K
- Bleeding from oesophageal varices

Table 7.39   Control of bleeding from oesophageal varices

- Blood transfusion
- Intravenous vasopressin
- Balloon tamponade (Sengstaken tube)
- Operation – transection of stomach
  portacaval anastomosis

Oedema and ascites

The measures which are helpful in controlling oedema and ascites associated with liver disease are shown in Table 7.40.

Intravenous infusions of albumin are of transient value only and have no place in routine maintenance treatment.

Table 7.40   Control of oedema and ascites

- Dietary salt restriction
- Frusemide 40–160 mg/day
- Spironolactone 100–400 mg/day

Hepatic encephalopathy

The management of this serious complication of liver disease is shown in Table 7.41.

Table 7.41 Treatment of hepatic encephalopathy

- Restriction of dietary protein (20–40 g/day)
- Neomycin orally 8 g initial dose; 2–4 g daily
- Lactulose 15–50 ml t.d.s.

Specific treatment

Steroids

The most valuable specific treatment is steroids. There are several important factors which will influence the decision as to whether steroids should be used (Table 7.42).

Table 7.42 Factors influencing decision on using steroids in chronic active hepatitis

- Presence of symptoms
- Age and sex
- Presence of auto-immune features
- HB_sAg status
- Bridging necrosis in the liver biopsy

Symptoms
There is no evidence that steroids are of value in asymptomatic patients.

Age and sex
Young females with chronic active hepatitis will usually respond better than older males with the disease. The reason is that the young female is more likely to have the auto-immune type of hepatitis.

Auto-immune features
The presence of extrahepatic manifestations indicates an auto-immune basis for the chronic hepatitis. The steroid response is therefore likely to be good.

HB_sAg status
In HB_sAg-positive patients the hepatitis is likely to be due to hepatitis B virus. This does not respond well to steroids.

Histology of liver
Chronic active hepatitis is unlikely to progress to cirrhosis or hepatic failure unless bridging necrosis is present. In these cases the prognosis is likely to be good anyway.

If bridging necrosis is present, steroids may well arrest its progress and so prevent cirrhosis and liver failure.

Dosage regime of steroids
Prednisolone is usually started in a daily dose of 60 mg. The dose is tapered

gradually over several weeks to a maintenance level of 20 mg daily.

If there is no satisfactory response within 3 months treatment is discontinued.

If improvement occurs, treatment is continued for a minimum period of 12 months and then slowly withdrawn. If this leads to a recurrence of activity, the prednisolone is reintroduced.

The patient is assessed monthly for signs of improvement (Table 7.43). Liver biopsy should be repeated every 6 months. During the regular check-ups, particular attention must be paid to detecting side-effects of long term steroid treatment (Table 7.44).

Table 7.43 Signs of improvement with steroids

- Reduction of symptoms
- Improvement in liver function tests (especially transaminases)
- Improvement in liver histology (especially bridging necrosis)

Table 7.44 Side-effects of long term steroids

- Weight gain
- Oedema
- Hypertension
- Hypokalaemia
- Diabetes
- Peptic ulcer
- Osteoporosis
- Mental disturbance
- Hirsutes

HB$_s$Ag-positive chronic active hepatitis

The value of steroids remains controversial in this type of hepatitis. It has been suggested that steroids may encourage growth of the virus and might also pre-dispose to development of primary carcinoma of the liver.

Steroids are not necessary if the patient is asymptomatic or has minimal symptoms only. In this type of case, the patient should be kept under regular observation with liver biopsy repeated every 6 months or every year. If the disease is progressive, steroids should be tried. If the patient has severe symptoms with markedly abnormal liver function tests and extensive inflammatory changes in the liver biopsy, a trial of prednisolone is indicated.

Regular reassessment of the clinical state, liver function tests and liver biopsy should show whether to continue treatment or withdraw.

Azathioprine

This immunosuppressive drug is of no value in chronic active hepatitis if given alone. It can, however, reduce the requirements of prednisolone when this is desirable (Table 7.45).

Addition of 50–100 mg of azathioprine daily will reduce prednisolone requirements to 30 mg initial daily dose and 10 mg daily maintenance dose.

The main hazard of azathioprine is bone marrow depression (Table 7.46).

Table 7.45 Indications for azathioprine in prednisolone-treated patients with chronic active hepatitis

- Elderly patients
- Side-effects with full dose prednisolone
- Inadequate control with prednisolone alone
- Associated diabetes mellitus

Table 7.46 Clinical effects of bone-marrow suppression by azathioprine

- Red cells   – anaemia
- White cells   – susceptibility to infection
- Platelets   – bleeding

NATURAL HISTORY OF CHRONIC ACTIVE HEPATITIS

Development from acute hepatitis

Approximately 10% of patients with acute type B hepatitis remain HB_sAg positive for more than 7 years.

Most of these will lose the antigen from their circulation over the subsequent few years, but a small number will remain carriers, and some of these will develop chronic active hepatitis HB_sAg-positive.

Chronic active hepatitis will occur in 3–5% of patients who have had acute type B hepatitis. It may also be a late complication of non-A non-B acute hepatitis, but is extremely rare after acute type A hepatitis.

The features in acute type B or non-A non-B hepatitis which indicate progression to chronic active hepatitis are shown in Table 7.47.

Table 7.47 Prognostic features in acute hepatitis indicating progression to chronic disease

- Failure of symptoms to resolve
- Persistence of hepatomegaly
- Bridging necrosis on liver biopsy
- Abnormal liver function tests persisting 6–12 months
- Persistence of HB_sAg longer than 6 months

Once chronic active hepatitis is established, the rate of progression varies considerably but the mean survival time is 5 years.

Prognosis

The prognosis in HB$_s$Ag-positive patients is favourable. It may persist for years without clinically overt liver disease and with very little in the way of symptoms.

The auto-immune type of chronic active hepatitis (HB$_s$Ag-negative) has a poorer prognosis and the fatality rate is high – 50–75% within the first few years.

The causes of death are shown in Table 7.48.

Table 7.48 Causes of death in chronic active hepatitis

- Liver failure
- Cirrhosis with variceal haemorrhage
- Intercurrent illness

Changes of cirrhosis will be found on liver biopsy in 30–50% of patients with chronic active hepatitis even in the early stages of the disease. Bridging necrosis on liver biopsy is a particularly bad prognostic sign.

CAN WE MODIFY THE NATURAL HISTORY?

The most effective way of modifying the disease is by prophylaxis.

Passive immunization

Immune serum globulins

Immune serum globulin contains antibodies to hepatitis B virus and is variably effective in modifying infection with the virus.

Hepatitis B immunoglobulins

A more efficient, but more expensive, preparation is obtainable from persons who are negative for hepatitis B surface antigen but have high levels of hepatitis B antibodies. This is the specific hepatitis B immunoglobulin preparation.

Indications for immunization

The recommended prophylactic use of these preparations is shown in Table 7.49.

Table 7.49 Recommended prophylactic use of hepatitis B immunoglobulin preparations

> • Staff in a haemodialysis unit
> • Institutional mentally-handicapped patients
> • Neonate from mother with recent hepatitis B infection

Non-A non-B immunization

Prophylactic immune serum globulin may be effective in modifying the progression of this type of acute hepatitis to chronic hepatitis. It should be given as soon as possible after infection.

Active immunization

Plasma from healthy carriers of the hepatitis B virus can be used to produce an active immunogenic vaccine. At present this is still under investigation and further developmental work is necessary before a safe and effective vaccine is available to the public.

Active immunization against non-A non-B hepatitis is not yet available.

Established chronic active hepatitis

Once the disease has become established, the only measure which will modify its progress to hepatic failure or cirrhosis is *steroid treatment*.

The beneficial effects of steroids are confined mainly to the patient with auto-immune type of chronic active hepatitis who does not carry the hepatitis B surface antigen.

The value of steroids in the HB_sAg-positive patient remains controversial. In these patients, it should, however, be always considered if such a patient is pursuing a relentless down-hill course.

Antiviral treatment

Vidarabine and *leukocyte interferon* are antiviral agents which reduce viral infectivity and may improve liver function. Their use is, so far, only experimental.

USEFUL PRACTICAL POINTS

- Chronic active hepatitis is a late complication in up to 5% of patients with acute type B hepatitis.

- Isoniazid, nitrofurantoin (Furadantin), methyldopa (Aldomet) and dantrolene (Dantrium) may also cause chronic active hepatitis.

- The definitive diagnostic test is liver biopsy which shows portal infiltration and fibrosis extending into the liver lobule (bridging necrosis), piece-meal necrosis of hepatocytes and rosettes of regenerating liver cells.

- The two main clinical types of the disease are HB_sAg-positive cases in older males with few symptoms and a good prognosis, and the auto-immune type in HB_sAg-negative young females with severe symptoms, systemic manifestations and a poor prognosis.

- Steroid treatment is of greatest value in the auto-immune HB_sAg-negative patient.

- Passive immunization with immune serum globulin is available and effective.
    Active immunization is still experimental.

8

Headache and fits

PRESENT HISTORY

A 46-year-old male patient presented with a long history of headache becoming worse over the last 12 months, and a recent fit.

Headache

The patient gave a history of headache going back to childhood.

The headache was dull and throbbing which usually affected one side of his head only, though it could be either side. It would tend to occur more frequently at times of stress.

The headache would usually last for several hours and ended frequently after a bout of vomiting.

The headache was invariably preceded by visual disturbances.

Visual disturbances

The patient always knew when a headache was coming on since it invariably started, and usually suddenly, with patchy blindness affecting one side of his field of vision. About 10 minutes later he would develop scintillating curved zigzag lights which lasted about 15–20 minutes and would always herald the onset of the throbbing headache.

Progress of the headache

The headache has decreased progressively in frequency over the years, so that up to 12 months ago, attacks were occurring only once every few months, usually at times of mental stress or after an excessive bout of drinking alcohol. The pattern of the symptoms had also changed with the years, in that the predominant visual symptoms were as prominent as ever but the headache had become much less severe and the vomiting had entirely disappeared.

However, over the past year he had noticed a recurrence of his headache which was getting steadily worse. It was still a dull throbbing headache but now localized always over the right side of his head.

At first, the headache occurred on waking in the morning and occasionally would wake him in the middle of the night. Then it became more frequent and more severe and occurred throughout the day also.

The pattern had also changed once more. He no longer had the visual disturbances prior to the headache, but the nausea had now returned and he was often sick with the headache but did not obtain the relief of the headache that the vomiting used to bring.

The fit

One week before the patient presented, he had a fit which was seen by his wife. He was sitting watching television and his wife noticed that his left hand was twitching. Immediately afterwards, he muttered something, half rose from the chair then fell back unconscious. His body went stiff for a short time and he then started to 'shake all over'.

The whole episode lasted about 10 minutes and when he came round he seemed confused for about half an hour afterwards. When his mind became clearer he complained of a severe headache and a sore tongue. When his wife looked at the tongue she saw some blood on it.

He had not been incontinent of urine.

There was no history of any previous fits.

Other relevant facts on direct enquiry

Personality change

When specifically asked about this, his wife thought that there had been a definite change in his personality in recent months.

He had become unusually aggressive and argumentative at home. At other times he seemed depressed and apathetic with loss of interest in ordinary day to day affairs concerning his home and family. He had difficulty, for the first time, in filling in his tax returns and was making obvious errors in his calculation.

Another symptom noticed by his wife was that he had lost all interest in sex.

Nervous system

He had not noticed any weakness of his arms or legs. He had, however, experienced uncomfortable tingling at times over the left side of his face and in his left arm.

He admitted also that there had been a recent deterioration in his vision. This was especially noticeable on reading a newspaper when the small print would often blur. This was also causing difficulty in his work as an office manager.

There had been no disturbance of his speech.

242

Respiratory system

He had a smoker's cough for many years. He would bring up a small amount of grey or white sputum most mornings. He had never coughed up blood.

Alimentary system

His appetite was becoming poor and he was losing interest in his food. He had lost nearly a stone (6·5 kg) in the past few months.

He had no indigestion and there had been no recent change in his bowel habits.

Past history

There was no past history of epilepsy.
There were no other serious illnesses.

FAMILY HISTORY

Both his mother and his sister had suffered from migraine.
There was no family history of fits or epilepsy.

PERSONAL HISTORY

He had been happy in his work as an office manager in a mail-order business up to about 9 months previously.

He was having increasing difficulty in coping with the work largely due to forgetfulness and inability to concentrate on the organizational work and the correspondence.

He was a heavy smoker – 30 cigarettes daily for many years.

His drinking was moderate – about 5 or 6 pints (3–3·5 litres) of beer at the weekend.

DRUG TREATMENT

The only drugs he had used recently were a variety of different analgesics to control his headache. Currently he was using dihydrocodeine (DF 118) but relief was very limited.

EXAMINATION

The abnormal physical signs are shown in Figure 8.1, and mainly involved the nervous system.

Mental state

The patient's manner was abnormal. He appeared to be quite indifferent to his problems and uninterested in the examination.

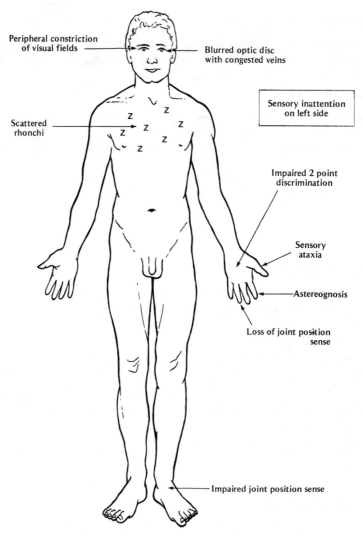

Peripheral constriction of visual fields

Blurred optic disc with congested veins

Sensory inattention on left side

Scattered rhonchi

Impaired 2 point discrimination

Sensory ataxia

Astereognosis

Loss of joint position sense

Impaired joint position sense

Figure 8.1　Abnormal physical signs

Central nervous system

Cranial nerves

The only abnormalities related to his eyes.

The visual acuity tested with a Snellen test card was only slightly impaired, 6/9 in each eye. Testing his visual fields by the confrontation technique showed some peripheral constriction of the fields.

The margins of both optic discs were blurred and the veins were congested; there were no retinal haemorrhages or exudates. Conjunctival sensation was intact and there was no sensory abnormality to pinprick or cotton wool in the face.

Motor system

No abnormality was detected in muscle tone, power or reflexes.

Sensory system

There was a loss of *joint position sense* in the left hand and considerable impairment in the left foot.

Two-point discrimination was impaired in the left hand. This was tested with compass points. The patient was unable to distinguish two separate points on the dorsum of the hand and foot until the points were at least 25 mm apart (normal 3–5 mm). With his eyes closed he was unable to recognize coins placed in his left hand (*astereognosis*).

He had difficulty in localizing cutaneous sensory stimuli in his left side. This was tested by asking him to point with his right forefinger to the site of stimulation on his left arm and leg – this was very inaccurate.

Sensory inattention (sensory extinction) was present in both the left arm and the left leg: when he was stimulated simultaneously with cotton wool or with a pin on both sides he was able to feel the stimulus on the right side only.

There was *no* loss of primary cutaneous sensation to pinprick or cotton wool; vibration sense was also quite intact.

Coordination

The finger–nose and heel–knee tests were quite satisfactory with his eyes open, but both tests became poor when his eyes were closed (*sensory ataxia*).

Murmurs

There were no carotid or intracranial murmurs.

Cardiovascular systems

The pulse was normal.
The blood pressure was 165/90.
The heart was normal with no murmurs.

Respiratory system

There was no finger clubbing.
There were no enlarged neck or axillary lymph nodes.
The only abnormality in the lungs was scattered high-pitched expiratory rhonchi.

Abdomen

There was no liver enlargement. No other abnormality was found.

ANALYSIS OF THE HISTORY

Headache

This was the main presenting symptom.

The pain-sensitive structures which cause headache are shown in Table 8.1. The common causes of headache are shown in Table 8.2.

Table 8.1   Pain-sensitive structures causing headache

- Basal intracranial arteries
- Intracranial venous sinuses
- Meningeal arteries
- Basal dura mater
- Scalp muscles

Table 8.2   Causes of headache

- Migraine
- Psychogenic ('tension' headache)
- Raised intracranial pressure
- Vascular disorders
    - hypertension
    - temporal arteritis
    - subarachnoid haemorrhage
- Trauma
- Local disease

Migraine

This is a frequent cause of headache. The typical features of migraine are shown in Table 8.3.

The patient's longstanding headache has all the characteristic features and undoubtedly indicates migraine.

The recent headache has different features (Table 8.4). This indicates an alternative cause for the headache.

Table 8.3   Typical features of migraine

- Throbbing headache
- Hemicranial or bilateral
- Lasts several hours to several days
- Nausea and vomiting common
- Visual disturbances (teichopsia)
- Trigger factors
    - mental stress
    - menstruation
    - alcohol (especially red wine)
    - foodstuffs

Table 8.4 Change of pattern in recent headache

- Localization to right side only
- Predominance on waking
- Disappearance of visual prodromata
- Loss of relief on vomiting

Psychogenic headache ('tension' headache)

This is very frequent and together with migraine accounts for the great majority of headaches encountered in clinical practice. The typical features are shown in Table 8.5.

Table 8.5 Features of 'tension' headache

- Character – 'pressure'
  'weight on the head'
  'band round the head'
- Site – often vertex
  sometimes occipital or temporal
  sometimes 'all over'
- Lasts for hours, days, weeks or months
- Related to periods of mental stress
- Other anxiety symptoms often present

Emotional stress is a frequent precipitating factor – related often to problems with marriage and children in women and problems with work or with finance in men.

The patient's chronic headache often occurred with emotional stress, which is a distinctive feature of migraine.

There was nothing in the history, however, to suggest a relationship between his recent headache and psychological tension.

Raised intracranial pressure

The characteristics of headache due to raised intracranial pressure are shown in Table 8.6.

Table 8.6 Characteristics of headache due to raised intracranial pressure

- Throbbing or bursting
- Worse on waking
- Worse on straining, coughing or sneezing
- Nausea and vomiting frequent
- Occipital – subtentorial lesion
- Fronto-parietal – supratentorial lesion

The patient's recent headache had all the features of raised intracranial pressure. The localization to the right hemicranium suggests a right-sided supratentorial space-occupying lesion.

Vascular disorders

Hypertension

The characteristics of a hypertensive headache are shown in Table 8.7. It occurs only in severe hypertension as with malignant hypertension or hypertensive encephalopathy.

Table 8.7 Characteristics of hypertensive headache

- Severe hypertension
- Throbbing
- Occipital
- Worse on waking

The majority of headaches in hypertensive patients develop after the diagnosis of high blood pressure has been disclosed and are of psychogenic origin.

The parietal localization of the patient's recent headache makes it unlikely to be of hypertensive origin.

The duration and benign course of the longstanding headache rule out severe hypertension as a cause.

Temporal arteritis

The features of this condition are shown in Figure 8.2.

The patient's relatively young age, the lack of temporal localization and the absence of arthralgia or myalgia exclude the diagnosis.

Subarachnoid haemorrhage

The features are shown in Table 8.8.

The picture is quite unlike the patient's presentation.

Table 8.8 Features of subarachnoid haemorrhage

- Dramatic onset
- Severe occipital pain
- Neck stiffness
- Double vision may occur due to oculomotor paresis

Trauma

Head trauma may be followed by continuous localized or generalized headache which may go on for weeks, months or years. This type is usually psychogenic.

There was no head trauma in the patient's history.

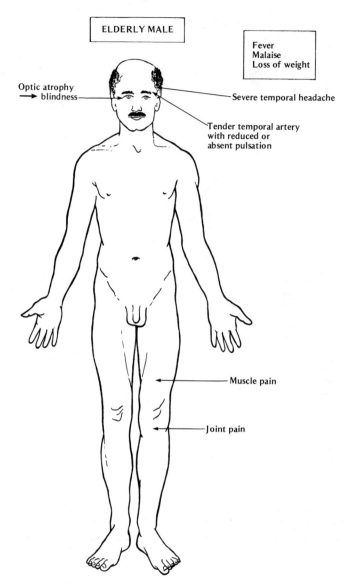

ELDERLY MALE

Fever
Malaise
Loss of weight

Optic atrophy
→ blindness

Severe temporal headache

Tender temporal artery
with reduced or
absent pulsation

Muscle pain

Joint pain

Figure 8.2 Features of temporal arteritis

Local disease

The local conditions which may cause headache are shown in Figure 8.3.

There was no past history of nose trouble or sinusitis.

There was no history of eye trouble previously and the patient's headache was parietal and not frontal.

The headache caused by cervical spondylosis is occipital and related to head

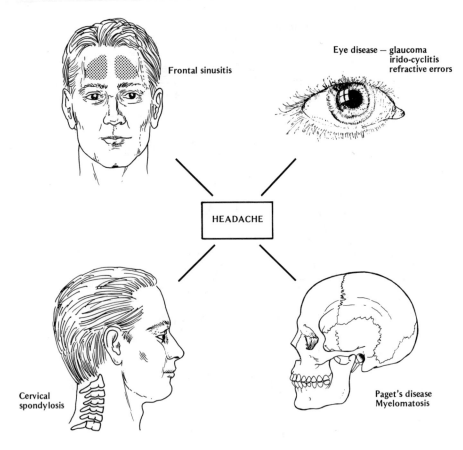

Eye disease — glaucoma
irido-cyclitis
refractive errors

Frontal sinusitis

HEADACHE

Cervical
spondylosis

Paget's disease
Myelomatosis

Figure 8.3   Local disease causing headache

turning: neither feature applied to the patient's headache.

The exclusion of Paget's disease of the skull and myelomatosis can not be made on the history. Skull X-rays are necessary to assess this further, if suspected.

The fit

The patient lost consciousness and had a fit.

The main differential diagnosis is between a *syncopal* attack followed by an anoxic convulsion and *epilepsy*.

Syncope

Syncope is a transient and critical fall in cerebral blood flow leading to loss of consciousness. The causes of syncope are shown in Table 8.9.

Table 8.9   Causes of syncope

• Cardiac	• Stokes–Adams attacks
	• Tachyarrhythmia
	• Myocardial infarction
	• Aortic or pulmonary stenosis
• Vasomotor	• Simple faint (vasovagal attack)
	• Prolonged standing
	• Hypotensive drugs
• Cough and micturition syncope	
• Hypoglycaemia	

Cardiac causes of syncope

Stoke–Adams attacks are due to sudden ventricular asystole (or rarely ventricular fibrillation) associated with heart block.

Since the usual cause of a Stokes–Adams attack is ischaemic heart disease, a history of angina or a heart attack is often obtained. There was no such history in the patient.

Definite exclusion of a Stokes–Adams attack can only be confirmed by an electrocardiogram recorded during an attack.

Tachyarrhythmias can so impair cardiac output that a critical fall in cerebral blood flow can occur.

There would usually be a complaint of palpitations at the onset of the attack. This was not felt by the patient before he lost consciousness.

The loss of consciousness with *aortic and pulmonary stenosis* occurs with exercise. There may also be a history of breathlessness or angina. These symptoms did not apply to the patient.

Vasomotor causes of syncope

A *vasovagal attack* causes loss of consciousness but only very exceptionally leads to a convulsion. The features are shown in Table 8.10.

Table 8.10   Features of a vasovagal attack

• Extreme emotion or stress
• Preceding nausea and sweating
• Sense of impending loss of consciousness
• Rapid recovery on lying flat

The differentiation between loss of consciousness caused by a faint and by epilepsy is shown in Table 8.11.

The nature of the patient's loss of consciousness was quite unlike a simple faint, and the subsequent convulsion is a very strong point against the diagnosis.

Table 8.11 Differentiation between a faint and epilepsy

	Epilepsy	*Simple faint*
Precipitation	Rare	Fear, grief, pain Prolonged standing
Speed of onset	Instantaneous	Over minutes
Sweating	Rare	Common
Injury	Frequent	Rare
Incontinence	Common	Rare
Tongue-biting	Common	Never
After-effects	Headache Drowsiness Confusion	'Exhaustion'

Postural syncope

The patient had not been standing at the time of his attack.
He was not on any hypotensive drugs.

Cough/micturition syncope

Cough syncope follows a bout of prolonged coughing and is due to obstruction to the venous return to the heart, a fall in cardiac output and consequent cerebrovascular insufficiency.

Micturition syncope usually occurs at night when a patient gets out of a warm bed to empty his bladder and is especially prone to occur when micturition is difficult due to an enlarged prostate gland.

Neither a bout of coughing nor micturition preceded the patient's attack.

Hypoglycaemia

This usually occurs in diabetic patients overtreated with insulin.
The patient was not a diabetic.

Epilepsy

A simple classification of epilepsy is shown in Table 8.12.

Table 8.12 Classification of epilepsy

• Grand mal	– generalized convulsions
• Minor epilepsy	• petit mal ('absences')
	• myoclonic
	• akinetic
• Focal epilepsy	• motor
	• sensory
	• psychomotor

Grand mal epilepsy

The classical pattern of the grand mal attack is shown in Table 8.13. The aura preceding the loss of consciousness may take several forms (Table 8.14).

Table 8.13 Pattern of grand mal epilepsy

• Aura
• Cry
• Loss of consciousness
• Tonic phase   – tongue-biting   incontinence
• Clonic phase

• After-effects   – headache
                         confusion
                         drowsiness
                         automatism (rare)

Table 8.14 Types of aura

• Vague abdominal then ascending discomfort
• Feeling of apprehension
• Olfactory   – bad smell
• Auditory   – bells ringing
• Visual   – alteration of form or shape   hallucination

The patient's attack had most of the features of grand mal epilepsy and this must therefore be regarded as the diagnosis.

Minor epilepsy

Petit mal occurs usually in childhood and adolescence. It produces a transient and very brief alteration in consciousness ('absence') and manifests as a sudden blankness, stare or cessation of talking lasting 5–10 seconds only.

Myoclonic epilepsy consists of a sudden brief episode of generalized muscle twitching not associated with alteration or loss of consciousness.

Akinetic epilepsy is a sudden transient generalized loss of muscle tone resulting in a sudden fall with immediate recovery afterwards.

The patient's attack in no way resembled any of these types of minor epilepsy.

Focal (partial) seizures

The presentation will depend on the site of the epileptogenic focus.

Partial motor seizure

Jacksonian epilepsy is an example of focal epilepsy. The epileptogenic focus is often in the hand area of the motor cortex (Figure 8.4).

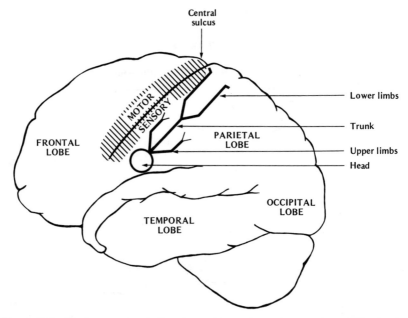

Figure 8.4 Body representation in motor and sensory cortex of the brain

As the seizure discharge spreads from the hand area to adjacent areas of the motor cortex, twitching of the thumb and index finger spreads up the arm to the same side of the face. If the discharge continues to spread across to the other side of the brain, consciousness will be lost and a generalized convulsion will occur.

Partial sensory seizure

This follows a similar pattern to Jacksonian epilepsy with a march of para-esthesiae from the tip of an extremity up to the trunk and face.

Psychomotor epilepsy

This is a partial seizure of complex type originating in the temporal lobe. Some of the symptoms which may occur are shown in Table 8.15.

Table 8.15 Symptoms of psychomotor epilepsy

- *Déjà-vu* phenomenon
- Intense emotional feeling
- Objects get smaller or larger
- Formed sensory hallucinations
- Unusual smells
- Lip smacking
- Aimless behaviour
- Automatic behaviour – may involve skill

There were no symptoms to suggest that the patient was having any of these types of focal epilepsy.

Causes of epilepsy

The common causes of epilepsy are shown in Table 8.16.

Table 8.16   Common causes of epilepsy

- Idiopathic
- Secondary
  - brain tumour
  - head injury
  - cerebrovascular disease
  - heart block
  - metabolic
    - hypoglycaemia
    - uraemia

Idiopathic epilepsy

The patient's late age of onset and the absence of a family history of epilepsy makes this diagnosis unlikely.

Brain tumour

This is a likely cause of the epilepsy in view of the headache which is very suggestive of raised intracranial pressure, and the personality change which occurs in brain tumours.

Head injury

There was no history of this.

Heart block

The absence of other symptoms of ischamic heart disease has already been mentioned, which makes this diagnosis unlikely.

Cerebrovascular disease

Epileptic fits due to cerebrovascular disease usually occur in elderly hypertensive patients with widespread arteriosclerosis causing scattered areas of cerebral ischaemia and infarction.

The patient was not elderly and there were no other symptoms to suggest widespread arteriosclerosis such as angina or intermittent claudication.

The patient did however, complain of paraesthesiae on the left side which could be due to cerebrovascular insufficiency.

This diagnosis therefore remains a possibility pending further investigation.

Hypoglycaemia

This occurs mainly in insulin-treated diabetics. The patient was not a diabetic.

Uraemia

There was no past history of kidney disease, there were no current urinary symptoms and no other symptoms of uraemia (Table 8.17).

Table 8.17 Symptoms of uraemia

- Loss of energy
- Weakness
- Nausea and vomiting
- Diarrhoea
- Thirst
- Polyuria

Personality change

Personality change can be caused by emotional disorders or by organic disease (Table 8.18). The mental manifestations are common to most of these disorders and are shown in Table 8.19.

Table 8.18 Causes of personality change

• Psychiatric	• Anxiety
	• Depression
	• Psychosis, e.g. schizophrenia
• Organic disease	• Cerebral arteriosclerosis
	• Chronic epilepsy
	• Brain tumour
	• Parkinson's disease
	• Myxoedema
	• Alcoholism
	• Systemic lupus erythematosus

Table 8.19 Mental manifestations of personality disorder

- Poor memory
- Faulty judgement and insight
- Indifference to family and friends
- Mental apathy and lack of concentration
- Confusion and disorientation
- Emotional lability

There was no past history of psychiatric disease.

Cerebral arteriosclerosis usually occurs in older patients and the onset is more gradual than in the patient's case.

The patient was not a chronic epileptic or an alcoholic.

There was no impairment of movement or tremor to suggest Parkinson's disease.

There were no symptoms of cold intolerance, increasing weight, constipation, voice change or loss of hair to suggest myxoedema.

Systemic lupus erythematosus occurs predominantly in young women and is

associated with polyarthritis, pleurisy, pericarditis, renal disease and polyneuropathy. The patient had no symptoms of this condition.

The recent onset of the personality change and the progressive headache of
raised intracranial pressure indicates clearly that the likely diagnosis is *brain
tumour*.

Paraesthesiae on the left side

The tingling affecting the left side of the face and the left arm suggests an
irritant focus in the lower part of the postcentral gyrus (sensory cortex) in the
right cerebral hemisphere (see Figure 8.4).

Deterioration of vision

The patient had recent deterioration of vision. Some causes which might be
responsible for this symptom are shown in Table 8.20.

Table 8.20 Causes of recent deterioration
of vision

• Glaucoma
• Retinal disease:
diabetes
hypertension
• Papilloedema
• Compression of optic chiasma
• Neuromyelitis optica
• Toxic damage to optic nerve:
methyl alcohol
quinine
lead poisoning
chloroquine and hydroxychloroquine
ethambutol

Glaucoma leads to painful eyes and a rainbow-coloured halo is seen around
lights. The patient had neither symptom.

Diabetic retinopathy is excluded because the patient is not a diabetic.

There was no history of *hypertension*, but the patient could still be an
asymptomatic hypertensive: recording the blood pressure will decide this
point.

Papilloedema is a very likely diagnosis in view of the headache which
indicated raised intracranial pressure.

Compression of the optic chiasma causes bitemporal hemianopia (Figure
8.5). This defect of visual field was not present.

Neuromyelitis optica is a rare demyelinating disease characterized by
bilateral optic neuritis, leading to impaired vision, and massive demyelination
of the spinal cord, resulting frequently in paraplegia, or severe ataxia. The
lack of symptoms of severe spinal cord involvement excludes this condition.

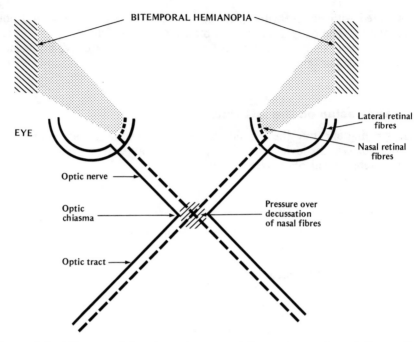

Figure 8.5 Bitemporal hemianopia caused by compression of the optic chiasma

The patient had not taken any of the *toxic substances* specified in Table 8.20, which excludes toxic damage to the optic nerves.

CONCLUSIONS FROM THE HISTORY

- There is not doubt that the patient has had longstanding migraine.

- The change in the type of headache and the associated vomiting and visual deterioration indicate raised intracranial pressure.

- The left-sided paraesthesiae and the epileptic fit suggest an irritant lesion in the lower part of the postcentral gyrus in the right parietal lobe.

- The recent change in personality suggests that the lesion is likely to be an infiltrating brain tumour.

ANALYSIS OF THE EXAMINATION

The main abnormalities were in the nervous system.

Papilloedema

The blurred disc margins and congested veins indicate papilloedema.
The causes of papilloedema are shown in Table 8.21.

Table 8.21 Causes of papilloedema

* Raised intracranial pressure
* Malignant hypertension
* Optic neuritis
* Blocked retinal veins
* Carbon dioxide retention

Raised intracranial pressure

The causes of raised intracranial pressure are shown in Table 8.22.

Table 8.22 Causes of raised intracranial pressure

• Space-occupying lesion	• abscess
	• haematoma
	• tumour
• Benign intracranial hypertension	
• Infections	• meningitis
	• virus encephalitis
• Subarachnoid haemorrhage	

Space-occupying lesions

The patient was not febrile and there were no symptoms relating to the usual causes of *brain abscess* (Table 8.23).

Table 8.23 Causes of brain abscess

• Ear infection	– painful discharging ear deafness
• Sinus infection	– frontal headache blocked nose
• Lung infection	– productive cough purulent sputum dyspnoea
• Infective endocarditis	– history of heart disease recent dental extraction malaise joint pains

A *haematoma* leading to raised intracranial pressure is either intracerebral, in which case the patient is seriously ill and often unconscious with a stroke, or subdural, associated with trauma to the head. Neither of these conditions was applicable to the patient.

Brain tumour remains a very likely cause of the raised intracranial pressure as indicated by the very suggestive history.

Benign intracranial hypertension

This condition occurs in women either at the menarche or at the menopause. Menstrual irregularity is often present.

It is a diagnosis of exclusion after space-occupying lesions, obstruction of the cerebral ventricles, intracranial infection and hypertensive disease have been excluded.

The patient's sex and the strong evidence of brain tumour makes this diagnosis irrelevant.

Infection

Meningitis and encephalitis are excluded by absence of the relevant symptoms (Table 8.24).

Table 8.24 Symptoms of intracranial infection

• Fever
• Constitutional disturbance
• Neck stiffness
• Alteration of consciousness

Subarachnoid haemorrhage

The absence of dramatic onset of occipital headache and neck stiffness excludes this diagnosis.

Malignant hypertension

The patient's normal blood pressure excludes this diagnosis.

Optic neuritis

The ophthalmoscopic appearance of optic neuritis is indistinguishable from papilloedema. The differentiation depends on the associated visual disturbance (Table 8.25).

Table 8.25 Visual disturbances in optic neuritis and papilloedema

	Optic neuritis	Papilloedema
Visual acuity	impaired	preserved
Visual field	central scotoma	peripheral constriction

The preservation of the patient's visual acuity and the peripheral constriction with lack of a central scotoma excludes optic neuritis.

Blocked retinal veins

Thrombosis of the central retinal vein is unilateral and has a distinctive retinal appearance (Figure 8.6).

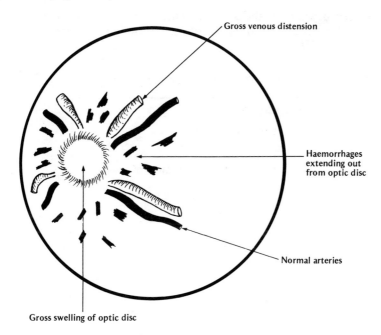

Figure 8.6   Fundal appearances in central retinal vein thrombosis

The bilateral involvement of the optic discs and the absence of retinal haemorrhages excludes this diagnosis.

Cavernous sinus thrombosis is a serious condition the features of which are shown in Table 8.26. The patient had none of these features.

Table 8.26   Features of cavernous sinus thrombosis

- Antecedent infection • face
  - • sinuses
  - • ear
- Bilateral proptosis
- Distended superficial veins in forehead
- Weakness or paralysis of external ocular muscles
- Impaired sensation over forehead

Carbon dioxide retention

This only occurs in patients with severe chronic obstructive lung disease causing marked respiratory insufficiency. There was no evidence of such disease in the patient.

Sensory abnormalities

The main sensory abnormalities found in the patient indicate impairment, not of primary cutaneous sensation, but of the discriminating aspects of sensory function (Table 8.27).

Table 8.27 Patient's sensory findings

• Discriminatory function abnormal
• Impaired two-point discrimination
• Astereognosis
• Impaired localization of sensory stimuli
• Sensory inattention (extinction)
• Loss of joint position sense
• Primary cutaneous sensation normal
• Pain
• Touch
• Temperature
• Vibration

This indicates a *parietal lobe lesion* which leads to this distinctive pattern of sensory abnormality.

The distinctive abnormalities produced by lesions in the various lobes of the brain are shown in Figure 8.7.

Coordination

The impairment of coordination tests produced by closing the eyes indicates sensory ataxia caused by loss of position sense.

The loss of joint sense and preservation of vibration sense excludes a lesion of the posterior columns of the spinal cord.

This pattern is one of the distinctive features of a parietal lobe lesion.

Respiratory system

The scattered rhonchi indicate widespread bronchitis, no doubt attributed to his smoking.

There were no signs of emphysema (Figure 8.8).

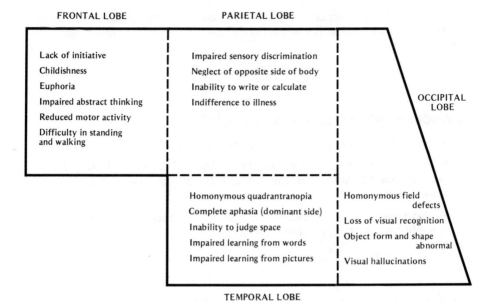

FRONTAL LOBE

Lack of initiative
Childishness
Euphoria
Impaired abstract thinking
Reduced motor activity
Difficulty in standing
and walking

PARIETAL LOBE

Impaired sensory discrimination
Neglect of opposite side of body
Inability to write or calculate
Indifference to illness

OCCIPITAL LOBE

Homonymous quadrantranopia
Complete aphasia (dominant side)
Inability to judge space
Impaired learning from words
Impaired learning from pictures

Homonymous field
defects
Loss of visual recognition
Object form and shape
abnormal
Visual hallucinations

TEMPORAL LOBE

Figure 8.7 Syndromes due to lesion of cerebral lobes

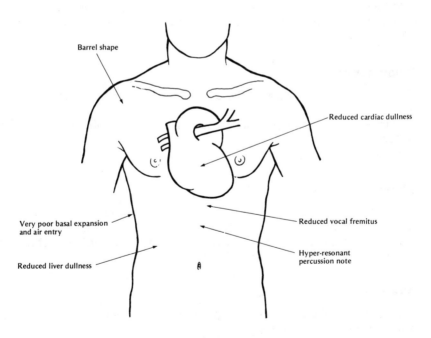

Barrel shape

Reduced cardiac dullness

Very poor basal expansion
and air entry

Reduced vocal fremitus

Reduced liver dullness

Hyper-resonant
percussion note

Figure 8.8 Physical signs of emphysema

263

The absence of finger clubbing and enlarged neck and axillary lymph nodes is against a diagnosis of bronchial carcinoma which might have metastasized to the brain.

CONCLUSIONS FROM THE EXAMINATION

- The papilloedema confirms raised intracranial pressure.

- The impairment of sensory discrimination and preservation of primary cutaneous sensation confirms a lesion in the right parietal lobe, most likely a brain tumour.

- There was no clinical evidence of primary bronchial carcinoma which might have metastasized to the brain.

INVESTIGATIONS FOR BRAIN TUMOUR

Computerized tomography (CT scan) is now the most important test in the diagnosis of brain tumour and supersedes all other tests. However, it is an expensive test and is at present available in relatively few centres in the United Kingdom. Accordingly, the more traditional methods of investigation will be discussed first, and more detailed reference to CT scanning made subsequently.

Blood count

This is of very little value in the diagnosis of the great majority of brain tumours.

There is a rare tumour of the cerebellum, a haemangioblastoma, in which there is polycythaemia.

The patient's blood count was normal.

Chest X-ray

Carcinoma of the lung is a frequent source of metastatic brain tumour. A chest X-ray is therefore always necessary in suspected brain tumour.

The patient's chest X-ray was normal with no evidence of either bronchial carcinoma or chronic obstructive lung disease.

Skull X-ray

X-ray of the skull may be helpful in the diagnosis of brain tumours and should always be carried out (Table 8.28).

The patient's skull X-ray was normal.

Table 8.28   The skull X-ray in the diagnosis of brain tumour

• Displacement of calcified pineal	
• Calcification	– meningioma
	craniopharyngioma
	oligodendroglioma
	astrocytoma
• Enlarged vascular channels	– meningioma
	angioma
• Bone erosion	– secondary carcinoma
	myelomatosis
• Increased bone density	– meningioma
• Eroded sella turcica	– pituitary lesion
• Eroded petrous temporal	– acoustic neuroma

Radio-isotope scan

This is carried out with technetium-99 m. It is a relatively simple and non-invasive test (apart from venepuncture). The main value of the test is in the localization and vascularity of certain tumours (Table 8.29).

Table 8.29   Radio-isotope scan in brain tumours

• Vascular tumours	• meningioma
	• angioma
	• glioma
• Cerebral metastases	– multiple 'avascular' defects

The patient's isotope scan showed an area of increased vascularity over the right parietal lobe.

Electroencephalogram

This is a non-specific investigation which may lateralize, and to a less extent localize, an irritant focus caused by a brain tumour. However, many patients with proven brain tumours have normal records.

The test was desirable in this patient because of the associated epilepsy. The result showed a generalized slow wave dysrhythmia with an occasional irregular burst of a fast spike discharge over the right side of the head – more precise localization was not possible.

Angiography

Angiography is of value in localizing brain tumours by showing displacement of the normal vascular pattern by an avascular tumour (Figure 8.9.)

It may also show an abnormal circulation in a vascular tumour (Figure 8.10).

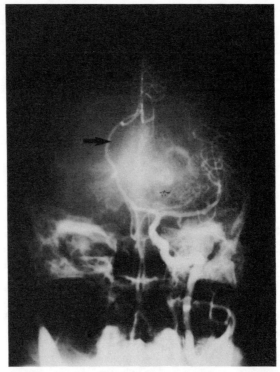

Figure 8.9 Cerebral angiogram showing avascular tumour

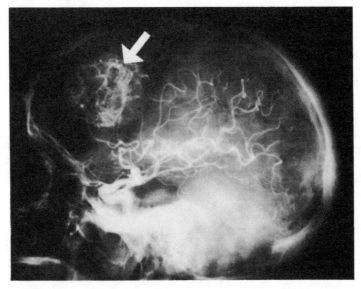

Figure 8.10 Cerebral angiogram showing vascular tumour

Air encephalogram and ventriculogram

This is an unpleasant and painful test.

It may be of value in detecting tumours which are difficult to pick up with CT scanning such as sellar, parasellar and third ventricle tumours.

It is a dangerous investigation if raised intracranial pressure is present because of the possibility of fatal 'coning'.

Lumbar puncture

This is of very limited value in the diagnosis of brain tumours, and is dangerous if raised intracranial pressure is present – it may lead to fatal herniation of either the uncus of the temporal lobe through the tentorial hiatus, or the cerebellar tonsil through the foramen magnum (coning).

Its only value is in the detection of the rare conditions of pinealoma, medulloblastoma and meningeal carcinomatosis, where exfoliative cytology may be diagnostic.

The raised intracranial pressure precluded lumbar puncture in the patient.

CT scan

This is a very effective means of detecting brain tumours and will pick up lesions as small as 1 cm in diameter.

When difficulty is encountered in visualizing tumours, as in the area adjacent to the sella turcica (pituitary fossa) and in the brain stem, where bony masses interfere with interpretation of the picture, the image of the tumour can be enhanced by intravenous injection of contrast material such as Conray.

The patient's CT scan showed a right-sided parietal meningioma.

INVESTIGATION OF EPILEPSY

The diagnosis of epilepsy should be made primarily on a detailed history of the seizure.

Electroencephalogram (e.e.g.)

The e.e.g. may be of help in confirming the clinical diagnosis of idiopathic epilepsy or in establishing a cerebral cause for symptomatic (secondary) epileptiform attacks.

A negative e.e.g. does not exclude epilepsy since a normal record is obtained between attacks in about one third of patients with undoubted epilepsy.

The e.e.g. may be of more value in the diagnosis of petit mal as the frequency of attacks is such that there is a good chance of recording an abnormal discharge.

The main disturbance of e.e.g. pattern is the paroxysmal spike discharge (fast waves of high amplitude) of grand mal or the alternating 3 per second spike and wave discharge of petit mal.

Focal seizures may be associated with either slow or fast wave abnormalities in the e.e.g. A slow wave is more suggestive of a structural lesion.

Investigations in symptomatic (secondary) epilepsy

Epilepsy may occur in various metabolic disturbances. The relevant investigations in these conditions are shown in Table 8.30.

Table 8.30 Investigations in symptomatic epilepsy

• Hypoglycaemia	blood sugar
• Uraemia	blood urea
• Hepatic encephalopathy	blood ammonia
• Hypocalcaemia	serum calcium

INVESTIGATION OF MIGRAINE

Investigations have very little part to play either in the diagnosis or management of migraine.

Very rarely, migraine may be associated with a vascular malformation of the cerebral vessels, such as an angioma. In these circumstances an intracranial murmur will be heard. It is only when such a murmur is present that radio-isotope scan and angiography are justifiable. There is no place for routine scanning in migraine.

MANAGEMENT OF BRAIN TUMOUR

This will involve *symptomatic* treatment and *specific* measures to eradicate the tumour itself (Table 8.31).

Table 8.31 Management of brain tumour

• Symptomatic	• Control of raised intracranial pressure
	• Anticonvulsant therapy
• Specific treatment	• Surgery
	• Radiotherapy
	• Chemotherapy

Symptomatic treatment

This is used to control raised intracranial pressure and to control seizures due to the tumour.

Treatment of raised intracranial pressure

This is necessary in patients with incapacitating headache and vomiting due to the raised intracranial pressure, especially when the tumour is inoperable. Both medical and surgical treatment are available.

Medical treatment of raised intracranial pressure

The drugs which may be of value are shown in Table 8.32.

Table 8.32   Drugs used in reducing intracranial pressure

• Intravenous	– mannitol 200 ml 20% in 20 minutes
	  glycerol
	  dexamethasone 16 mg

• Oral	– dexamethasone 4 mg 6 hourly

The *intravenous preparations* are used when urgent reduction of the raised intracranial pressure is required, as in threatened 'coning'. Their use is also of value in gaining time for essential investigations to be completed or preparation made for operation.

Oral *dexamethasone* is used to reduce oedema of the brain cells when pressure reduction is less urgent, or with an inoperable tumour.

Oral therapy may be effective for as much as several months. However, if it is used long-term, attention should be paid to possible side-effects, especially haematemesis and melaena.

Surgical treatment of raised intracranial pressure

This is based on shunting operations which bypass the obstruction to the flow of cerebrospinal fluid in the brain.

In one type of operation a tube is passed from the lateral ventricle in the cerebrum to the cisterna magna (Figure 8.11).

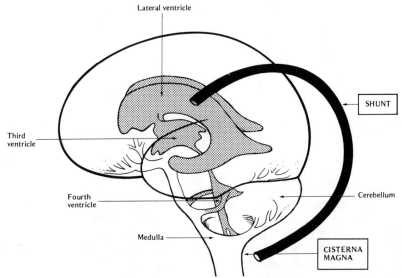

Figure 8.11   Surgical relief of raised intracranial pressure by shunt from lateral ventricle to cisterna magna

Another operation links the lateral ventricle with the superior vena cava or right atrium by a subcutaneous tube (Figure 8.12).

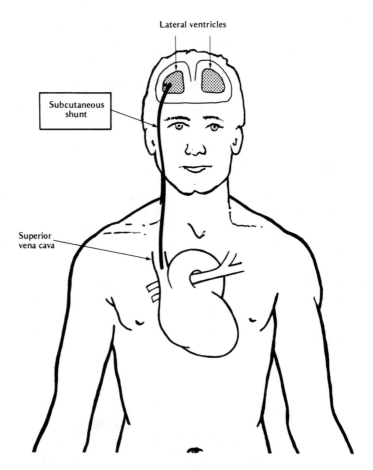

Figure 8.12 Surgical relief of raised intracranial pressure by shunt between lateral ventricle and superior vena cava

Treatment of seizures

Anticonvulsants are required in patients who have epilepsy pre-operatively, and are usually continued for up to 12 months after operation.

Many neurosurgeons will also use postoperative prophylactic anticonvulsant therapy even when there has been no previous epilepsy, since there is a risk of development of epilepsy following craniotomy for 12 months after the operation.

The drug most commonly used is phenytoin, 300 mg daily in adults.

Specific treatment of the brain tumour

The aim of treatment is complete eradication of the tumour by surgery, radiotherapy or chemotherapy.

Before deciding on the type of treatment required it is necessary to establish the pathology of the tumour. This is done either by needle biopsy through a burr-hole, or by exploratory craniotomy.

Surgery

Complete surgical removal of the tumour is desirable. Sometimes however, this involves either serious hazard to life or very severe residual disability and, in these circumstances, partial removal may be carried out and combined with subsequent radiotherapy and/or chemotherapy.

The operability of the more common brain tumours is shown in Table 8.33.

Table 8.33 Operability of common brain tumours

• Total removal possible	• Meningioma
	• Neurofibroma
	• Pituitary tumour
	• Angioma
	• Cerebellar astrocytoma
• Total removal not possible	• Glioblastoma
	• Other gliomas
	• Metastatic carcinoma (unless solitary)

Radiotherapy

Radiotherapy is indicated postoperatively for most malignant brain tumours, especially as complete removal is usually not possible.

Radiotherapy may also be of value in treating benign tumours which cannot be removed completely by operation.

The most radio-sensitive tumours are shown in Table 8.34.

Table 8.34 Radiosensitive brain tumours

• Malignant	• Glioma
	• Medulloblastoma
	• Ependymoma
• Benign	• Pituitary adenoma
	• Craniopharyngioma
	• Meningioma

Chemotherapy

Cytotoxic drugs have been used for treating gliomas, either as primary treatment in inoperable cases where it may be combined with radiotherapy, or postoperatively after complete or partial removal.

The drugs used are shown in Table 8.35. There are significant side-effects with these drugs (Table 8.36). The results of chemotherapy in brain tumours remain uncertain.

Table 8.35   Cytotoxic drugs used in brain tumour

> • Carmustine
> • Lomustine
> • Procarbazine

Table 8.36   Side-effects of cytotoxic drugs

> • Bone marrow suppression
> • Gastrointestinal upset
> • Alopecia
> • Infertility
> • Acute myeloid leukaemia

Immunotherapy has been tried in brain tumour but at present is an area of research only.

MANAGEMENT OF EPILEPSY

Treatment of epilepsy involves general measures, symptomatic control of the seizures and specific treatment where there is a primary cause, such as a brain tumour, which can be removed by surgery.

General measures

Education

Epilepsy still causes a social stigma. A clear and simple explanation of the condition to the patient and his family may help to alleviate anxiety.

The particular points which may be helpful in this explanation are shown in Table 8.37.

Table 8.37   Points to make in explaining epilepsy

> • Epilepsy is a non-specific condition
> • There is usually no structural brain disease
> • Anyone can develop a fit in appropriate circumstances
>   • low blood sugar
>   • oxygen deprivation
>   • stimulant drugs
> • The seizures can be controlled
> • There is only slight increased risk of passing it on

Work

Epileptics should be encouraged to undertake any normal work provided that a fall or loss of consciousness would not be dangerous to themselves or to others.

Some professions, such as nursing, teaching, police force, will not usually accept epileptics.

Driving

An ordinary driving licence is given to an epileptic if he has had no attacks during waking for at least 3 years.

Attacks confined to sleep during the 3 year period do not preclude granting of the licence.

An epileptic cannot hold a Heavy Goods Vehicle licence or Public Service Vehicle licence.

Precautionary measures at home

Fires should be well-guarded. Gates should be used to prevent falls downstairs.

An epileptic mother can bath her baby if someone else is around to supervise.

Schoolchildren

The minimum of restriction should be placed on schoolchildren. They should be allowed to participate in all the usual school activities.

Swimming is a special case but can be allowed if a supervisor is present.

Pregnancy

Pregnancy may either increase or reduce the frequency of seizures.

Care should be taken to avoid hydantoins and sodium valproate in the first 6 or 8 weeks of pregnancy because of the possibility of fetal abnormality (mainly facial, e.g. cleft palate).

Symptomatic treatment of epilepsy

The aim of treatment is to use anticonvulsant drugs to reduce the seizures as far as possible, and ideally, completely abolish them. The choice of drugs is influenced by the type of seizure (Table 8.38). The doses in Table 8.38 refer to adults, and the appropriate reduction must be made for children according to body weight.

Treatment should be started with a single drug. If the seizures are not controlled, the dose should be progressively increased up to the maximum permitted unless toxic side-effects occur. Blood levels of the drug are helpful in assessing whether the therapeutic levels are reached and whether toxicity is likely.

Table 8.38   Choice of anticonvulsant drugs

Condition	Drugs	Dose
Petit mal	Sodium valproate (Epilim)	200–800 mg t.d.s.
	Ethosuximide (Zarontin)	0.5–2 g daily
	Clonazepam (Rivotril)	4–8 mg daily
Grand mal	Phenytoin (Epanutin)	150–300 mg b.d.
	Sodium valproate	200–800 mg t.d.s.
Grand mal + petit mal	Ethosuximide and phenytoin	
Partial seizures	Carbamezepine (Tegretol)	100–600 mg b.d.
	Phenytoin (Epanutin)	150–300 mg b.d.
	Sodium valproate (Epilim)	200–800 mg t.d.s.
	Primidone (Mysoline)	125–500 mg b.d.
	Sulthiame (Ospolot)	100–200 mg t.d.s.
	Phenobarbitone (Luminal)	90–600 mg at night

Drug combinations should be avoided unless necessary to control seizures not controllable on maximum dose of one drug alone.

The side-effects of the anticonvulsant drugs in general use are shown in Table 8.39.

Table 8.39   Side-effects of anticonvulsant drugs

• Excessive sedation	– Phenobarbitone (Luminal) Primidone (Mysoline)
• Skin rashes	– Phenobarbitone (Luminal) Phenytoin (Epanutin)
• Alopecia	– Sodium valproate (Epilim)
• Hyperventilation paraesthesiae	– Sulthiame (Ospolot)
• Gingival hyperplasia	– Phenytoin (Epanutin)
• Ataxia	– Phenobarbitone (Luminal) Phenytoin (Epanutin)
• Macrocytic anaemia	– Phenobarbitone (Luminal) Phenytoin (Epanutin)
• Fetal abnormality	– Phenytoin (Luminal) Sodium valproate (Epilim)

SPECIFIC TREATMENT OF EPILEPSY

The only specific treatment is to remove the epileptogenic focus. The indications for surgery in epilepsy are shown in Table 8.40.

Table 8.40   Indications for surgery in epilepsy

• Brain tumour	
• Idiopathic epilepsy	• Poor seizure control
	• All anticonvulsants tried
	• Single focus identified

Up to half the patients selected for surgery on these criteria lose their seizures completely.

MANAGEMENT OF MIGRAINE

General measures in treating migraine

Patient education

As in any potentially chronic and disabling condition, in which the aetiology is largely unknown, it helps to establish a good and sympathetic relationship with the patient and his family by giving a clear and simple explanation of the nature of the condition and the benefits and limitations of treatment.

Trigger factors

Migraine may be precipitated by a variety of factors (Figure 8.13).

Psychological stress

This depends more on a patient's personality than external stressful factors.
Sympathetic discussion of the patient's feelings of anger, hostility, rage etc. may be of some value in alleviating the stress.
Avoidance of stressful situations is desirable if feasible.

Hormonal changes

Migraine often occurs in the premenstrual week, possibly due to fluid retention caused by hormonal changes.
A loop diuretic such as frusemide (Lasix) or bumetanide (Burinex) during this week may help to prevent the attacks.
The use of the contraceptive pill, or the use of oestrogens for menopausal symptoms, should be discouraged in migraine sufferers.

Food and drink

If the patient can identify the offending food or drink, it can be avoided.

Drugs

Any drug causing peripheral vasodilatation should be avoided.

Specific drugs in treating migraine

Drugs afford symptomatic control only since the aetiology of migraine is unknown. Drug treatment has two aims:

(1) prevention of attacks
(2) treatment of the attack itself.

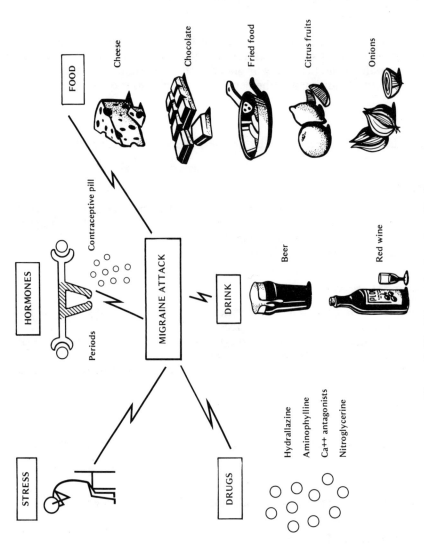

Figure 8.13 Trigger factors in migraine

Preventive treatment

The drugs which are of value are shown in Table 8.41.

Table 8.41   Drugs used in prevention of migraine

Drug	Dose
Diazepam (Valium)	2 mg t.d.s.
Clonidine (Dixarit)	50–70 µg b.d.
Pizotifen (Sanomigran)	0.5 mg once daily to start maximum 2 mg t.d.s.
Methysergide (Deseril)	1–2 mg t.d.s.
Propranolol (Inderal)	40–80 mg t.d.s.

With regard to methysergide (Deseril), there is one potentially hazardous side-effect, retroperitoneal fibrosis, when the drug is used for a period of months. This will present with urinary symptoms since the ureters are often involved, leading to obstructive uropathy. An intravenous pyelogram will be of help if retroperitoneal fibrosis is suspected.

Treatment of the acute attack

The drugs used to control the attack of migraine are shown in Table 8.42. The side-effects of ergot preparations are shown in Table 8.43.

Table 8.42   Drugs used in the acute migraine attack

Drug	Dose
Ergotamine	
Oral Cafergot	1–2 mg at onset repeat every 30 min if necessary maximum 6–8 mg/attack; 12 mg/week
Suppository Cafergot	2 mg at once repeat in 1 h if necessary maximum 6–8 mg/attack; 12 mg/week
Aerosol Medihaler-ergotamine	360 µg at onset repeat in 5 min if necessary
Sublingual lingraine	2 mg at onset
Isometheptene (Midrid)	1–2 capsules up to 6 times daily maximum 8 daily
Dihydroergotamine (Dihydergot)	2–3 mg at onset repeat every 30 min if necessary maximum 10 mg daily
Metoclopramide (Maxolon)	5–10 mg up to t.d.s.

277

Table 8.43 Side-effects of ergot preparations

- Nausea and vomiting
- Abdominal pain
- Muscle cramps
- Gangrene
- Mental disturbance
- Withdrawal symptoms

Metoclopramide (Maxolon) may help in the acute attacks. It can control the nausea and vomiting, and can also increase the retarded absorption of analgesic which occurs because of the gastric stasis in an attack of migraine. The metoclopramide should be given 10 minutes before the analgesic (e.g. paracetamol) is given.

Combined preparations are popular in the treatment of the acute attack to control both headache and vomiting (Table 8.44).

Table 8.44 Combined proprietary preparations in the treatment of an acute attack of migraine

Migraleve –	buclizine
	paracetamol
	codeine
	dioctyl sodium sulphonate
Migravess –	metoclopramide
	aspirin
Paramox –	metoclopramide
	paracetamol
Migril –	ergotamine
	cyclizine
	caffeine

Cluster headache (migrainous neuralgia)

This is a distinctive type of migraine, the features of which are shown in Figure 8.14.

An intramuscular injection of 1–2 mg of ergotamine is usually very effective in controlling the acute symptoms.

THE NATURAL HISTORY OF BRAIN TUMOURS

Prevalence

The incidence is 5–10 per 100 000 of the population.

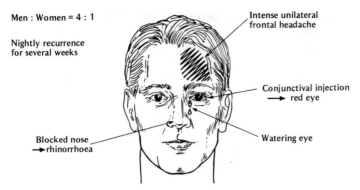

Figure 8.14 Features of cluster headache

There are two age peaks of incidence – children under 10 years and adults aged 40–60 years.

There is a slight male preponderance with most tumours.

Types of brain tumour

The majority of brain tumours are primary.
The frequency of the different types of tumour is shown in Figure 8.15.

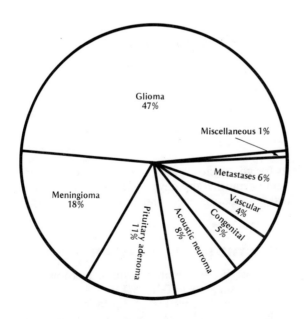

Figure 8.15 Frequency of brain tumours

279

The distribution of tumours in children and adults is shown in Table 8.45.

Table 8.45 Distribution of brain tumours in children and adults

• Children	• Medulloblastoma: posterior fossa
	• Ependymoma: posterior fossa
	• Cerebellar astrocytoma
	• Glioma of brain stem
• Adults	• Cerebral glioma
	• Cerebral metastases
	• Meningioma
	• Pituitary adenoma

Prognosis of brain tumour

This will depend on the malignancy of the tumour and its location. If surgical removal is not possible, almost all brain tumours will end fatally.

The highly malignant glioblastoma, medulloblastoma and metastases will end life within a few months, while the slow-growing meningioma and astrocytoma allow survival for many years.

Postoperatively there is complete cure of the more benign tumours (Table 8.46).

Table 8.46 Postoperative cure of brain tumour

• Meningioma
• Craniopharyngioma
• Acoustic neuroma
• Pinealoma

The prospects for glioblastoma after operation are very poor (Figure 8.16). Radiotherapy and chemotherapy have added little to survival.

Just over 2000 patients die each year in the United Kingdom from brain tumours.

CAN WE MODIFY THE NATURAL HISTORY?

The aetiology of most brain tumours is quite unknown. Several possible mechanisms have been suggested (Table 8.47).

In the absence of firm knowledge of causation there is no means yet available to modify the natural history other than surgery, radiotherapy and possibly chemotherapy.

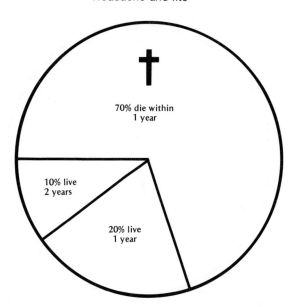

Figure 8.16   Postoperative prognosis of glioblastoma

Table 8.47   Possible aetiological factors in brain tumour

- Toxoplasma infection
- Head injury
- Industrial exposure
    rubber
    petrochemicals
- Therapeutic radiation
- Genetic factors
    certain gliomas
    haemangioblastoma
    neurofibroma

THE NATURAL HISTORY OF IDIOPATHIC EPILEPSY

Prevalence

Epilepsy occurs in 1:200 of the population.

Prognosis

The prognosis of adult epilepsy has been studied over a 20 year period in a typical family practice by John Fry (Figure 8.17).

Relapse of epilepsy will occur in 30% of patients whose treatment has been withdrawn after a seizure-free period of 3 years.

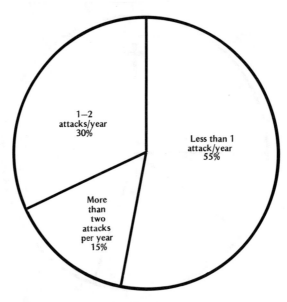

Figure 8.17   Twenty year prognosis of adult epilepsy in a family practice (from survey by John Fry)

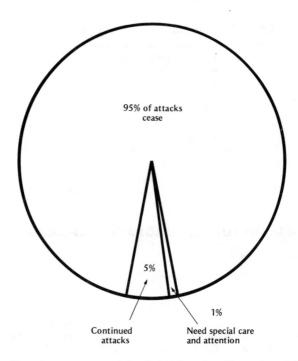

Figure 8.18   Twenty year prognosis of childhood epilepsy in a family practice (from survey by John Fry)

Febrile convulsions

About 3% of all children between 6 months and 5 years of age develop epileptiform convulsions in response to a raised temperature. The convulsions often recur in the same child.

The prognosis depends in the frequency and duration of the convulsions. The risk of subsequent epilepsy in a child who has had a single febrile convulsion is about 1:100, twice that in the normal population. This risk increases to 1 in 20 when the convulsions are frequent and prolonged.

In a 20 year survey of his family practice, John Fry found the overall prognosis excellent, since 95% cease by the age of 5 years and do not herald adult epilepsy (Figure 8.18).

Can we modify the natural history of epilepsy?

The only established aetiological factors in idiopathic epilepsy are a genetic predisposition and febrile convulsions in childhood.

Genetic aspects

40% of siblings of epileptic patients will have an epileptiform type of spike and wave discharge in their e.e.g., even in the absence of overt attacks. Screening of these siblings by e.e.g. therefore offers the possibility of prevention of epilepsy by prophylactic continuous anticonvulsant treatment.

Since it is not clear how many of these siblings will develop frank epilepsy and the e.e.g. abnormality lessens with the passage of time, it is probably better to delay treatment until clinical epilepsy occurs rather than subject an otherwise asymptomatic individual to possibly unnecessary lifelong treatment with the attendant drug hazards and social implications.

Febrile convulsions

Similar considerations apply to children with frequent febrile convulsions, who stand a 1 in 20 chance of developing epilepsy in adult life.

It is even more desirable to allow a child to live a normal active life than an adult. The child could be kept under periodic observation and treatment started only if frank epilepsy develops.

THE NATURAL HISTORY OF MIGRAINE

Prevalence

The incidence of migraine in the general population is between 5% and 10%.

Age and sex

The majority of sufferers are between the ages of 10 years and 30 years. Females predominate by 2 to 1.

Prognosis

The amount of incapacity caused by the migraine has been shown clearly by John Fry in a survey of his family practice (Figure 8.19). With the passage of time, he further found that the prognosis was quite favourable (Figure 8.20).

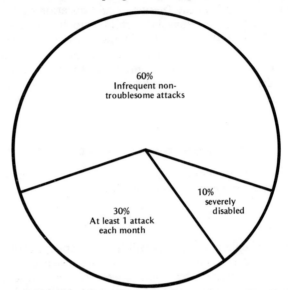

Figure 8.19 Incapacity caused by migraine in a family practice (from survey by John Fry)

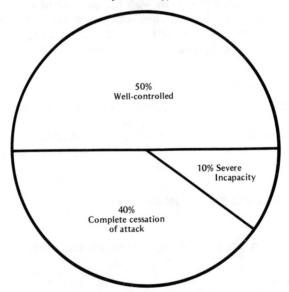

Figure 8.20 Twenty-five year prognosis of migraine in a family practice (from survey by John Fry)

Can we modify the natural history of migraine?

As in idiopathic epilepsy, the only established aetiological factor is a genetic predisposition.

Avoidance of any trigger factors will obviously help to reduce the number of attacks but some attacks will still continue.

Apart from prolonged prophylactic drug therapy, there is no other method yet available to modify the natural history.

USEFUL PRACTICAL POINTS

- If a migrainous headache always occurs on the same side of the head, the possibility of underlying structural brain disease should be considered.

- The combination of recent headache, personality change and fits is strongly suggestive of brain tumour.

- Localized supraorbital headache with a watery red eye and a blocked nose indicates migrainous neuralgia (cluster headache). This responds well to intramuscular ergotamine.

- The most valuable test in the diagnosis of brain tumour is a CT scan. It supersedes all other diagnostic measures.

- Treatment of idiopathic epilepsy should be based on using a single anti-convulsant drug to its maximum potential.
  Blood levels of the drug are helpful in deciding therapeutic and toxic doses.

- The prognosis of febrile convulsions in childhood is very good: 95% will have no further fits after the age of 5 years.

9

Dizziness

PRESENT HISTORY

A 65-year-old man complained of attacks of dizziness and falling over the previous year which were gradually getting more frequent.

Dizziness

This usually consisted of a feeling of faintness or light-headedness lasting for a few minutes only. It would sometimes occur on getting out of bed in the morning. He had also noticed that turning his head sharply to the side or looking up often caused the dizziness. The other occasions on which he had become dizzy were if he was undertaking any strenuous activity like digging the garden or sometimes while he was doing woodwork, especially sawing wood, which was his hobby.

The falls

These would usually occur while he was walking. They came on suddenly without warning when he would fall without any loss of consciousness. He was able to get up within a few seconds and would feel all right though sometimes a little light-headed after the attack. He had never noticed any palpitations before the attacks.

Vertigo

In addition to the attacks of faintness, he had occasionally had more severe dizziness during which he felt as if the room was 'going round'. When asked specifically, he also admitted to ringing in his ears during these attacks. He thought also that his hearing had not been so good in recent months. He denied any past history of ear trouble.

Other relevant facts on direct enquiry

Visual disturbance

He had been worried once or twice in the previous few months by a brief loss of vision in the right eye. It lasted only for a few seconds but it felt 'like a curtain coming down over his eye'. On other occasions, he had noticed some blurring of vision during which he had seen double for a few minutes.

Central nervous system

He had no headache.
He had no speech disturbance.
He had not noticed any limb weakness.
He had never had paraesthesiae over the face or limbs.

Cardiovascular system

He did not get chest pain on exertion.
He had no calf pain on walking.

PAST HISTORY

Over the previous few years he had been getting *bronchitis* during the winter months which usually cleared up after a course of antibiotics.

He also had a history of a *'stomach ulcer'* about 7 years earlier which had eventually cleared up with various medicines and tablets – he had not had any indigestion for several years.

Family history

There was nothing relevant.

Personal history

He was a retired clerk who had worked in a Wages Office. He smoked *30 cigarettes daily* for most of his life. He was a very moderate drinker, about 2–3 pints (1–1.7 litres) of beer weekly, though not every week.

EXAMINATION

The abnormal physical signs are shown in Figure 9.1.

General

He was a thin fit-looking 65-year-old man who had a well-marked *arcus senilis*.

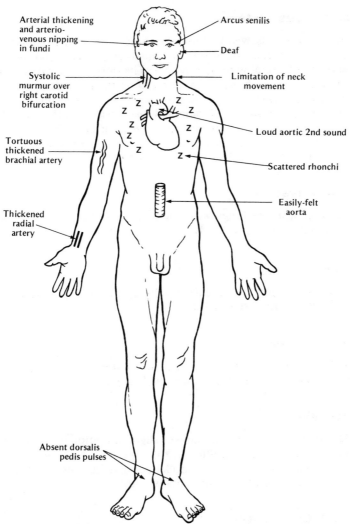

Arterial thickening
and arterio-
venous nipping
in fundi

Arcus senilis

Deaf

Systolic
murmur over
right carotid
bifurcation

Limitation of neck
movement

Loud aortic 2nd sound

Tortuous
thickened
brachial artery

Scattered rhonchi

Easily-felt
aorta

Thickened
radial
artery

Absent dorsalis
pedis pulses

Figure 9.1 Abnormal physical signs

Cardiovascular system

The pulse rate was normal but the pulse on the right seemed poorer than that
on the left. The radial artery was thickened and there was a tortuous *brachial
artery.* The blood pressure was 230/95 on the left side but only 170/90 on the
right.

The apex beat was normal.

The *aortic second sound was loud* and there was a soft blowing midsystolic
murmur over the base of the heart, only poorly conducted towards the apex.

There was a *loud blowing systolic murmur over the right carotid bifurcation*
in the upper part of the neck, though pulsation was not reduced compared
with the left side.

Central nervous system

Fundal examination showed tortuous arterioles and *arteriovenous nipping*. There was no evidence of arteriolar obstruction. External oculomotor movements were normal with no diplopia. The only abnormal cranial nerve was the auditory nerve: *hearing was reduced* on the left side; the *Weber test* was referred to the right ear; the *Rinne test* showed equal diminution of air and bone conduction on the left side and was normal on the right. The ear drums were clearly seen on both sides and were normal.

No abnormality was found in the peripheral motor system or sensory system and cerebellar coordination was unimpaired.

Respiratory system

The main finding in the lungs was a few scattered high-pitched *expiratory rhonchi* over both sides posteriorly.

Abdomen

On abdominal examination he relaxed well and the aortic pulsation was easily felt. No other abnormality was found.

Peripheral vessels

Examination of the pulses in the feet showed that both posterior tibial pulses were present but neither of the *dorsalis pedis pulses*.

Cervical spine

Examination of neck movements showed slight limitation of extension, which produced dizziness, some limitation of rotation to the right but most marked limitation with lateral flexion of the neck in both directions, which the patient found quite uncomfortable if not actually painful.

ANALYSIS OF THE HISTORY

Dizziness

The main complaint was dizziness. It is important to establish precisely what is meant by this complaint (Table 9.1).

Table 9.1 Possible meanings of the complaint of dizziness

• Vertigo
• Impending faint
• Loss of balance
• Light-headedness

Vertigo

Vertigo is a sense of rotation either of the patient or his surroundings. It is caused by a disorder of the vestibular system which may be peripheral in the labyrinth or in the central connections in the brainstem. Further discussion of vertigo follows on page 293.

Faint

In a faint there is a sense of impending loss of consciousness often accompanied by sweating, nausea and dimness of vision. Recovery is rapid on lying down. It is usually due to a transient critical fall in cerebral blood flow (syncope); the common causes are shown in Table 9.2.

Table 9.2   Common causes of syncope

• Cardiac	• Stokes–Adams attacks
	• Myocardial infarction
	• Aortic or pulmonary stenosis
• Vasomotor	• Simple faint (vasovagal attack)
	• Prolonged standing
	• Hypotensive drugs
• Cough and micturition syncope	
• Hypoglycaemia	

Loss of balance

A complaint of loss of balance without associated vertigo usually indicates a neurological disorder involving the sensory, motor or cerebellar systems. The dizziness is based on focal neurological signs according to the part of the nervous system involved.

Light-headedness

This patient specified the meaning of dizziness as being '*light-headedness*'. This particular symptom accounts for over half of all complaints of dizziness and may have an organic or psychiatric basis (Table 9.3).

Table 9.3   Causes of 'light-headedness'

• Cerebrovascular insufficiency
• Anaemia
• Post-tussive dizziness and syncope
• Anxiety state
• Hyperventilation

Cerebrovascular insufficiency

The relationship of the light-headedness to getting out of bed suggests *postural hypotension* leading to cerebrovascular insufficiency. This may occur with cerebral arteriosclerosis alone but is most frequent when hypotensive drugs are being used in elderly patients.

The occurrence of the light-headedness on sharply turning the head is typical of *vertebrobasilar insufficiency associated with cervical spondylosis*, where the atherosclerotic vertebral artery is compressed by the osteophytic intervertebral joints as it traverses the vertebral canal.

The development of dizziness on vigorous use of the right arm, as in sawing wood, suggests the *'subclavian steal syndrome'*. This is caused by atheromatous ibstruction in the right subclavian artery proximal to the origin of the vertebral artery (Figure 9.2): during vigorous exercise in the affected arm, blood is diverted by retrograde flow from the basilar system in the arm which results in basilar ischaemia and dizziness.

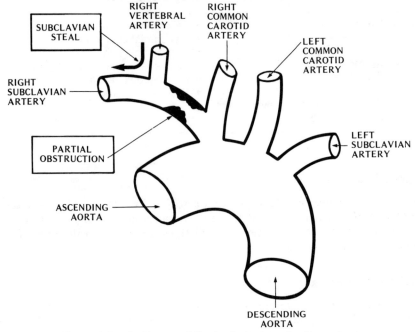

Figure 9.2   Anatomy of the 'subclavian steal' syndrome

Anaemia

Light-headedness due to anaemia is usually accompanied by other symptoms of anaemia, such as breathlessness, palpitations, pallor and excessive tiredness. The patient was not clinically anaemic.

Post-tussive dizziness

Post-tussive dizziness occurs after a prolonged bout of coughing usually in the chronic bronchitic patient. It may lead to loss of consciousness ('cough epilepsy'). The mechanism is based on the reduction of venous return to the heart produced by the prolonged expiration during coughing, which leads to a fall in cardiac output resulting in cerebrovascular insufficiency. The patient's light-headedness was not related to coughing.

Anxiety state

An anxiety state is often associated with vague and often bizarre complaints of 'swimming sensations' or 'light-headedness'. This may occur in panic situations. Hyperventilation may be a factor here too. Other manifestations of an anxiety state may be present such as palpitations, left inframammary chest pain, tremor, excessive fatigue, inability to take a deep breath etc. There was no evidence of an anxiety state in this patient.

Vertigo

The patient has attacks of vertigo as well as the light-headedness. The causes of vertigo are shown in Table 9.4.

Table 9. 4   Causes of vertigo

- Vertebrobasilar insufficiency
- Ménière's disease
- Middle-ear disease
- Vestibular neuronitis
- Benign positional vertigo
- Drug therapy

The patient's light-headedness already indicates vertebrobasilar insufficiency. However, the association of *tinnitus* and *deafness* with the vertigo clearly indicates that the patient has a peripheral labyrinthine disorder also (Table 9.5); tinnitus and deafness are extremely rare in vertigo of central origin. The most likely cause of his labyrinthine disturbance is Ménière's disease.

Table 9.5   Classical triad of symptoms in peripheral labyrinthine disorder

- Vertigo
- Tinnitus
- Deafness

Ménière's disease

This is a condition of unknown aetiology in which there is an increased amount of endolymph in the membranous labyrinth in the inner ear which controls balance and hearing. It is characterized by recurrent attacks of vertigo associated with tinnitus as well as a gradually progressive deafness.

The disease is very disabling and may last for years. In some cases the attacks of vertigo diminish as the deafness becomes more established.

Middle-ear disease

There was no past history of ear disease, which makes middle-ear disease very unlikely.

Vestibular neuronitis

Vestibular neuronitis tends to occur in young people and is self-limiting. This excludes the condition in this patient.

Drugs

Drugs causing vertigo are shown in Table 9.6.
The patient was not taking any of these.

Table 9.6   Drugs causing vertigo

- Salicylates
- Phenytoin
- Quinine
- Antibiotics – streptomycin
- Gentamicin

Benign positional vertigo

Benign positional vertigo most often occurs in bed on changing position. This distinguishes it from vertebrobasilar insufficiency which is more frequent on standing.

The falls

The conditions which may lead to the sudden falls experienced by the patient are shown in Table 9.7.

Table 9.7   Causes of sudden falls

- Stokes–Adams attack
- Vertebrobasilar insufficiency
- Akinetic type of minor epilepsy

Stokes–Adams attack

A Stokes–Adams attack, due to sudden complete atrioventricular heart block, often occurs in a patient who already has other manifestations of coronary artery disease, such as angina or a previous heart attack. The sudden fall is usually accompanied by loss of consciousness and may go on to cyanosis, stertorous breathing and convulsions. The electrocardiogram may show some evidence of impaired conduction or, if recorded during the attack, will show complete ventricular asystole (Figure 9.3).

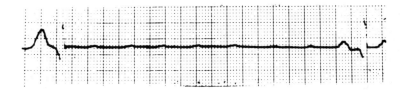

Figure 9.3 Electrocardiogram showing ventricular asystole in a Stokes–Adams attack

Minor epilepsy

The *akinetic type of minor epilepsy* is very unlikely in this patient since it occurs almost always in children. In cases of doubt an electroencephalogram may help.

Drop attack

The type of fall in this patient is the typical drop attack of vertebrobasilar ischaemia. The fall is due to a sudden loss of all muscle tone resulting from ischaemia in the pontine region. It is not accompanied by loss of consciousness and lasts a few seconds only, and the patient is back to his usual self immediately afterwards.

Visual disturbance

The patient describes two types of visual disturbance – transient monocular loss of vision and episodes of blurred vision with diplopia.

Transient loss of vision

The transient loss of vision in one eye is very suggestive of a *transient ischaemic attack* due to embolic blockage of the retinal artery. The usual cause of this type of blockage is a platelet embolus, and the usual site of origin is from an atheromatous plaque in the carotid artery in the neck.

The other possible site of origin is in the heart (Table 9.8). There was no evidence of heart disease in this patient.

Table 9.8 Cardiac causes of embolism

• Atrial fibrillation	– left atrial thrombus
• Myocardial infarction	– mural thrombus
• Valvular heart disease	– rheumatic
	infective endocarditis
	prosthesis
• Left atrial myxoma	– very rare

Blurred vision and diplopia

The episodes of blurred vision with diplopia could also be due to transient ischaemia involving the external ocular muscle nuclei and the accommodation reaction pathway in the midbrain and pons.

The usual clinical manifestations of transient ischaemic attacks are shown in Table 9.9.

Table 9.9 Clinical manifestations of transient ischaemic attacks

• Visual	– Temporary loss of monocular vision (amaurosis fugax)
	Double vision
	Hemianopia
• Speech	– Dysarthria
	Dysphasia
• Sensory	– Paraesthesiae face (especially circumoral)
	Paraesthesiae limbs
• Motor	– Weakness of facial muscles
	Weakness of limbs
• Amnesia	

Past history

The only condition relevant to his current symptoms is the past history of stomach trouble. This may influence the choice of treatment and will be discussed on pp. 307, 308, in the section on Management.

Personal history

The heavy cigarette smoking is very relevant as it is a major contributory factor in the development of arterial disease.

CONCLUSIONS FROM THE HISTORY

- The postural dizziness indicates cerebrovascular insufficiency.

- The dizziness precipitated by head movement indicates vertebrobasilar insufficiency due to cervical spondylosis.

- The precipitation of dizziness on strenuous use of the arms suggests a 'subclavian steal syndrome'.

- The falls are due to drop attacks resulting from vertebrobasilar insufficiency.

- The vertigo, tinnitus and deafness indicate a peripheral labyrinthine lesion, probably Ménière's disease

- The visual disturbances suggest transient ischaemic attacks.

- The heavy cigarette smoking is a major factor causing his arterial disease.

ANALYSIS OF THE EXAMINATION

Arcus senilis

Arcus senilis is associated with hypercholesterolaemia and arterial disease.

It is more significant in a young man, when it indicates premature atherosclerosis.

Cardiovascular system

There was clear evidence of widespread arteriosclerosis (Figure 9.4).

The weaker right radial pulse suggests obstruction higher up in the artery and this is supported by the lower systolic pressure in the right arm compared with the left. This difference between the two arms supports the diagnosis of stenosis of the subclavian artery which is responsible for the *'subclavian steal'* *syndrome* (Table 9.10).

Table 9.10   Typical features of the 'subclavian steal' syndrome

> - Dizziness on strenuous use of arm
> - Unequal radial pulses
> - Systolic pressure difference of at least 20 mmHg between the two arms
> - Systolic murmur over the supraclavicular fossa

The high systolic pressure in the left arm, which is the true systolic pressure, is attributable to the *generalized arteriosclerosis*.

The aortic second sound was increased due to the systolic hypertension. The soft systolic murmur over the base of the heart was probably caused by atherosclerotic involvement of the aortic valve and is of no clinical significance.

The loud systolic murmur over the right carotid artery indicates *stenosis* of the artery. Palpation of the artery is a less reliable guide to stenosis. The carotid artery stenosis is the likely source of the emboli causing his transient ischaemic attacks.

Abdomen

The palpable aortic pulsation is due to the large pulse pressure and is of no clinical significance. However, if the pulsating area is large, aneurysmal dilatation should be considered. In these circumstances the pulsation may be expansile, unless the aneurysm is partly filled with blood clot.

The lungs

There is evidence of mild bronchitis only. There was no associated emphysema.

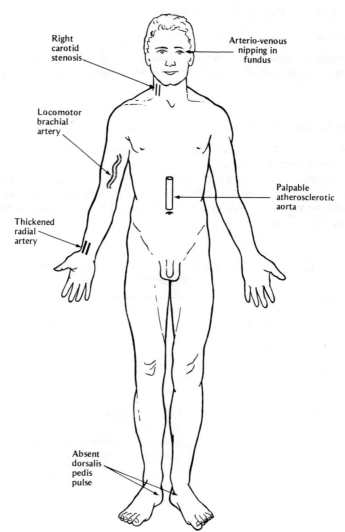

Figure 9.4 The arteriosclerotic changes in the patient

Nervous system

The main finding was the poor hearing in the left ear.

Simple clinical testing with the Weber and Rinne tests may help to indicate whether the deafness is due to middle-ear disease (conductive deafness) or inner-ear disease (nerve or perceptive deafness). The *Weber* test is based on placing a tuning fork centrally over the forehead and finding whether the sound is heard centrally or on one side. The *Rinne* test compares air conduction with bone conduction in each ear. Interpretation of the results is shown in Table 9.11.

Table 9.11 Interpretation of Weber and Rinne tests in distinguishing middle-ear from inner-ear disease

Disease	Weber test	Rinne test
Middle ear	Better affected side	bone > air
Inner ear	Better on normal side	air > bone
		but both reduced

In this patient, the results showed inner-ear disease on the left side. The normal ear drum confirmed the absence of middle-ear disease.

Neck movement

The limitation of movement and the discomfort on movement clearly indicates *cervical spondylosis*.

The dizziness produced by neck extension confirms vertebrobasilar ischaemia caused by compression of the vertebral arteries in the vertebral canal in the cervical vertebrae.

CONCLUSIONS FROM THE EXAMINATION

- He has evidence of generalized arteriosclerosis.

- The weak right radial pulse indicates obstruction of the right subclavian artery and confirms 'subclavian steal' syndrome.

- The systolic murmur over the right carotid artery in the neck confirms stenosis of the artery. This is very likely to be the source of the platelet emboli causing the transient ischaemic episodes affecting vision.

- The hearing tests confirm inner-ear disease on the left side, the basis of the Ménière's disease.

- He has evidence of bronchitis due to the heavy smoking.

- The limitation of neck movements confirms cervical spondylosis.

INVESTIGATIONS

Vertebrobasilar insufficiency and transient ischaemic attacks

X-ray of the cervical spine

The patient's X-ray is shown in Figure 9.5. This confirms the cervical spondylosis. It also shows carotid calcification indicating advanced carotid atherosclerosis.

An X-ray of the cervical spine is not really necessary to make the diagnosis of cervical spondylosis in this patient, since the clinical findings are conclusive. Additionally, cervical spondylosis is frequently seen as an incidental finding in

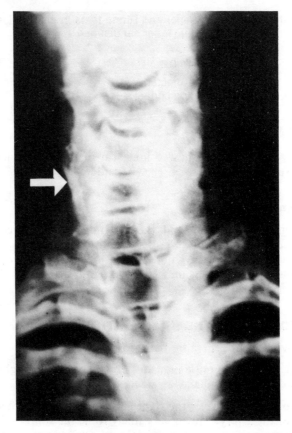

Figure 9.5   X-ray of the cervical spine showing spondylosis and calcification
of the carotid arteries

otherwise asymptomatic middle-aged and elderly individuals. It should not,
therefore, be considered of clinical significance unless there are accompanying
clinical manifestations (Table 9.12).

Table 9.12   Clinical manifestations of cervical
spondylosis

- Symptoms of vertebrobasilar insufficiency
- Pain in the back of the neck or occiput
- Root pain in the shoulder or arm
- Undue restriction of neck movement, e.g. driving

There is one additional advantage of a neck X-ray. It may show carotid
calcification, as in this patient.

300

Blood count

Anaemia and polycythaemia may contribute to cerebrovascular insufficiency and are correctable.

The patient's blood count was normal.

Blood lipids

There is no point in estimating cholesterol and other lipids in a patient of this age. It is irrelevant diagnostically and has no significance for therapy, since there is no evidence that reduction of a high blood cholesterol at this age produces any clinical benefit whatsoever.

It may be more relevant in a younger man who may not yet have advanced atherosclerotic changes.

Electrocardiogram

Cardiac dysrhythmias may lead to vertebrobasilar insufficiency.

The e.c.g. however, is unlikely to be helpful in detecting transient dysrhythmias unless recorded fortuitously when an attack is occurring.

If there is a definite reason to suspect a cardiac dysrhythmia, such as the association of palpitations with the episode of ischaemia, then 24h ambulatory tape monitoring of heart rhythm is more likely to be helpful.

Arteriography

This is the definitive investigation in transient ischaemic attacks with particular reference to establishing carotid artery stenosis (Figure 9.6). The requirements for ateriography are shown in Table 9.13.

Table 9.13   Requirements for carotid arteriography in transient ischaemic attacks

• Medical treatment has failed
• The ischaemic attacks are incapacitating
• There is no significant hypertension (diastolic <110 mmHg)
• There is a possibility of surgery
• The patient is otherwise fit for surgery
• There is an experienced radiologist
• There is an experienced anaesthetist
• There is an experienced carotid artery surgeon

In skilled hands, both morbidity (hemiplegia) and mortality from carotid arteriography are less than 1%.

If a radiologist experienced in this investigation is not available, it should not be considered.

Vertebral arteriography is rarely necessary since the possibility of effective surgery is much more limited.

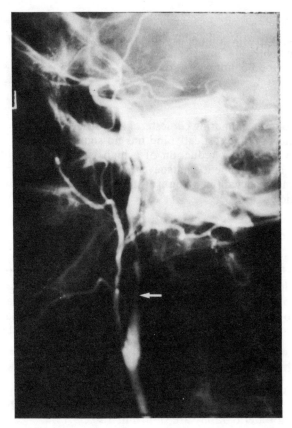

Figure 9.6 Arteriogram showing carotid artery stenosis

Phonoangiography and pulsed Doppler ultrasonic imaging

There are advanced newer non-invasive techniques using sound waves to detect the presence and degree of carotid artery stenosis. The tests are only available in a highly specialised neuroradiology unit.

Miscellaneous investigations

There may be conditions other than carotid disease responsible for transient ischaemic attacks. Some of the investigations necessary for these conditions are shown in Table 9.14.

Table 9.14 Investigations for other conditions causing transient ischaemic attacks

• Echocardiography	– rheumatic heart disease
	infective endocarditis
• Blood culture	– infective endocarditis
• Cardiac enzymes	– myocardial infarction
• Temporal artery biopsy	– temporal arteritis

Investigation of 'subclavian steal' syndrome

The only relevant investigation is arteriography to show the site and the degree of subclavian obstruction.

Investigation of Ménière's disease

Assessment of labyrinthine function requires audiometric testing which is only available in an audiological unit, either in a Health Centre or a hospital ENT department.

MANAGEMENT OF VERTEBROBASILAR INSUFFICIENCY

The usual clinical manifestations of vertebrobasilar insufficiency are shown in Table 9.15.

Table 9.15 Clinical manifestations of vertebrobasilar insufficiency

• Dizziness
• Vertigo
• Loss of vision in both eyes
• Drop attacks
• Generalized unsteadiness

General measures

These are outlined in Table 9.16.

If control of hypertension is necessary because of a high diastolic pressure (>110 mmHg) or because of target organ damage, the pressure should not be reduced below the level at which disabling dizziness occurs – the desirable level is the lowest compatible with absence of dizziness.

The patient has an abnormally elevated systolic pressure only. There is no evidence yet that lowering the systolic pressure at this age produces any clinical benefit.

Direct peripheral vasodilators and adrenergic neurone-blocking drugs should be *avoided* because they encourage postural hypotension (Table 9.17).

303

Table 9.16 General measures in the management of vertebrobasilar insufficiency

- Correction of anaemia
- Control of hypertension
    not too low
    not too rapid
    avoid peripheral vasodilators
    avoid adrenergic neurone-blocking drugs
- Control of cardiac arrhythmia
- Avoid standing up suddenly
- Lie down if dizziness coming on
- Avoid potent diuretic which may lower the blood pressure too much

Table 9.17 Hypotensive drugs to be avoided in vertebrobasilar insufficiency

• Peripheral vasodilators	• hydrallazine (Apresoline)
	• prazosin (Hypovase)
	• minoxidil (Loniten)
• Adrenergic neurone-blocking drugs	• guanethidine
	• bethanidine
	• debrisoquine

The best drugs to use for blood pressure control in patients with vertebro-basilar insufficiency are shown in Table 9.18.

Table 9.18 Best hypotensive drugs in vertebrobasilar insufficiency

- Thiazides
- β-receptor blockers
- Methyldopa

Specific treatment

Plastic collar

The most effective measure is a well-fitting *plastic collar* to immobilize the neck.

This is of greatest value when severe cervical spondylosis is present, but should always be tried even when spondylosis is minimal. The collar should be worn continuously during the day for at least several weeks. Withdrawal of use thereafter is on a 'trial and error' basis.

Antihistamines

These drugs are sometimes of value in controlling the dizziness associated with vertebrobasilar insufficiency when the patient is unable to tolerate a plastic collar or finds the collar ineffective.

The antihistamines probably exert their beneficial effect in dizziness by blocking H-receptors in the medulla that are involved in mediating the dizziness reaction. A choice of antihistamines is shown in Table 9.19.

Table 9.19 Antihistamines for symptomatic control of dizziness due to vertebrobasilar insufficiency

Drug	Dose
Prochlorperazine (Stemetil)	5–10 mg t.d.s
Betahistine (Serc)	8–16 mg t.d.s
Cinnarizine (Stugeron)	15–30 mg t.d.s

Surgery

In severe and incapacitating cases where mechanical compression of the vertebral artery by osteophytes can be identified on arteriography, and no relief is obtained with a plastic collar, surgical removal of the osteophytes and decompression of the vertebral canal is possible.

MANAGEMENT OF TRANSIENT ISCHAEMIC ATTACKS

General measures

The measures recommended for vertebrobasilar insufficiency are equally applicable with transient ischaemic attacks.

Specific treatment

Treatment may be medical or surgical.

Medical treatment is based on the use of three important drugs to inhibit thrombus formation (Table 9.20).

Table 9.20 Drugs used in the treatment of transient ischaemic attacks

- Aspirin
- Dipyridamole (Persantin)
- Anticoagulants (Warfarin)

Medical treatment

Aspirin

The clumping together of blood platelets is often the starting stimulus for the development of a blood clot in an artery. This platelet aggregation is very much influenced by two *prostaglandins – thromboxane A2* which is produced by the platelets themselves and encourages clumping and *prostacyclin* which is produced by the vascular endothelium and inhibits clumping.

The action of aspirin is based primarily on the inhibition of the synthesis of thromboxane A2 by inactivation of the enzyme prostaglandin cyclo-oxygenase (Figure 9.7). Unfortunately, this will also prevent the formation of the desirable prostaglandin, prostacyclin, which inhibits the clumping of platelets. To obtain maximum inhibition of thromboxane A2 and minimum inhibition of prostacyclin, it is necessary to use only a very small dose of aspirin amounting to no more than 150 mg.

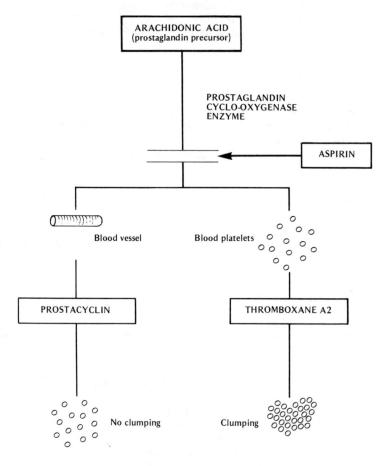

Figure 9.7 Formation of prostaglandins and inhibition by aspirin

There is one other consideration in relation to aspirin therapy in this patient, the history of peptic ulcer. However, as he has had no indigestion for several years it would be worth trying the aspirin. The smallness of the dose makes it unlikely to lead to a recurrence of the indigestion or to bleeding, but if this does occur, the aspirin could always be stopped.

Dipyridamole (Persantin)
Dipyridamole inhibits the clumping of platelets in a different way to aspirin (Figure 9.8). It prevents the action of the enzyme phosphodiesterase which breaks down cycle adenosinemonophosphate (cAMP) inside the platelets: the higher the level of cyclic cAMP, the less likely the platelets are to clump together.

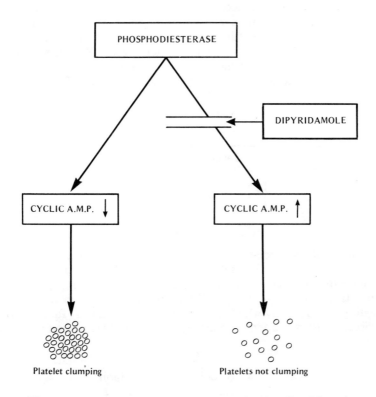

Figure 9.8   Inhibition of platelet clumping by dipyridamole

The dose is 100–200 mg four times daily.
The side-effects are shown in Table 9.21.

307

Table 9.21 Side-effects of
dipyridamole

- Nausea
- Diarrhoea
- Throbbing headache
- Hypertension

Anticoagulants

Anticoagulants are used when aspirin and dipyridamole fail to control the transient ischaemic attacks.

Warfarin is the drug of choice and acts by antagonizing the action of vitamin K which is necessary for the formation of prothrombin. To achieve effective anticoagulation it is necessary to maintain the prothrombin time – the measure of blood prothrombin level – at $2-2\frac{1}{2}$ times the normal control level. Treatment is continued for a minimum period of 1 year and then can be slowly withdrawn. If the transient ischaemic attacks recur, Warfarin can be re-introduced or alternative treatment such as surgery considered.

The contraindications to Warfarin therapy are shown in Table 9.22.

Table 9.22 Contraindications
to Warfarin therapy

- Severe hypertension
- Active peptic ulcer
- Bleeding disorders
- Liver disease

The only significant side-effect of Warfarin is excessive bleeding which may occur in different organs (Table 9.23). With minor bleeding, all that is usually necessary is to omit Warfarin for several days. Major bleeding, however, may require intravenous vitamin K (10–20 mg) or even blood transfusion.

Bleeding is more likely when certain drugs are also taken (Table 9.24) or in liver disease. *Elderly* patients are also more susceptible to bleeding.

Table 9.23 Bleeding due to warfarin

- Minor – Haematuria
  Bruising in the skin
- Major – Muscle
  Bowel – melaena
  Retroperitoneal
  Brain – stroke
  Placenta – fetal death

Table 9.24   Drugs which enhance bleeding
due to Warfarin

- Phenylbutazone (arthritis)
- Aspirin (analgesic)
- Clofibrate (hyperlipidaemia)
- Phenobarbitone withdrawal (epilepsy)

Surgical treatment

Carotid endarterectomy is only justifiable if the risks of future stroke and
death are clearly reduced and the risk of operation is slight. The benefits still
remain controversial.

The circumstances under which carotid surgery might be considered are
shown in Table 9.25. The contraindications are shown in Table 9.26.

Table 9.25   Indications for carotid endarterectomy in transient
ischaemic attacks

- Failure of medical treatment
- Frequent and incapacitating ischaemic attacks
- Substantial carotid obstruction on arteriography (>60%)
- Experienced carotid surgeon available
- No contraindications

Table 9.26   Contraindications to carotid
endarterectomy

- Myocardial infarction within 6 months
- Unstable angina
- Severe pulmonary insufficiency
- Too old and feeble

The long-term prognosis after surgery remains poor, with a 25% recurrence
rate of neurological symptoms and a 30% mortality within 5 years.

MANAGEMENT OF SUBCLAVIAN STEAL SYNDROME

If symptoms of vertebrobasilar insufficiency are severe even with minor effort
involving the arms, endarterectomy of the subclavian artery ought to be
considered.

MANAGEMENT OF MÉNIÈRE'S DISEASE

Medical

The best treatment for the prolonged severe attack is *bed-rest*.

The other medical measures which may be of value are shown in Table 9.27; when antihistamines are used, the patient should be warned of the possible side-effects (Table 9.28).

Table 9.27   Medical treatment of Ménière's disease

• Antihistamines   • Dimenhydrinate (Dramamine) 50–100 mg 3–6 times daily (oral, intramuscular or intravenous) • Betahistine (Serc) 8–16 mg t.d.s. • Prochlorperazine (Stemetil) 5–10 mg t.d.s.
• Control of salt and water intake
• Diuretics

Table 9.28   Side-effects of antihistamines

• Drowsiness
• Impairment of driving ability
• Enhanced effects of alcohol
• Enhanced effects of tranquillizers

Surgery

If medical treatment is unsuccessful and the condition interferes with work and social life, surgery could be considered (Table 9.29).

Table 9.29   Surgery for Ménière's disease

• Endolymphatic drainage
• Subarachnoid shunt
• Labyrinthectomy
• Section of vestibular division of auditory nerve

NATURAL HISTORY OF TRANSIENT ISCHAEMIC ATTACKS

Incidence

The incidence of transient ischaemic attacks is 0.3–1.3/1000 adults/year in the Western population.

Stroke development

Approximately one in three patients will develop a stroke within 5 years of initial presentation (Figure 9.9). At least 20% of strokes will occur within the first month and 50% within the first year. After this the annual incidence is 5% which is five times greater than in a control population. The time interval from initial presentation is therefore an important factor in determining the occurrence of a stroke.

310

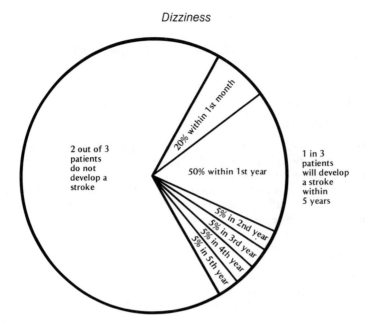

Figure 9.9   Prognosis of transient ischaemic attacks

It is thought that the prognosis is worse with attacks in the carotid territory than those in the vertebrobasilar system.

CAN WE MODIFY THE NATURAL HISTORY?

The problem of preventing or delaying cerebrovascular disease (including transient ischaemic attacks) is essentially the problem of controlling the atherosclerotic process itself.

A number of risk factors have been identified which can predict the likelihood of atherosclerotic heart disease and brain disease. Although there is little doubt of the risk potential of these factors in the development of the disease, there is as yet much less evidence of the beneficial effects of modifying these factors on the subsequent clinical progress of the disease once it has been established.

Table 9.30   Risk factors in the development of atherosclerotic disease

• Major	• Cigarette smoking
	• Hypertension
	• Raised blood cholesterol
• Minor	• Diabetes
	• Obesity
	• Physical inactivity
	• 'Soft water'
	• Contraceptive pill
	• ?Personality type

311

The risk factors can be divided into those of major significance and those of minor significance (Table 9.30).

Major risk factors

Cigarette smoking

The close relationship between the number of cigarettes smoked and cerebro-vascular disease is well established. By age 45 years the excess risk of all atherosclerotic disease in male smokers is 70%.

Stopping smoking has been clearly shown to reduce the risk of clinical coronary events, including sudden death, but a similar clearcut change in the incidence of cerebrovascular events has yet to be demonstrated.

Hypertension

The beneficial effects of reducing severe hypertension on the incidence of stroke has also been clearly shown.

Recent studies have also shown that control of mild hypertension favourably influences the development of subsequent stroke (US Public Health Service Study, Australian National Blood Pressure Study and US Hypertension Detection and Follow-up Study – reviewed *Lancet*, 6 Jan 1982).

The risk potential of hypertension relates to both systolic and diastolic pressure. It remains unclear whether control of an elevated systolic pressure in the elderly will be beneficial.

Hyperlipidaemia

While there is again an undeniable and close relationship between elevated blood lipids, especially cholesterol, and the incidence of atherosclerotic disease, there is no convincing evidence that reduction of blood lipids will result in clinical improvement in patients with cerebrovascular disease.

Minor risk factors

Diabetes

Poorly-controlled diabetes is associated with increased atherosclerotic disease. Control of diabetes, though necessary for its own sake, has yet to be shown to reduce the incidence of cerebrovascular disease.

The lack of convincing benefit may be due to our present inability to maintain consistently normal blood sugar levels in the diabetic patient. The development and introduction of sophisticated insulin pumps may improve the results.

Obesity

Obesity itself does not appear to be an independent risk factor for athero-sclerosis. Its risk depends on several associated factors (Table 9.31).

Table 9.31 Atheroma risk factors associated
with obesity

- Hypertension
- Diabetic tendency
- Hyperlipidaemia (mainly triglycerides)
- Physical inactivity

Control of obesity is a perennial problem in many fields of medicine. Perhaps the most important aim is to not to put the patient temporarily 'on a diet' but to alter the eating habits permanently. Motivation and will-power to persist are essential. The financial difficulties involved in buying appropriate food may well be an important factor.

Physical inactivity

A sedentary life may encourage cardiovascular events but the role of exercise in primary and secondary prevention remains far from clear.

'Soft' water

The adverse influence of 'soft' water in the atherosclerotic process is ill-understood and the place of manipulation of the chemical content of the water in the management of cardiovascular disease remains to be established.

Contraceptive pill

The use of the contraceptive pill encourages the development of ischaemic stroke. Death from stroke occurs five times more frequently when the pill is used than in age-matched controls. The risk is greater in older women, especially smokers, but there is also a significant increase in the frequency of ischaemic stroke in younger women especially during pregnancy.

It is not clear whether the mechanism is based on accelerated development of atherosclerosis of the cerebral vessels or on the increased incidence of thrombosis and embolism caused by modification of platelet behaviour by the oestrogen.

The use of the contraceptive pill must obviously depend on medical and socio-economic considerations. Its use in the older woman who is also a smoker should, however, be discouraged.

Personality type

An aggressive obsessional personality (Type A) seems to predominate in patients with coronary disease, compared with the placid, easygoing personality (Type B). A similar distinction in cerebrovascular disease has yet to be shown.

In any case, if personality is shown to be a relevant factor, it is unlikely that personality type is amenable to correction apart from stopping smoking, altering dietary habits and as far as possible avoiding stressful situations.

Conclusions on control of atheroma

In the absence of clearcut evidence of clinical benefits from control of the various risk factors associated with atherosclerosis, probably the most useful preventive measures are *control of hypertension*, especially in males under 60 years old, and avoidance of the use of the *contraceptive pill* in older women who are smokers.

USEFUL PRACTICAL POINTS

These are as follows.

- Vertebrobasilar insufficiency produces a generalized disturbance of neurological function, such as dizziness, ataxia, and drop attacks, while a transient ischaemic attack causes a focal neurological abnormality, such as monocular blindness, diplopia, speech disturbance, monoparesis or hemiparesis or unilateral limb paraesthesiae.

- Cervical spondylosis is a frequent association with, and an important contributory factor to, vertebrobasilar insufficiency.

- It is important to consider a transient cardiac dysrhythmia as a cause of a transient ischaemic attack, since it is correctable.

- A systolic murmur heard over the carotid artery in the neck suggests the source of the platelet emboli causing the transient ischaemic attack.

- In the present state of knowledge and experience it is preferable to try medical treatment first for transient ischaemic attacks. The drugs used are low-dose aspirin (not >150 mg/day), dipyridamole or Warfarin.

- The simplest and most effective treatment of vertebrobasilar insufficiency, especially when associated with cervical spondylosis, is a plastic collar.

- Carotid arteriography should be considered only if medical treatment has failed to control the transient ischaemic attacks and there is a real possibility of surgery by an experienced surgeon in a patient with no contraindication to operation.

10

Difficulty in walking

PRESENT HISTORY

A 32-year-old lady presented with a history of increasing difficulty in walking for about 6 weeks, associated with problems of balance.

Difficulty in walking

Her right leg had started to feel 'heavy' about 6 weeks earlier. Over the course of the next week or two, the heaviness had become progressively worse and was interfering with her walking. The right foot was tending to drag and she would occasionally trip over floor mats.

The leg now felt very weak and unable to support her so that she had to hold on to furniture with her right hand to get about the house.

She had not noticed any weakness in the left leg while she was walking but she did say that once or twice her left leg had felt a bit 'heavy' after she had a hot bath: this would improve in a few hours.

Loss of balance

As well as the difficulty in walking caused by the weakness in her right leg, she also complained that her 'balance was going'. By this, she meant that she felt unsteady when she stood up and also when she was walking. Occasionally, she said she seemed to 'bump into things' on her right side because of the lack of balance.

Clumsiness

Another complaint was that her right hand seemed a bit clumsy recently, and didn't seem to go where she wanted it to go. On one occasion a fortnight previously she had dropped a tea cup from her right hand, broken the cup and made a mess of the carpet. She didn't really know why this had happened, as she had never noticed any weakness in the right hand or difficulty in holding things.

315

Other relevant facts on direct enquiry

When asked specifically about her *balance at night* or in poor light, she thought it was *a bit worse*, and cited getting up at night to go to the toilet as one of the instances when she was more unsteady than usual.

She admitted to occasional *blurring of vision* over the last few years, usually lasting no more than a few hours. However, she did have one bad attack of blurred vision about 18 months earlier which had lasted about a week. During this attack, her left eye had been very painful.

She had never had double vision.

She had not noticed any numbness or tingling in her limbs.

She had never had any episodes of vertigo.

She had not had any difficulty with her speech.

She had not noticed any muscle twitching.

She was not subject to headaches and had not had any recent headache.

There had been no difficulty in passing urine or controlling micturition.

Her weight had remained steady.

She had not had any recent cough or haemoptysis.

There were no gastrointestinal symptoms.

PAST HISTORY

About 3 months earlier she had an attack of shingles which had caused a painful rash on the left side of her chest. The rash had since gone but she was still getting some pain over the affected area.

There were no other relevant illnesses.

FAMILY HISTORY

Her father, aged 57 years, had a heart attack when he was 49 years old which has left him handicapped by angina.

Her mother, aged 55 years, had been treated for hypertension for the past 10 years.

PERSONAL HISTORY

She had never *smoked*.

Alcohol consumption was very moderate – an occasional glass of lager at weekends.

She had two children aged 7 and 9 years and had been able to manage normally at home until the last 6 weeks or so.

DRUG HISTORY

Apart from analgesics, for the recent attack of shingles she had not taken any drugs.

CLINICAL EXAMINATION

General

Her mental state was normal.
There was no abnormality of speech.
There was no arcus senilis or xanthelasma.
The abnormal findings were confined to the nervous system (Figure 10.1).

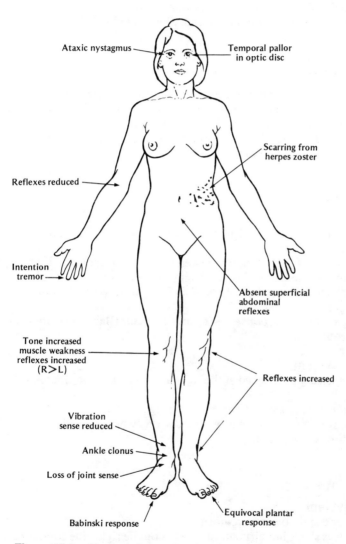

Ataxic nystagmus

Temporal pallor
in optic disc

Scarring from
herpes zoster

Reflexes reduced

Intention
tremor

Absent superficial
abdominal
reflexes

Tone increased
muscle weakness
reflexes increased
(R>L)

Reflexes increased

Vibration
sense reduced

Ankle clonus

Loss of joint sense

Babinski response

Equivocal plantar
response

Figure 10.1 Abnormal examination findings in the patient

Central nervous system

Balance

When she stood with her feet together she was slightly unsteady, and this became worse when she closed her eyes (*Romberg's sign*).

Walking

Her walking was unsteady and she tended to veer to the right. The right leg was held rather stiffly with restricted flexion at the hip and knee. She was also inclined to catch her toe on the ground. She had difficulty stopping and almost fell over to the right.

Cranial nerves

Fundal examination showed *temporal pallor* in the left optic disc.

Nystagmus was present. It was a coarse jerky nystagmus which was most marked in the abducting eye: the slow phase of the nystagmus was towards the centre and the quick phase towards the direction of the gaze.

The other cranial nerves were normal.

Lower limbs

Motor system
Muscle tone was increased in the right lower limb and *ankle clonus* was obtained.

There was *weakness* of all the movements in the right lower limb, especially dorsiflexion of the ankle. There was no weakness on the left side.

The *reflexes* were abnormally *brisk* in both the lower limbs but especially so on the right.

The *right plantar response* was clearly *extensor* (Babinski response) and the left was equivocal.

Sensory system
Vibration sense was reduced at the right ankle and knee compared with the left side.

Joint position sense was absent in the right foot.

There was no abnormality of cotton wool sensation, pinprick or temperature sense in either leg.

Upper limbs

Motor system
Muscle tone and power were normal.

There was slight impairment of reflexes on the right side compared with the left.

Hoffman's sign – a sign of pyramidal involvement – was negative.

318

Sensory system
Sensation was intact for all modalities.

Cerebellar system

In the upper limbs, the finger-nose test was poor on the right: the patient repeatedly showed a slight intention tremor and past-pointing. This was not significantly worse when the patient's eyes were closed.

In the lower limbs, the heel–knee test was difficult to carry out on the right because of the considerable weakness and stiffness of the right leg. Even so, it was evident that there was *difficulty in coordinating* the movement of the right leg down the left shin. When the test was repeated with the patient's eyes closed, the incoordination became a lot worse.

Cardiovascular system

The pulse and blood pressure were normal.
There was no arterial thickening.
There was no abnormality on palpation and auscultation of the heart.
The fundal arteries looked normal.

Respiratory system

There was evidence of healed shingles in the dermatome distribution of the eighth thoracic to the twelfth thoracic nerve on the left side.
The lungs were quite clear.

Abdominal examination

The superficial abdominal reflexes were absent in all four quadrants. No abnormality was otherwise found.

The spine

There was no local tenderness over any vertebra.
Mobility was free and painless.

ANALYSIS OF THE HISTORY

Difficulty in walking

Difficulty in walking can be due to general disorders or specific disease of the systems involved in walking (Table 10.1).

Table 10.1 Causes of difficulty in walking

- Debility following prolonged bed-rest
- General disorders
    - anaemia
    - malignancy
    - hypokalaemia
- Disease of muscle
- Disease of joints
- Disease of nervous system

General conditions

There was no previous history of prolonged bed-rest.

To interfere with walking, anaemia would have to be severe, and in this case other symptoms would be likely (Table 10.2). Additionally, the difficulty in walking would affect both legs. The absence of symptoms of anaemia, and the limitation of the weakness to one leg, exclude this diagnosis.

Table 10.2 Symptoms of anaemia

- Breathlessness
- Palpitations
- Dizziness
- Severe fatigue
- Pallor
- Ankle swelling

There were no symptoms to suggest a primary site of malignancy, although this does not of course exclude the diagnosis. Muscle wasting associated with malignancy is likely to be bilateral. The absence of loss of weight, and the unilateral leg weakness, make this diagnosis unlikely.

Hypokalaemia also causes symmetrical muscle weakness affecting all four limbs. The localization of the weakness to one leg and the absence of diuretic treatment – the commonest cause of hypokalaemia – or the other causes of hypokalaemia (vomiting, renal disease) make this diagnosis very unlikely.

Muscle disease

The types of muscle disease which can cause difficulty in walking are shown in Table 10.3

Table 10.3 Muscle disease causing difficulty in walking

• Muscular dystrophy	• Pseudohypertrophic (Duchenne)
	• Facio-scapulo-humeral (Landouzy–Déjerine)
	• Dystrophia myotonica
• Myasthenia gravis	
• Myositis	• Dermatomyositis
	• Polymyalgia rheumatica
• Endocrine	• Thyrotoxic myopathic
	• Diabetic amyotrophy
	• Cushing's syndrome – muscle breakdown
	• Steroid therapy – muscle breakdown
• Malignancy	

Muscular dystrophy is hereditary and usually starts in childhood or early adolescence: it is usually symmetrical. The lack of a family history, the late onset and the unilateral leg involvement makes muscular dystrophy a highly unlikely diagnosis.

Myasthenia gravis leads to progressive weakness of the muscles after repetitive use. It will also frequently affect the eyelids, the pharynx and the larynx causing drooping eyelids, dysphagia and dysarthria. It is very unlikely that walking alone will be affected in the absence of involvement of the cranial muscles. Because of this, and the absence of the typical pattern of weakness coming on only after repeated use, myasthenia gravis is excluded.

The clinical features of *dermatomyositis* are shown in Table 10.4. None was present in the patient.

Table 10.4 Clinical features of dermatomyositis

• Wasting of proximal muscles
• Lilac coloured rash
• Raynaud's phenomenon
• Subcutaneous calcification
• Bronchial carcinoma common

The clinical features of *polymyalgia rheumatica* are shown in Table 10.5. None was present in the patient.

Table 10.5 Clinical features of polymyalgia rheumatica

• Usually elderly males
• Pain and stiffness in shoulders and thighs
• Headache with scalp tenderness
• Temporal arteritis common
• Polyarthralgia common

The *endocrine disorders* associated with myopathy or muscle breakdown all produce a symmetrical picture of muscle involvement. The asymmetrical weakness, and the absence of any of the general symptoms of the respective endocrine disorders, exclude endocrine disease as a cause of the walking difficulty in this patient.

Joint disease

Arthritis affecting the hip and knee can interfere with walking. There was no pain or swelling of either of these joints in the patient.

Neurological disease

Neurological disorders can interfere with walking in various ways (Table 10.6).

Table 10.6   Neurological disorders interfering with walking

• Motor	• Pyramidal tracts
	• Lower motor neurone
	• Peripheral nerves
• Sensory	• Afferent pathways from joints and muscles
• Cerebellum and its connections	
• Basal ganglia	

Motor system
Involvement of the upper motor neurone (pyramidal tract), lower motor neurone and the peripheral nerves must all be considered.

Pyramidal tracts
Involvement of the corticospinal tracts anywhere in their course from the motor cortex to the anterior horn cells in the spinal cord will cause muscle weakness and interfere with walking (Figure 10.2).

A left-sided *cortical lesion* affecting the leg area in the precentral gyrus produces a contralateral monoplegia. This remains a possible site of disease in the patient and will be reviewed subsequently in the light of other manifestations.

A common site of involvement of the pyramidal tracts is in the internal capsule between the basal ganglia. The effects of a lesion in this area are shown in Table 10.7.

An *internal capsular lesion* is therefore very unlikely in this patient since there are no symptoms of hemianaesthesia or visual field defect.

A *brain stem lesion* is associated with the features shown in Table 10.8.

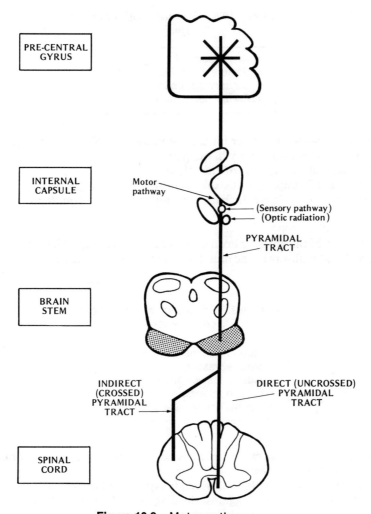

Figure 10.2 Motor pathway

Table 10.7 Effects of internal capsular lesion

- Hemiplegia
- Hemianaesthesia
- Hemianopia

The absence of hemiplegic manifestation, sensory symptoms and cranial nerve involvement make this diagnosis unlikely.

A localized lesion on one side of the *spinal cord*, below the outflow of the

323

Table 10.8 Features of brain
stem lesion

- Hemiplegia
- Bilateral hemiplegia
- Sensory disturbance
- Cranial nerve involvement

pyramidal fibres to the upper limbs, can produce weakness of the ipsilateral leg. This is a likely possibility in the patient.

The transient 'heaviness' of the left leg after a hot bath may indicate an early pyramidal lesion on this side also. The relationship to an increase in temperature produced by the bath is highly suggestive of *multiple sclerosis*.

Lower motor neurone
Involvement of the anterior horn cells in the spinal cord, which represent the final common pathway to the muscles, results in several manifestations (Table 10.9).

Table 10.9 Effects of anterior horn
cell disease

- Muscle weakness or paralysis
- Muscle wasting
- Muscle fasciculation
- Loss of reflexes
- Normal plantar response

The two commonest causes of anterior horn cell disease are *poliomyelitis* and *motor neurone disease*.

The absence of fasciculation, which is experienced by the patient as muscle twitching, is a strong point against the diagnosis of anterior horn cell disease.

Peripheral nerves
The common causes of *peripheral neuritis* are shown in Table 10.10.

Peripheral neuritis usually produces symmetrical involvement of the limbs; since the patient's complaint of weakness is in one leg only, the possibility of peripheral neuritis will only apply in those conditions causing a lesion of isolated nerves (Table 10.11).

Diabetes is excluded by absence of the classical triad of symptoms (Table 10.12).

The symptoms associated with polyarteritis are shown in Table 10.13. The female patient (polyarteritis usually occurs in males) and the absence of any of the symptoms, excludes the diagnosis of polyarteritis nodosa.

The symptoms of systemic lupus erythematosus are shown in Table 10.14. The absence of any of the symptoms excludes the diagnosis in this patient.

Table 10.10 Causes of peripheral neuritis

- Diabetes
- Vitamin B_{12} deficiency
- Acute infective polyneuritis
- Carcinomatous neuropathy
- Chronic alcoholism
- Polyarteritis nodosa
- Acute porphyria

Table 10.11 Causes of mononeuritis multiplex

• Vascular	• Diabetes
	• Polyarteritis nodosa
	• Systemic lupus erythematosus
	• Rheumatoid arthritis
• Inflammatory	• Sarcoidosis
	• Leprosy
• Infiltration	Amyloidosis
• Carcinoma	

Table 10.12 Clinical triad of symptoms in diabetes mellitus

- Thirst
- Polyuria
- Loss of weight

Table 10.13 Symptoms of polyarteritis nodosa

- Constitutional symptoms – fever, anorexia, weight loss
- Pains in joints and muscles
- Pleuritic pain
- Precordial pain – pericarditis
- Abdominal pain

Table 10.14 Symptoms of systemic lupus erythematosus

- Constitutional – fever, anorexia, weight loss
- Skin rashes
- Polyarthralgia
- Abdominal pain
- Pleurisy
- Pericarditis pain
- Symptoms of anaemia
- Alopecia

The symptoms of sarcoidosis are shown in Table 10.15. Again the absence of any of these symptoms excludes the diagnosis.

Table 10.15   Symptoms of sarcoidosis

• Skin rashes	• erythema nodosum lupus pernio
• Respiratory	• dyspnoea cough
• Glandular enlargement	
• Polyarthralgia	
• Eye symptoms	• iridocyclitis

There was no joint involvement in the patient to indicate rheumatoid arthritis.

The diagnosis of leprosy is obviously not relevant in the patient.

Amyloidosis is either primary, often associated with myelomatosis, or secondary to chronic suppurative conditions (e.g. bronchiectasis) or inflammatory conditions (e.g. rheumatoid arthritis). The absence of an underlying condition, and the lack of symptoms of involvement of the gut (diarrhoea) or kidneys (oedema) excludes secondary amyloidosis. Similarly, in primary amyloidosis the lack of relevant symptoms excludes this diagnosis (Table 10.16).

Table 10.16   Symptoms of amyloidosis

• Gut	– diarrhoea
• Kidneys	– oedema
• Heart	– palpitations heart failure
• Lungs	– dyspnoea cough
• Joints	– polyarthralgia joint swelling
• Skin	– rashes
• (Myelomatosis	– symptoms of anaemia bleeding susceptibility to infection back pain pathological fractures)

Peripheral neuritis is one of the non-metastatic neurological complications of carcinoma (Table 10.17). The mononeuritis which may occur with carcinoma is usually mixed motor and sensory, or less commonly pure sensory. It would therefore produce sensory symptoms such as paraesthesiae or numbness, which the patient did not have. Additionally, the absence of loss of weight is against a diagnosis of carcinoma.

Table 10.17 Non-metastatic neurological complications of carcinoma

- Pure sensory neuropathy
- Mixed motor and sensory neuropathy
- Cerebellar degeneration
- 'Motor neurone disease' syndrome
- Dementia

Sensory system

Difficulty in walking may be due not only to muscle weakness but also to impairment of coordination of muscle movement owing to lack of proprioceptive sensory information from the muscles, joints and tendons.

The deterioration in the patient's balance in poor light is a characteristic feature of sensory ataxia, since vision is an important compensatory factor in maintaining balance when proprioceptive information is lacking.

Cerebellar system

The characteristic feature of impairment of cerebellar control of walking is the veering or lurching to the side of the cerebellar lesion.

If both cerebellar hemispheres are affected, the gait tends to be broad-based and reeling. It has been likened to a drunken gait, but the main distinguishing feature is that a drunk, however unsteady, usually maintains upright balance, while a cerebellar patient could easily fall.

The patient tended to veer to the right side when she walked, suggesting a right-sided cerebellar lesion. The complaint of clumsiness of the right hand and dropping the tea cup also suggests cerebellar involvement.

The history therefore suggests that the patient has both sensory ataxia and cerebellar ataxia.

Basal ganglia

Involvement of the basal ganglia produces the very characteristic disturbance of gait of *Parkinson's disease*. The patient has difficulty starting to walk, but when walking has difficulty stopping. The steps are short and shuffling with the body inclined forward, the arms still at the sides and the face expressionless.

There was no suggestion of a Parkinsonian walk in this patient.

Loss of balance

The other major complaint by the patient was unsteadiness and loss of balance. The important causes of loss of balance are shown in Table 10.18.

Table 10.18 Causes of loss of balance

- Peripheral labyrinthine lesion
- Loss of proprioceptive sense
- Cerebellar disease

Labyrinthine lesion

The characteristic features of a labyrinthine lesion are shown in Table 10.19. Apart from the unsteadiness, the patient had none of these symptoms.

Table 10.19 Features of a labyrinthine lesion

- Loss of balance
- Attacks of vertigo
- Tinnitus
- Deafness

Loss of proprioceptive sense

The deterioration of the patient's balance in poor light indicates loss of proprioceptive sense.

Cerebellar ataxia

The patient showed evidence of a right-sided cerebellar lesion by the veering to the right during her walking.

Visual disturbance

The patient had one bad attack of blurred vision with pain in the left eye. This is highly suggestive of *retrobulbar neuritis*. The important causes of retrobulbar neuritis are shown in Table 10.20.

Table 10.20 Causes of retrobulbar neuritis

- Multiple sclerosis
- Neurosyphilis
- Diabetes
- Vitamin B_1 deficiency
- Vitamin B_{12} deficiency
- Chemical
  - lead
  - alcohol
  - quinine
  - tobacco

There were no symptoms of tabes dorsalis (Table 10.21) thus excluding neurosyphilis.

Diabetes is excluded by the absence of thirst, polyuria and loss of weight.

Her diet was normal, thus excluding vitamin B_{12} deficiency.

Although there were no symptoms of anaemia which might be associated

Table 10.21 Symptoms of tabes dorsalis

- Paraesthesiae – especially feet
- 'Lightning' pains
- Visceral crises
  - gastric
  - vesical
  - rectal
  - laryngeal
- Loss of sphincter control
- Impotence
- Double vision

with vitamin B_{12} deficiency, neurological complications, such as peripheral neuritis and subacute combined degeneration of the cord, can occur in the absence of associated anaemia. In these circumstances, however, paraesthesiae in the limbs are very common, especially a complaint of 'walking on cotton wool'. This was not one of the patient's symptoms, and together with the lack of symptoms of anaemia, makes B_{12} deficiency a very unlikely diagnosis.

There was no contact with lead. She was not an alcoholic. She did not smoke. She has not taken quinine.

Past history

The attacks of *shingles, (herpes zoster)* may be relevant, since shingles is associated occasionally with neurological complications (Table 10.22).

Table 10.22 Neurological complications of shingles

- Transverse myelitis
- Encephalitis
- Polyneuritis

Transverse myelitis can lead to difficulty in walking and ataxia. However, sensory symptoms such as paraesthesiae and numbness are common in transverse myelitis, and usually spread up from the feet towards the trunk up to the level of involvement of the spinal cord. This presentation did not occur in the patient.

Family history

The only relevance of the family history is that both parents suffered from *cardiovascular disease*. This suggests that the patient may be susceptible to vascular disease also, and offers a possible basis for ischaemic disease affecting either the brain or the spinal cord.

Drug history

This is irrelevant.

CONCLUSIONS FROM THE HISTORY

The neurological involvement evident from the history includes:

- retrobulbar neuritis in the past
- pyramidal involvement of the legs
- posterior column involvement of the legs
- cerebellar involvement of the legs and right arm.

The 'dissemination' of these lesions in 'space' in the nervous system and in their time relationships makes the *diagnosis of multiple sclerosis ('disseminated' sclerosis) a virtual certainty.*

ANALYSIS OF THE EXAMINATION

To help in the analysis of the abnormal physical signs, which are confined to the nervous system in the patient, Figure 10.3 shows a cross-section through the spinal cord.

Pyramidal involvement

The signs which indicate pyramidal involvement are shown in Table 10.23.
The common causes of pyramidal disease are shown in Table 10.24.

Table 10.23   Signs of pyramidal involvement
in the patient

- Spastic gait
- Increased muscle tone right leg
- Muscle weakness right leg
- Increased reflexes both legs R > L
- Babinski response both feet
- Absent superficial abdominal reflexes

Table 10.24   Causes of pyramidal disease

- Multiple sclerosis
- Spinal cord compression
- Cerebrovascular disease
- Subacute combined degeneration
- Motor neurone disease
- Spinal vascular disease

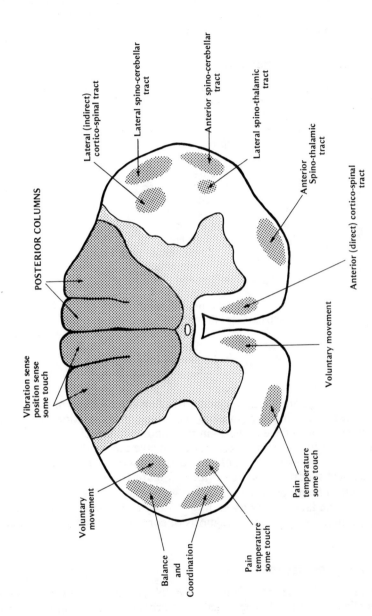

Figure 10.3 Transverse section of the spinal cord

Multiple sclerosis

This is a common cause of pyramidal involvement of one or both lower limbs and this type of presentation is one of the most common in the disease.

This diagnosis is high on the list of likely diagnoses.

Compression of the spinal cord

Difficulty in walking may be the initial presentation of this condition. The common causes of cord compression are shown in Table 10.25.

Table 10.25   Causes of compression of the spinal cord

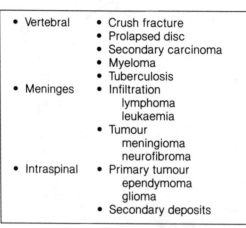

• Vertebral	• Crush fracture
	• Prolapsed disc
	• Secondary carcinoma
	• Myeloma
	• Tuberculosis
• Meninges	• Infiltration
	lymphoma
	leukaemia
	• Tumour
	meningioma
	neurofibroma
• Intraspinal	• Primary tumour
	ependymoma
	glioma
	• Secondary deposits

Pain over the vertebrae or in a root distribution is frequently present and it is made worse by straining, e.g. sneezing, coughing or defaecation. Numbness and paraesthesiae also develop early in the condition, especially in the lower limbs, and then usually ascend upwards to involve the trunk.

If the cord compression is confined to one side of the spinal cord, the Brown–Sequard syndrome may be evident (Figure 10.4).

The absence of any pain, either in the vertebrae or of root distribution, together with the lack of any ascending sensory symptoms, such as paraesthesiae or numbness, makes the diagnosis of cord compression very unlikely.

Cerebrovascular disease

Cerebrovascular disease most commonly involves the internal capsule in the basal ganglia (Figure 10.5). The effects of internal capsular lesions are shown in Table 10.26.

None of these features was evident in the patient, which excludes an internal capsular lesion.

However, a cerebrovascular lesion involving the *motor cortex* can produce a

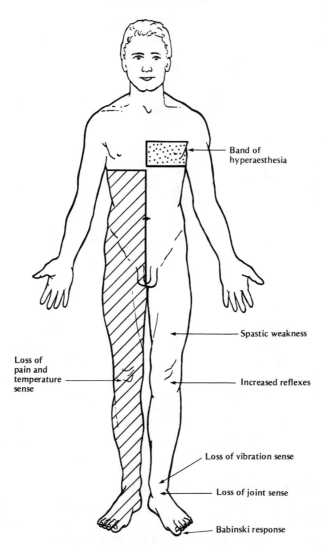

Band of hyperaesthesia

Spastic weakness

Loss of pain and temperature sense

Increased reflexes

Loss of vibration sense

Loss of joint sense

Babinski response

Figure 10.4 Brown–Sequard syndrome

Table 10.26 Effects of internal capsular lesions

- Hemiplegia
- Hemianaesthesia
- Paralysis of lower face
- Homonymous hemianopia

333

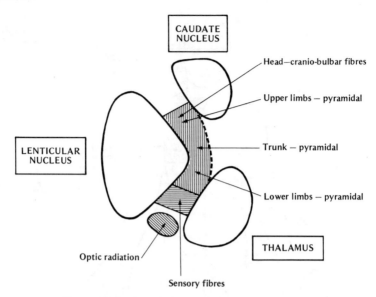

Figure 10.5 Internal capsule in the basal ganglia

spastic monoplegia affecting one leg. The likelihood of this diagnosis must be considered in the light of the other neurological findings.

Vascular disease affecting the *brain stem* usually produces bilateral pyramidal involvement and is very frequently associated with cranial nerve paralysis. The particular diagnostic feature is that the cranial nerve paralysis is on the opposite side to that of the hemiplegia ('crossed paralysis'). This was not evident in this patient.

Subacute combined degeneration of the cord

The features of this condition are shown in Table 10.27.

Although the patient has evidence of posterior column and pyramidal involvement, the lack of paraesthesiae and other sensory changes, as well as the absence of symptoms of anaemia, makes the diagnosis very unlikely.

Table 10.27 Features of subacute combined degeneration of the spinal cord

• Pyramidal involvement	– Spastic weakness legs
• Posterior column involvement	– Position sense lost
	Vibration sense lost
• Peripheral neuritis	– Paraesthesiae
	Sensory changes
• Anaemia	

Motor neurone disease

The distinctive features of this degenerative disease of the nervous system are shown in Table 10.28. The main clinical types of motor neurone disease are shown in Table 10.29.

Table 10.28 Distinctive features of motor neurone disease

- Unknown aetiology
- May be familial
- Affects upper and lower motor neuron
- Muscle fasciculation common
- No sensory changes

Table 10.29 Clinical types of motor neurone disease

- Bulbar palsy
- Progressive muscular atrophy
- Amyotrophic lateral sclerosis

In *bulbar palsy* an important feature is progressive involvement of speech and swallowing. This was not evident in this patient.

Progressive muscular atrophy causes wasting of the small muscles of the hand, producing a 'claw-hand' (Figure 10.6): pyramidal signs in the legs are a late development. The absence of wasting of the hands and fasciculation excludes the diagnosis.

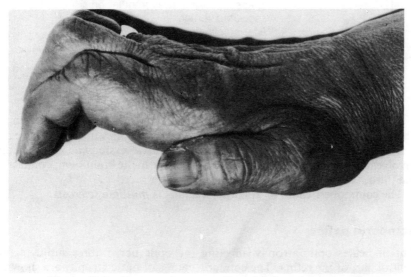

Figure 10.6 Progressive muscular atrophy – 'claw-hand'

In *amyotrophic lateral sclerosis* both upper motor neurone and lower motor neurone signs exist together: this causes wasting of the hands and pyramidal signs in the legs. Again the absence of wasting in the hands and fasciculation excludes the diagnosis.

Spinal vascular involvement

Occlusion of the anterior spinal artery affects predominantly the anterior half of the spinal cord. This will lead to pyramidal involvement of the lower limbs but also involvement of the spinothalamic tract with loss of pain and temperature sense. The absence of such sensory change excludes spinal artery thrombosis.

Nystagmus

The causes of nystagmus are shown in Table 10.30. The characteristics of the nystagmus caused by the various types of lesion are shown in Table 10.31.

Table 10.30   Causes of nystagmus

> • Labyrinthine lesion
> • Cerebellar lesion
> • Brain stem lesion

Table 10.31   Characteristics of different types of nystagmus

• Labyrinthine	– Conjugate Horizontal or rotatory Increased looking away from lesion Associated vertigo
• Cerebellar	– Wider amplitude Increased looking towards lesion Horizontal only
• Brain stem	– Horizontal or vertical May be ataxic – increased in abducting eye

The patient's nystagmus was very distinctive – it was more marked in the abducting eye, so that looking right increased nystagmus in the right eye and vice versa. This type of nystagmus is called *ataxic nystagmus* and indicates involvement of the posterior longitudinal bundle in the brain stem, connecting the third, fourth and sixth cranial nerve muscles.

The commonest cause of ataxic nystagmus is *multiple sclerosis*.

Temporal pallor

This indicates optic atrophy affecting the optic nerve fibres supplying the central part of the retina. The common causes of optic atrophy are shown in Table 10.32.

Table 10.32   Causes of optic atrophy

- Glaucoma
- Chronic papilloedema
- Retinal disease
- Retrobulbar neuritis
- Pressure on optic nerve
  - tumour
  - aneurysm
  - Paget's disease

There was no evidence of glaucoma, papilloedema or retinal disease on examination of the eye.

Pressure on the optic nerve is likely to produce permanent impairment of vision, and not for just a week as in the patient.

The history of severe pain in the eye with blurring of vision for 1 week in the absence of evidence of glaucoma is highly suggestive of *retrobulbar neuritis.*

An attack of retrobulbar neuritis followed by temporal pallor of the optic disc due to optic atrophy is a typical manifestation of multiple sclerosis.

Posterior column involvement

The loss of joint position sense and vibration sense indicates involvement of the posterior columns of the spinal cord. The important causes of posterior column involvement are shown in Table 10.33.

Table 10.33   Causes of posterior column involvement

- Multiple sclerosis
- Subacute combined degeneration of the cord
- Tabes dorsalis
- Friedreich's ataxia
- Peroneal muscular atrophy

Multiple sclerosis

This is a very likely cause in view of the retrobulbar neuritis.

Subacute combined degeneration

This has already been discussed and considered very unlikley due to the absence of paraesthesiae and symptoms of anaemia.

Tabes dorsalis

The symptoms have been shown in Table 10.21. The patient has none of these.

The signs of tabes dorsalis are shown in Figure 10.7. None was evident in the patient.

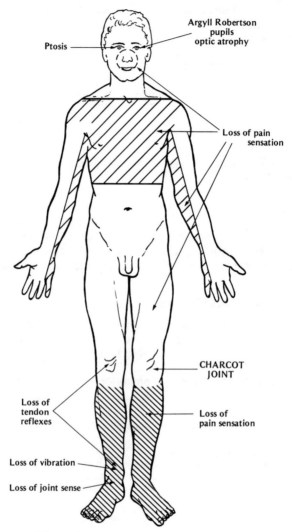

Figure 10.7   Signs of tabes dorsalis

Friedreich's ataxia

The features of Friedreich's ataxia are shown in Figure 10.8. The lack of a family history and an onset in childhood, and the absence of the skeletal and cardiac features of the disease, make this diagnosis very unlikely.

Peroneal muscular atrophy (Charcot-Marie-Tooth disease)

The features are shown in Figure 10.9. The lack of a family history, the

338

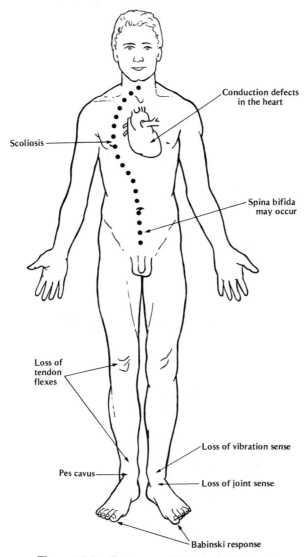

Figure 10.8   Features of Friedreich's ataxia

absence of an equinovarus deformity and the 'inverted champagne bottle' appearance (due to distal muscular atrophy), the absence of pain and temperature loss and the presence of reflexes in the patient all serve to exclude this diagnosis.

Cerebellar ataxia

The signs of cerebellar disease are shown in Table 10.34 and these signs were present in the patient.

339

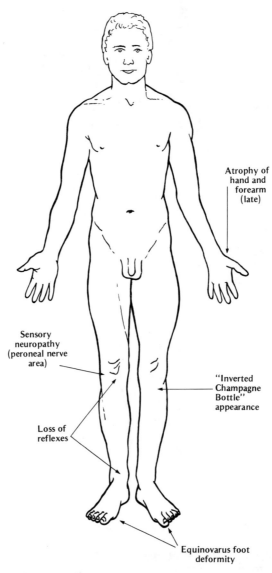

Figure 10.9 Features of Charcot–Marie–Tooth disease (peroneal muscular atrophy)

Table 10.34   Signs of cerebellar dysfunction

• Hypotonia	
• Alteration of reflexes	– reduced
	pendular
• Incoordination	– intention tremor
	past-pointing
	dysdiadochokinesis
• Disturbance of gait	– veering to side of lesion
• Nystagmus	

The important causes of cerebellar ataxia are shown in Table 10.35.

Table 10.35   Causes of cerebellar ataxia

- Multiple sclerosis
- Posterior fossa tumour
- Carcinoma (non-metastatic)
- Drugs – phenytoin, alcohol
- Myxoedema
- Hereditary degeneration

Multiple sclerosis

Again, this is obviously the most likely diagnosis.

Posterior fossa tumour

This gives rise early to the signs of raised intracranial pressure (Table 10.36). None of these symptoms was present in the patient.

Table 10.36   Signs of raised intracranial pressure

- Headache
- Vomiting
- Confusion
- Drowsiness
- Papilloedema

Non-metastatic manifestation of carcinoma

These manifestations are shown in Table 10.17 (p. 327).

There is no indication of a primary site of carcinoma in the patient and no weight loss. It is very unlikely therefore that the cerebellar dysfunction is attributable to carcinoma.

Drugs

The patient was not taking phenytoin and was a very moderate alcohol drinker.

Myxoedema

The absence of any of the typical features of myxoedema (Table 10.37) excludes this diagnosis.

Table 10.37   Features of myxoedema

- Increasing weight
- Mental and physical slowing
- Cold intolerance
- Hoarseness of voice
- Dryness of skin and hair
- Increasing constipation
- Puffy face
- Delayed relaxation of ankle joints

Hereditary degeneration

This is typified by Friedreich's ataxia. This has already been excluded.

CONCLUSIONS FROM THE EXAMINATION

The abnormal findings were:

- optic atrophy (following retrobulbar neuritis)
- pyramidal signs
- posterior column signs.
- cerebellar signs

This combination of signs is diagnostic of multiple sclerosis.

INVESTIGATIONS

The investigations relevant to a diagnosis of multiple sclerosis are a *lumbar puncture* and *visual-evoked reflex measurement*.

Cerebrospinal fluid

The characteristic abnormalities in multiple sclerosis are shown in Table 10.38. The patient's CSF result is shown in Table 10.39.

Table 10.38 Cerebrospinal fluid abnormalities in multiple sclerosis

- Mild lymphocytosis 10–15 cells/mm³
- Mild increase in protein 40–80 mg/100 ml
- Increase in γ-globulin
- Lange curve paretic (first zone rise)
- Negative Wassermann reaction

Table 10.39 The patient's c.s.f. result

	Result	Normal range
Cells	11 lymphocytes/mm³	(up to 4)
Protein	70 mg/100 ml	up to 40)
γ-Globulin	14 mg/100 ml	(up to 5)
Lange	2221000000	(0000000000)

Visual-evoked reflex

This test is based on the slowing of conduction along the optic nerve as a result of loss of myelin caused by the multiple sclerosis. Figure 10.10 shows how the test is done.

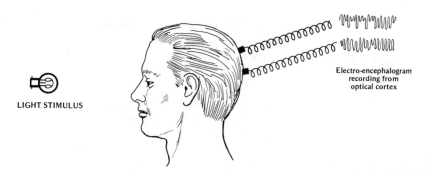

LIGHT STIMULUS

Electro-encephalogram recording from optical cortex

Figure 10.10 Visual-evoked reflex test

Prolonged response time between light stimulus and electroencephalographic recording to over 115 milliseconds indicates an optic nerve abnormality. This suggests the possibility of multiple sclerosis but is not pathognomonic, since other conditions can impair nerve conduction (Table 10.40).

Table 10.40   Prolongation of visual evoked reflex line

- Multiple sclerosis
- Glaucoma
- Compression of optic pathway by tumours
- Degenerative conditions of the optic pathway

The test was not considered necessary in the patient since the diagnosis of multiple sclerosis could be made confidently on clinical grounds.

MANAGEMENT OF MULTIPLE SCLEROSIS

The important factors to keep in mind in the management of this difficult disease are:

- An awareness and understanding of the difficult problems of the patient and his family in a progressively disabling and unpredictable disease.

- The need for whatever measures are available to control the symptoms of the disease.

- A healthy scepticism towards the many new curative treatments advocated.

General measures

Physiotherapy

Well-planned physiotherapy has an important part to play (Table 10.41).

Table 10.41   Aims of physiotherapy in multiple sclerosis

- Development of alternative muscle strengths
- Prevention of contractures of the limbs
- Maintenance of joint mobility
- Improvement in walking by coordination exercises
- Stretching and active resistance exercises to reduce spasticity
- Swimming in cold water to improve muscle weakness

Control of infection

Since a relapse of multiple sclerosis may be precipitated by an infection which causes pyrexia, prompt and effective control of infection is essential.

In this context, regular dental care is important as a prophylactic measure.

Aids for walking

There are several walking aids available for the handicapped patient who wishes to continue walking (Table 10.42).

Table 10.42 Walking aids

- Leg iron for foot drop
- Knee cage for hyperextensibility
- Tetrapod
- Walking frame

When such an aid is used, the hope is that the patient does not become so dependent on it that he or she is reluctant to give it up if the disease remits.

Wheelchairs

When a wheelchair becomes necessary, it is important to 'tailor' the chair to the desired requirements, e.g. for house use, outdoor use etc. The goal is always maximum independence for the patient.

The advice of a physiotherapist and occupational therapist is valuable when choosing the right wheelchair.

Bed-ridden patient

When the patient is totally disabled and bed-ridden, regular visits by the district nurse are essential. The hazards of prolonged bed-rest are well-known and particularly relevant in this type of patient (Table 10.43).

Table 10.43 Hazards of prolonged bed-rest

- Respiratory infections
- Urinary tract infection
- Bed-sores
- Leg vein thrombosis

In view of the very considerable burdens imposed by such a patient on his or her family, alternative long term arrangements may need to be considered, such as transfer to a long stay unit for the young chronic sick or even to a Cheshire Home.

If no long term arrangement can be made, short term accommodation in the local hospital, to relieve the family temporarily, may be feasible – e.g. for a holiday fortnight.

Psychological support

Dealing with a chronic, unpredictable and often progressively disabling disease, the cause of which is unknown and the available treatment for which is limited, is depressing and frustrating for both the patient and the doctor.

Marital breakdown is frequent and financial hardships ever-present. The family is often exhausted physically and mentally by the efforts to cope with the disease. As a result both the patient and his or her family may direct their feelings of anger and frustration at their medical advisers.

Understanding, sympathy and honesty are helpful in coping with the patient and the family. Although an optimistic outlook is desirable from the doctor, overenthusiastic optimism is to be avoided. It is to be hoped that patients and their families will respond to an explanation of the disease in terms fully comprehensible to them. A discussion of what can be done to help at every stage of the disease is valuable. Reassurance that intensive research is constantly undertaken into the disease will offer a realistic note of optimism.

Psychotropic drugs are of very little value and may produce the additional burden of undesirable side-effects.

Support groups

Joining the Multiple Sclerosis Society may be of great value to the patient. The benefits are shown in Table 10.44.

Table 10.44 Benefits of Multiple Sclerosis Society

- Improves knowledge of the disease
- Support by sharing problems with fellow sufferers
- Regular participation in social events
- Encourages optimism by emphasis on research
- Financial help to support research

Symptomatic treatment

Spasticity

The drugs available to reduce spasticity are shown in Table 10.45.

Table 10.45 Drugs to reduce spasticity

Drug	Dose
Baclofen	initial 5 mg t.d.s.
	maximum 100 mg daily
Dantrolene	initial 25 mg daily
	maximum 100 mg q.d.s.
Diazepam	initial 2–15 mg daily (t.d.s.)
	maximum 60 mg daily

The best of these three drugs is probably *baclofen*. The dose is critical, and exceeding the dose results in flaccidity which may impair walking even more.

Dantrolene is occasionally associated with the development of chronic aggressive hepatitis.

Urinary disturbances

Table 10.46 shows the disturbances which may occur and the drugs which may help.

Table 10.46   Urinary disturbances and their treatment in multiple sclerosis

Disturbance	Drug	Dose
Retention	Methyldopa	250 mg once or twice daily
	Phenoxybenzamine	10 mg once or twice daily
Incontinence	Pro-Banthine	7.5–15 mg one to four times daily
	Cetiprin	200 mg t.d.s.
Urgency	Ephedrine	15 mg once to three times daily
Infection	Appropriate antibiotic	

Constipation

This is a very frequent symptom in multiple sclerosis. The measures which may be helpful are shown in Table 10.47.

Table 10.47   Measures to help constipation

- High fibre diet (fruit, leafy vegetables)
- Bran products
- Stool softener – liquid paraffin

Stimulant laxatives are best avoided because of associated colic.

Impotence

This is commonest in the male, but frigidity may occur in the female because of a loss of sexual sensation. Testosterone is useless, and there is no other specific treatment.

A trained sex counsellor may help the relationship.

Trigeminal neuralgia

This is a rare complication of multiple sclerosis. The treatment available is shown in Table 10.48.

Table 10.48   Treatment for trigeminal neuralgia

- Phenytoin   – 100 mg t.d.s.
- Carbamazepine   – 200 mg t.d.s.
- Neurosurgery   – Alcohol injection
                    Trigeminal nerve section

Specific treatment

The only specific treatment which has so far stood the test of time is *steroid therapy*.

The only indication for effective steroid treatment is an acute relapse of multiple sclerosis. It is of no value in long term prophylaxis.

In the United Kingdom, most experience has been obtained from adreno-corticotrophic hormone. The treatment schedule is shown in Table 10.49. The short term side-effects are shown in Table 10.50.

Table 10.49 ACTH treatment in multiple sclerosis

First week	– 60 units daily
Second week	– 40 units daily
Third week	– 20 units daily

Table 10.50 Short term side effects of ACTH

• Fluid retention	– weight gain
	oedema
	hypertension
• Hypokalaemia	
• Hyperglycaemia	
• Mental disturbance	

Daily weighing is very helpful in detecting fluid retention.

Because hypokalaemia is so common, prophylactic administration of a potassium-retaining diuretic, such as amiloride or triamterene is desirable.

PREGNANCY

Multiple sclerosis is not a complete bar to pregnancy.

There may be a slightly increased risk of relapse but the long term prognosis is unaffected.

There is a slightly increased risk of multiple sclerosis in the offspring.

A large family is undesirable owing to the difficulty in the mother coping.

SURGERY

If surgery is required, the slight risk of relapse should not influence the decision.

NATURAL HISTORY OF MULTIPLE SCLEROSIS

The prevalence in the United Kingdom is about 50/100 000 population. This means four or five cases in a group practice of four GPs or one case per GP.

Migration from an area of different incidence of the disease will only alter the risk if the migration occurs in childhood.

The average duration of life from onset is 20 years.

Overall mortality is about 25% in 25 years; the distribution of those deaths is shown in Table 10.51.

Table 10.51 Mortality in multiple sclerosis

- 1% die within 5 years
- 5% die within 10 years
- 8% die within 15 years
- 11% die within 25 years

Seventy per cent of patients will improve after the initial event. With the passage of time, however, recovery after the relapse becomes less complete and the disease pursues a steady downhill course.

About 50% of the patients will be able to carry out their domestic and work commitments 10 years after the onset. This number reduces to 25% after 20 years.

The features which help in assessing prognosis are shown in Table 10.52.

Table 10.52 Prognostic features in multiple sclerosis

• Good prognosis	– Onset younger than 40 years of age Onset with sensory symptoms or retrobulbar neuritis Long interval between 1st and 2nd attack Infrequent relapses
• Bad prognosis	– Onset over 40 years of age Onset with brain stem involvement Less than 1 year between 1st and 2nd attack Frequent relapses

Seventy per cent of patients will have a benign course but 30%, usually older than 45 years at onset, will not improve between frequent and successive relapses. Factors which may trigger off a relapse are shown in Table 10.53.

The commonest causes of death are shown in Table 10.54.

Table 10.53 Factors causing relapses in multiple sclerosis

- Infection with pyrexia
- Emotional trauma
- Physical injury
- Pregnancy
- Surgical operation

Table 10.54 Commonest causes of death in multiple sclerosis

- Urinary tract infection
- Pneumonia
- Pressure sore with infection

CAN WE MODIFY THE NATURAL HISTORY?

The aetiology of multiple sclerosis is unknown. The theories which have been suggested are shown in Table 10.55.

Table 10.55 Aetiological theories in multiple sclerosis

- Familial predisposition
- Auto-immune disease
- Delayed sensitivity to virus infection
    e.g. measles
- Nutritional deficiency
    copper
    linoleic acid

Since the aetiology is unknown, there is as yet no effective means of preventing or delaying the onset of the disease in the United Kingdom.

While steroids are of value in treating an acute relapse, they have no effect on the long term prognosis.

USEFUL PRACTICAL POINTS

- Neurological involvement of the optic nerve, brain stem and spinal cord make multiple sclerosis a very likely diagnosis.
  Remissions and exacerbations make the diagnosis certain.

- If the patient presents with retrobulbar neuritis or sensory symptoms, the prognosis is good.

- An onset after 45 years of age, especially with brain stem involvement, indicates a very poor prognosis.

- The most helpful investigation in multiple sclerosis is c.s.f. analysis, which shows a mild lymphocytosis, a slight increase in protein, especially γ-globulin, and a paretic type of Lange curve.

- The only specific treatment available is a course of steroids, and it is effective only in dealing with an acute relapse of the disease (including retrobulbar neuritis).

11

Brain failure

PRESENT HISTORY

A 58-year-old company director presented with a year's history of increasing forgetfulness and alteration in behaviour.

The patient himself had been reluctant to attend the doctor as he maintained that there was nothing really wrong with him. It was only after the continued insistence of his wife that he agreed to come.

He was accompanied by his wife and the details of the history were obtained mainly from her.

Behaviour at business

His altered behaviour had first manifested itself in his work. His wife had learned the details from his fellow director and close friend who had become increasingly concerned about the patient's work.

The patient and his friend had established a small light-engineering business about 20 years ago and had been steadily more successful. Both men had devoted a lot of time to the business and they had worked very well together in building the business up.

Over the last year or so, however, he had been *losing interest* in the business. He had become increasingly *forgetful* and as a result had missed some important appointments which had resulted in loss of orders for the firm. His letters to clients had also been vague, imprecise and unduly repetitious. He had become *unpunctual* in attending the office which was very unlike his previous meticulous time-keeping. He was tending to misplace files and make serious errors in dealing with accounts.

When confronted with these problems, the patient was reluctant to accept that he was doing anything wrong and would explain the difficulty by blaming the expansion of business and the increasing work load. He would admit, however, that he was getting a bit more forgetful and put it down to his age.

Altogether, his fellow director felt that the patient seemed not to care very much about the problems or even about the business itself.

Behaviour at home

His wife was very concerned about the way her husband had changed in the past year.

He had become *untidy* in his dress and appearance and didn't seem to worry about the way he looked. He sometimes forgot to shave, didn't seem to bother very much about having a regular bath and would wear a dirty shirt for several days if it was not spotted by his wife.

His *memory had become poor*. He would forget to carry out tasks he had promised to do and when reminded would deny he had ever been asked. He had become subject to *outbursts of anger* especially if challenged about jobs he had forgotten to do.

Marital disharmony

The change in the patient's behaviour had imposed severe strains on the marriage.

His wife had been further upset by his recent and totally unfounded accusation by her husband that she was having an affair with the fellow director.

The patient had also lost all interest in sexual relations, a part of their marriage which had been satisfactory for many years.

Driving difficulties

The patient's driving ability had been deteriorating steadily over the past year.

He had a spate of minor accidents. He seemed to have difficulty in parking the car when they went shopping. On several occasions, he appeared confused on driving along a familiar route and had lost his way.

Other relevant facts on direct enquiry

Nervous system

He denied headache.
There had been no deterioration in his vision.
He had no limb weakness or paraesthesiae.

Cardiovascular system

He had no angina.
There was no calf or thigh pain on walking.

Respiratory system

He had no recent cough or sputum, and in particular had not coughed up blood.

Alimentary system

There was no recent indigestion.
There was no recent change in bowel habits.
The weight was steady.

Urinary system

There was no recent frequency, dysuria or haematuria.

PAST HISTORY

He had not suffered a head injury prior to the change in his behaviour.
There had been no past history of liver or kidney disease.
He had not had arthritis.
He had no previous psychiatric disorder.

FAMILY HISTORY

The patient's younger sister, aged 52 years, had suffered with 'mental trouble' for some years. Although neither the patient nor his wife knew the precise nature of the mental problem, they did know that her memory had become very poor.

The patient's grandfather had died in a mental institution which he had entered at the age of 50 years.

PERSONAL HISTORY

The patient had never been a heavy drinker, and only took alcohol on social occasions, perhaps once every 1 or 2 months.
He did not smoke.

DRUG HISTORY

He was not having any regular medication.

CLINICAL EXAMINATION

Physical assessment

General

There was no arcus senilis or xanthelasma.
He did not look myxoedematous.
Temporal artery pulsation was normal.
There was no facial rash.
He was not anaemic.
He did not have an atrophic glossitis.
There were no spider naevi, liver palms, finger clubbing or white nails.

Cardiovascular system

The pulse rate was normal.
The radial and brachial arteries were not thickened.
The blood pressure was 150/90.
The heart sounds were normal.
The peripheral pulses in the feet were normal.

Respiratory system

There were no enlarged axillary or neck glands.
   Chest examination was normal and in particular there were no focal abnormalities in the lungs.

Abdomen

The liver and spleen were not enlarged.
There were no masses.
The superficial veins were not dilated and ascites was not present.

Nervous system

There were no carotid artery or intracranial murmurs.
   The fundi were normal with no evidence of papilloedema.
   The only abnormality in the cranial nerves was a rather *halting speech disturbance* in which the patient appeared to have difficulty in finding the right word.
   Muscle power and reflexes were normal with normal plantar responses.
   There was no sensory abnormality.
   Cerebellar coordination tests (finger–nose and heel–knee) were normal.

Mental assessment

This assessment was based on a systematic psychological approach (Table 11.1).

General

Attitude
He seemed unconcerned about his problems and tried to deny them.

Attentiveness
His attention would repeatedly wander.

Mood
He was amiable, friendly and cooperative but his attention had to be brought back repeatedly to the discussion.

Table 11.1 Approach to psychological assessment of the patient

• General	• Attitude
	• Attentiveness
	• Mood
	• Dress
• Insight	
• Orientation	• Place
	• Time
• Memory	• Remote
	• Recent
	• Immediate
• Reasoning	• Calculation
	• Logical
	• Abstract
• Speech function	• Sensory
	• Motor

Dress

There was nothing remarkable about his dress or appearance at the consultation. However, his wife said that she had asked him to bathe, shave and put on a clean shirt as she was sure he would have done none of these things if she had not insisted.

Insight

He appeared to have very little insight into the problems of his work and marriage. He consistently denied that there was anything wrong and said that his wife was exaggerating.

Orientation

Personal
He knew his name and address and the nature of his work. He knew that he was married.

Place
He knew he was seeing a doctor but could not remember whether he or his wife had driven to the doctor.

Time
He was unable to state the day or the date, but knew the month and year.

Memory

Remote
He had no difficulty recalling remote events. He knew his mother's maiden

name and the year he married. He could remember the names of his two children and their ages but could not recall their actual birthdays. He remembered the name of the Queen and all her children.

Recent
He could not remember what he had for breakfast that day. Nor could he recall the news headlines though he had looked at the newspaper.

Immediate
He was unable to remember the doctor's name and address after 5 minutes though he repeated them correctly immediately after he was given them.

Reasoning

Calculation
He had difficulty with simple addition and subtraction. This was most evident with sequential subtraction of 7 from 100.

Logical
When asked to explain relationships between members of a family, e.g. uncle, niece, great-grandfather, he became confused.

Abstract
His performance was worst in this aspect. He was quite unable to explain the meaning of simple proverbs like 'too many cooks spoil the broth' or 'a stitch in time saves nine'.

Speech

Difficulty in speech was a notable feature.

His sentences tended to be hesitant and faltering as if he had to stop and search for words. Occasionally he would abandon the sentence before it was finished and start another one.

He had no difficulty in responding to simple verbal requests to carry out an action, e.g. 'put out your tongue'.

He was asked to name common objects such as a comb, pen, wrist watch, key. He had some difficulty with the names but was able to describe the use without any difficulty.

ANALYSIS OF THE HISTORY

The important symptoms in the history are shown in Table 11.3.

The symptoms indicate memory loss and intellectual deterioration in a patient with normal level of consciousness. Conditions which may cause deterioration of intellect with unimpaired consciousness are shown in Table

The first requirement is to distinguish *pseudo-dementia* from *true dementia* since some of the conditions leading to pseudo-dementia may be reversible while true primary dementia is quite irreversible.

356

Table 11.2   Summary of patient's symptoms

• Work	– Loss of interest
	Forgetfulness
	Unpunctuality
	Difficulty with accounts
• Home	– Untidyness in dress
	Deteriorating personal hygiene
	Forgetfulness
	False accusations of wife's infidelity
	Quick temper
	Loss of libido
• Driving	– Deteriorating skill
	Loss of sense of direction
	Difficulty in parking

Table 11.3   Causes of deteriorating intellect with normal consciousness

- Dementia due to primary cerebral degeneration
- Pseudo-dementia due to other organic disease
- Pseudo-dementia due to drugs
- Psychiatric disorder • Depression
  - Obsessive–compulsive states
  - Schizophrenia
  - Mental subnormality

Pseudo-dementia due to organic disease

Some points which may help to differentiate pseudo-dementia from true dementia are shown in Table 11.4.

Table 11.4   Differentiation between pseudo-dementia and true dementia

	Pseudo-dementia	True dementia
Onset	Short and abrupt	Long and insidious
Attitude	Inattentive	Facile
	Distressed	Unconcerned
Learning ability	Good	Poor
Memory	Complains of memory loss	Does not complain of memory loss
Affective disturbance	Anxiety/depression	Very little
Mental testing	Variable performance	Consistently poor

The types of organic disease causing pseudo-dementia are shown in Table 11.5.

Table 11.5   Organic disease causing pseudo-dementia

- Cerebral
    - Inflammatory   – Neurosyphilis
                                      Giant-cell arteritis
                                      SLE
                                      Associated with carcinoma
                                      Multifocal leukoencephalopathy
    - Space-occupying   – Tumour
                                      Subdural haematoma
    - Hydrocephalus
- Systemic disease • Hypothyroidism
    - Vitamin B_{12} deficiency
    - Hypocalcaemia
    - Porphyria
    - Hepatic failure
    - Chronic renal failure
    - Malabsorption
    - Chronic hypoglycaemia
    - Alcoholism

Cerebral inflammation

Neurosyphilis
Dementia occurs in general paralysis of the insane (GPI).

The dementia is due to degeneration of the cortical neurones caused by endarteritis obliterans. The clinical features of the condition are shown in Table 11.6.

Table 11.6   Clinical features of GPI

- Progressive dementia – delusions of grandeur
- Tremor of the tongue and hands
- Unsteadiness
- Transient focal cerebral upsets
    - Hemiplegia
    - Hemianopia
    - Dysphasia
- Epileptic fits

The patient had no delusions of grandeur, no focal cerebral symptoms and no fits, which makes the diagnosis very unlikely.

Giant-cell arteritis (temporal arteritis)
The dementia is due to a generalized arteritis of the cerebral vessels. The symptoms are shown in Figure 11.1.

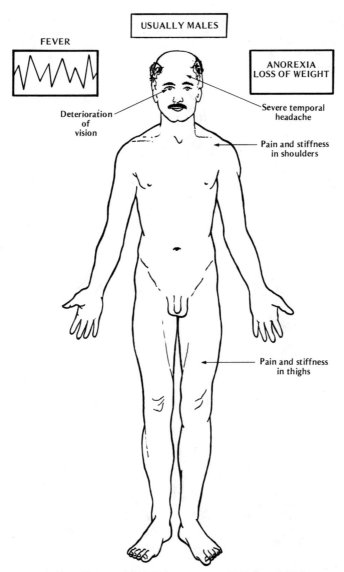

Figure 11.1 Symptoms of giant cell arteritis

The patient had no headache, muscle pain, visual disturbance, or weight loss, which excludes giant-cell arteritis.

Systemic lupus erythematosus (SLE)
The dementia is probably due to widespread micro-infarcts in the cerebral circulation. The symptoms occurring in SLE are shown in Figure 11.2.

359

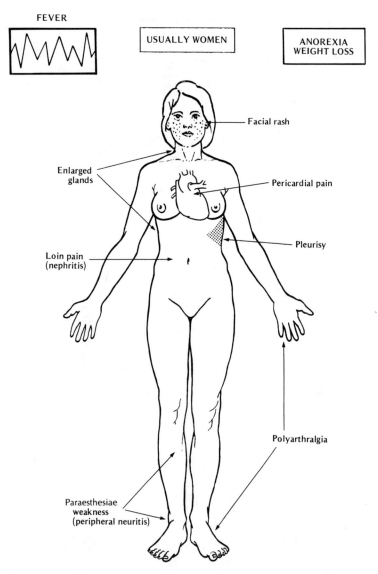

Figure 11.2   Symptoms in systemic lupus erythematosus

The absence of joint pains, pleurisy, pericarditic pain, enlarged glands and limb paraesthesiae or weakness excludes this diagnosis.

Carcinoma
The cause of the dementia associated with carcinoma is a diffuse non-metastatic involvement of the cerebral cortex by subacute encephalomyelitis.

The precise mechanism is unknown. The condition occurs with several types of carcinoma (Figure 11.3).

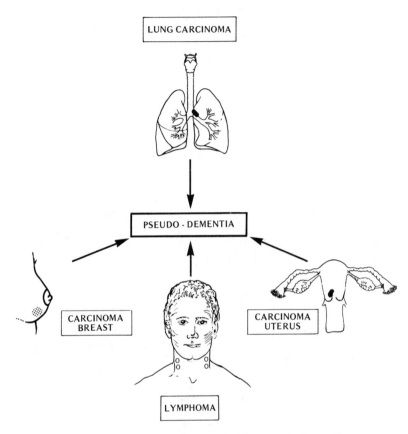

Figure 11.3 Neoplasms associated with pseudodementia

There were no symptoms referable to the lungs and no gland enlargement, which makes carcinoma unlikely in the patient. Further investigation is necessary to exclude these diagnoses with more certainty.

Multifocal leukoencephalopathy (MLE)

This is a rare disorder which occurs with other conditions (Table 11.7). The cause of the dementing process is widespread demyelination producing destructive foci throughout the cerebral cortex. As well as dementia, focal neurological disturbances occur (Table 11.8).

361

Table 11.7 Conditions associated with multifocal leukoencephalopathy

- Myeloproliferative disease
- Lymphoproliferative disease
- Tuberculosis
- Sarcoidosis

Table 11.8 Focal neurological disturbances in MLE

- Hemiparesis
- Visual field defects
- Dysarthria
- Ataxia

Although the patient had a speech defect, he had no limb weakness, visual impairment or unsteadiness, which makes the condition unlikely. Even more important, however, in excluding this diagnosis is that death occurs almost invariably within 6 months of the onset of the dementia.

Cerebral space-occupying lesions

Brain tumour
The typical triad of symptoms of brain tumour are shown in Table 11.9. The tumours which affect mental function early to cause pseudo-dementia are shown in Table 11.10.

Table 11.9 Symptoms of brain tumour

- Headache
- Vomiting
- Fits

Table 11.10 Brain tumours leading to early impairment of mental function

- Corpus callosum
- Right temporal lobe
- Frontal lobe

As the patient had no headache vomiting or fits, brain tumour is excluded as a cause of his dementia.

Subdural haematoma

The clinical features are shown in Table 11.11.

Table 11.11 Clinical features of subdural haematoma

- History of head injury
- General
  - Headache
  - Giddiness
  - Drowsiness
  - Slowness of thought
- Focal
  - Fits
  - Hemiplegia
  - Hemianaesthesia
  - Homonymous hemianopia

There was no history of head injury, though this may be absent or too trivial to have been noticed.

The absence of headache, drowsiness and focal neurological symptoms make subdural haematoma unlikely in this patient.

Hydrocephalus

Progressive deterioration of intellectual function can result from 'normal-pressure hydrocephalus'. In this condition, the formation of cerebrospinal fluid has reached equilibrium with its resorption, although a pressure gradient still exists between the intraventricular cavity and the subarachnoid space. The conditions which may lead to this type of hydrocephalus are shown in Table 11.12. In one third of the patients, however, the cause is unknown.

There is a characteristic triad of symptoms in this condition (Table 11.13).

Table 11.12 Conditions causing 'normal-pressure' hydrocephalus

- Subarachnoid haemorrhage
- Meningitis
  - tuberculous
  - syphilitic
  - pyogenic
- Paget's disease at base of skull

Table 11.13 Symptoms of 'normal-pressure' hydrocephalus

- Impairment of mental function
- Slowly progressive gait disorder
- Urinary and faecal incontinence

The abnormality of mental function is reversible with shunting operations to relieve the hydrocephalus.

The patient did not have any disturbance of his walking and was quite continent, which excludes this condition.

Systemic disease causing pseudo-dementia

Hypothyroidism ('myxoedema madness')

This is a very important cause of dementia since the mental disturbance is entirely reversible. The typical symptoms are shown in Table 11.14.

None was evident in the patient.

Table 11.14 Symptoms of hypothyroidism

• Increasing weight
• Physical and mental slowing
• Cold intolerance
• Increasing constipation
• Hoarseness of voice

Vitamin B$_{12}$ deficiency

This is another important cause of pseudo-dementia because of its reversibility. The intellectual deterioration which occurs is due to degeneration of the central white matter in the brain following vitamin B$_{12}$ deficiency. The symptoms are shown in Table 11.15.

Table 11.15 Symptoms of vitamin B$_{12}$ deficiency

• Anaemia	– Breathlessness
	Palpitations
	Excessive tiredness
	Dizziness
	Ankle swelling
• Polyneuritis	– Paraesthesiae in limbs
• Spinal cord	– Weakness of legs
degeneration	Unsteadiness

The patient did not have any symptoms of anaemia, paraesthesiae, limb weakness or unsteadiness on standing or walking. There is therefore no symptomatic evidence of vitamin B$_{12}$ deficiency to account for the patient's mental deterioration.

Hypocalcaemia

The mental abnormality is probably due to the lack of the calcium which is essential for normal function of central, as well as peripheral, nerve tissue. The clinical features are shown in Figure 11.4.

Apart from intellectual deterioration, the patient had none of these symptoms.

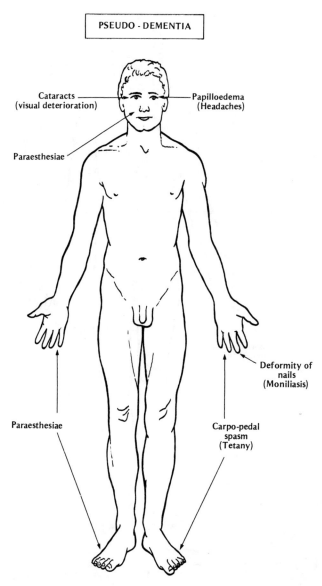

Figure 11.4   Clinical features of hypocalcaemia

365

Porphyria

Severe mental disturbance occurs in acute intermittent porphyria, the features of which are shown in Figure 11.5. The absence of abdominal colic, paraesthesiae, limb weakness and fits excludes this diagnosis.

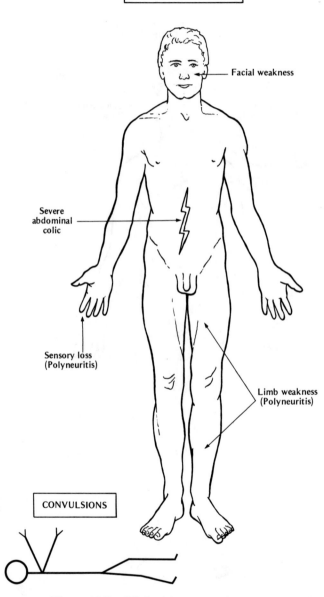

Figure 11.5   Clinical features of acute porphyria

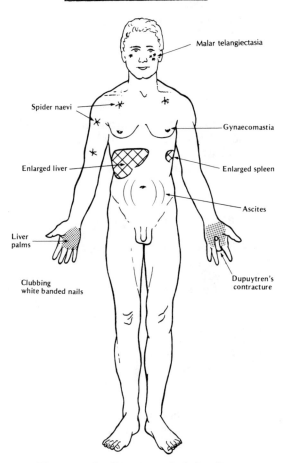

HISTORY OF ALCOHOLISM

Malar telangiectasia

Spider naevi

Gynaecomastia

Enlarged liver

Enlarged spleen

Ascites

Liver palms

Dupuytren's contracture

Clubbing white banded nails

Figure 11.6 Features of cirrhosis

Hepatic failure

Hepatic encephalopathy can cause mental dullness, apathy and confusion. If it persists for months, a mild dementia may ensue. The other manifestations of chronic hepatic encephalopathy are shown in Table 11.16.

Hepatic encephalopathy occurs in patients with cirrhosis, the features of which are shown in Figure 11.6. There was no evidence of cirrhosis or hepatic encephalopathy in the patient.

Uraemic encephalopathy

Cerebral symptoms manifesting in confusion and stupor can occur episodically in chronic renal failure or only when chronic haemodialysis is established.

367

Table 11.16 Manifestations of chronic hepatic encephalopathy

> - Mild dementia
> - Grimacing
> - Speech difficulty
> - Tremor
> - Unsteady gait
> - Choreo-athetotic movements

The mechanism remains uncertain in chronic renal failure but may be due to the effects of retention of organic acid and phosphate on the brain.

In chronic haemodialysis the cause of the encephalopathy has been established: it is due to the aluminium used in the water for dialysis.

The features of chronic renal failure are shown in Table 11.17.

Table 11.17 Features of chronic renal failure

> - Past history of kidney disease
> - Polyuria
> - Polydipsia
> - Loss of energy
> - Gastrointestinal   – nausea and vomiting
>   – diarrhoea
> - Hiccoughs
> - Twitching
> - Bleeding tendency
> - Polyneuritis

The absence of a past history of renal disease and the lack of urinary symptoms, vomiting and diarrhoea, twitching, hiccoughs, bleeding and paraesthesiae all serve to exclude uraemia as the cause of the mental deterioration in the patient.

Malabsorption

Chronic malabsorption can lead to mental changes caused by deficiency of proteins and vitamins.

The distinctive symptom in malabsorption is diarrhoea accompanied by large pale offensive stools which float and are difficult to flush away.

The absence of diarrhoea and abnormal stools excludes this diagnosis.

Chronic hypoglycaemia

This is a rare condition which leads to gradual deterioration of intellectual function. The causes of chronic hypoglycaemia are shown in Table 11.18 and are associated with the excess production of insulin or insulin-like substance. The only condition which is potentially reversible is islet cell tumour of the pancreas.

Table 11.18 Causes of chronic hypoglycaemia

- Islet cell tumour of the pancreas
- Carcinoma of the stomach
- Carcinoma of caecum
- Hepatoma
- Fibrous mesothelioma

Chronic hypoglycaemia is difficult to diagnose as a cause of dementia because the other typical symptoms of acute hypoglycaemia are minimal or absent (Table 11.19). Accurate diagnosis requires the measurement of blood sugar and insulin-like activity in the blood.

Table 11.19 Symptoms of hypoglycaemia

- Sweating
- Palpitations
- Tremor
- Weakness
- Dizziness
- Headache
- Feeling of hunger

It is not possible therefore to exclude the diagnosis in this patient on history alone.

Alcoholism

An *alcoholic* is an excessive drinker whose drinking impairs his health and interferes with his work or marriage and who is unable to stop.

The diagnostic clues which may help in the diagnosis are shown in Table 11.20. The main neuropsychiatric complications of alcoholism are shown in Table 11.21. There are many associated physical disorders (Figure 11.7).

Table 11.20 Diagnostic clues in alcoholism

- Family history of alcoholism
- Occupational hazard — Drink or catering trades
  Business executive
  Seamen
  Commercial travellers
  Doctors, actors, entertainers
- History of accidents
- Work problems — Declining efficiency
  Unpunctuality
  Extended meal breaks
- Marital problems
- Recurrent depression
- Attempted suicide

Table 11.21 Neuropsychiatric complications of alcoholism

• Korsakow's psychosis	– Memory poor for recent events Invention (confabulation)
• Wernicke's encephalopathy	– Difficulty in concentration Slowness of thought and speech Ophthalmoplegia Diplopia and nystagmus Disturbed balance Impaired walking

• Delirium tremens	– Clouded consciousness
	Disorientation in time and place
	Poor recent memory
	Perceptual disturbance
	Hallucinations
	Severe agitation
	Gross tremor
	Autonomic
	    fever
	    sweating
	    tachycardia

The patient drank very little alcohol which excludes this diagnosis.

Pseudo-dementia due to drugs

The chronic use of drugs, especially in the elderly, may produce a confused or depressed patient who might be mistaken for a patient with early dementia. The drugs which are associated with this condition most frequently are shown in Table 11.22.

Table 11.22 Drugs causing mental impairment

• Depression	• Reserpine
	• Methyldopa
• Confusion	• Digoxin
	• Barbiturates
	• Anti-Parkinsonian drugs
	• Tricyclic antidepressants
	• Phenothiazines
	• Anticonvulsants
	• Night sedatives

The reasons for drug toxicity in the elderly are shown in Table 11.23. The patient had not taken any of the drugs listed in Table 11.22.

Table 11.23 Drug toxicity in the elderly

- Reduced renal function
- Reduced protein binding (low serum albumin)
- Impaired detoxication in the liver

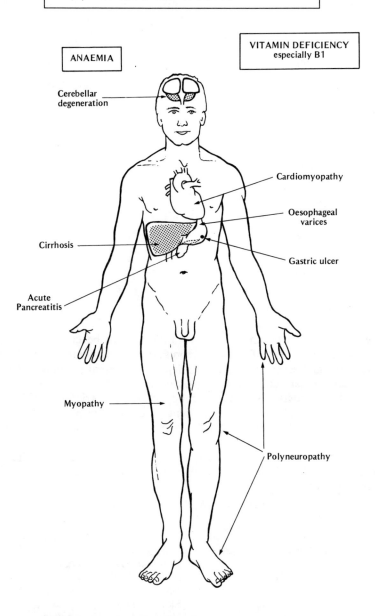

ANAEMIA

VITAMIN DEFICIENCY
especially B1

Cerebellar
degeneration

Cardiomyopathy

Oesophageal
varices

Cirrhosis

Gastric ulcer

Acute
Pancreatitis

Myopathy

Polyneuropathy

Figure 11.7 Physical manifestations of alcoholism

Pseudo-dementia due to psychiatric disease

Depression

This is the most frequent and most difficult psychiatric disorder to distinguish from true dementia, since poor concentration, forgetfulness and apathy in a severely depressed patient may closely simulate dementia. Some of the points which may help in the differentiation are shown in Table 11.24.

Table 11.24 Differentiation between depression and dementia

Depression	Dementia

Self-depreciation
    hopelessness
    unworthiness
    guilt
	No self-depreciation

Abnormality of mood	Abnormality of intellect
Emotional blunting early	Emotional blunting late
No focal neurological signs	Focal signs may occur

Somatic symptoms
    insomnia
    early waking
    anorexia
    weight loss
    constipation
    lack of energy	

Antidepressants improve	Antidepressants ineffective

The distinction between the two conditions may be confounded by the occasional development of a severe depression in a demented patient. Unless the previous intellectual ability of the depressed patient is known, it may be very difficult to distinguish the two conditions.

If real doubt exists, the most useful approach is a trial of antidepressive treatment (Table 11.25). If the patient is depressed he should improve significantly, but the treatment will have no effect on a purely demented patient.

Severe depression is a very unlikely diagnosis in this patient since he had no symptoms of self-depreciation and none of the typical somatic symptoms of a depressed patient.

Table 11.25 Antidepressive drugs

Drug	Dose
Amitriptyline (Tryptizol)	Start 30–75 mg daily Maintain 50–100 mg daily
Imipramine (Tofranil)	Start 30–75 mg daily Maintain up to 300 mg daily
Dothiepin (Prothiaden)	Start 75 mg daily Maintain up to 150 mg daily

Obsessive–compulsive neurosis

This is a condition dominated by obsessions and compulsions. Patients are obsessed by imperative and distressing thoughts and impulses which lead to compulsive ritualistic acts and behaviour, and they are powerless to control such acts.

The confusion which may arise with dementia is that after the neurosis has persisted for a long time, the patient becomes chronically depressed by his inability to control his troublesome thoughts and he then becomes apathetic and loses all interest in life.

The most helpful differentiating factor in distinguishing this type of neurosis from dementia is that the neurotic patient retains insight into his condition while the dement loses his insight.

The lack of obsessive thoughts and behaviour in the patient together with the loss of insight excludes neurosis and points to dementia.

Schizophrenia

A chronic schizophrenic may manifest:

- emotional blunting
- lack of drive
- self-neglect
- social withdrawal.

In these circumstances confusion with dementia is understandable. Some helpful differentiating factors are shown in Table 11.26.

Table 11.26 Differentiation between schizophrenia and dementia

	Schizophrenia	Dementia
Onset	young	middle-age or elderly
Delusions	frequent	rare
Hallucinations	frequent	never
Memory	unaffected	always impaired
Thought-broadcasting	frequent	never

The patient's age, the absence of hallucinations and thought-broadcasting and the deterioration of memory all exclude schizophrenia.

Mental subnormality

Though mental subnormality is not strictly a psychiatric disorder, a mentally subnormal individual who cannot cope with life may simulate a demented patient.

The most helpful distinguishing feature is the lack of memory loss, especially for recent events, in the mentally abnormal patient. Another helpful approach is to follow the patient up, to see whether further and progressive mental deterioration occurs. This would be expected in the demented patient but not in the retarded patient.

There was nothing to suggest mental abnormality in this patient who, up to 1 year before, had led an active intellectual life.

Primary dementia

A number of conditions directly cause cerebral degeneration leading to dementia (Table 11.27).

Table 11.27 Causes of primary cerebral degeneration with dementia

- Multiple cerebral infarcts
- Parkinson's disease
- Pick's disease
- Huntington's chorea
- Jakob–Creutzfeld disease
- Wilson's disease
- 'Punch-drunk' syndrome
- Multiple sclerosis
- Chronic epilepsy
- Alzheimer's disease

Multi-infarct dementia

This results from cerebral arteriosclerosis and occurs in older patients. It accounts for 15% of all patients with dementia encountered in practice.

The condition progresses in a *stepwise* fashion with repeated episodes of cerebral infarction leading to recurrent focal neurological disturbances.

The history of repeated slight strokes is the most helpful factor in diagnosing multiple infarcts as the cause of the dementia.

Another helpful diagnostic feature in these patients is the presence of associated clinical conditions attributable to arteriosclerosis (Figure 11.8).

The clues to the diagnosis of multi-infarct dementia are summarized in Table 11.28.

Table 11.28 Clues to diagnosis of multi-infarct dementia

- Abrupt onset
- Fluctuating course
- History of strokes
- Evidence of atheroma
- Focal neurological signs

There was no past history of repeated small strokes or a heart attack, and no current angina, claudication or 'mesenteric angina' in the patient, thus excluding this diagnosis.

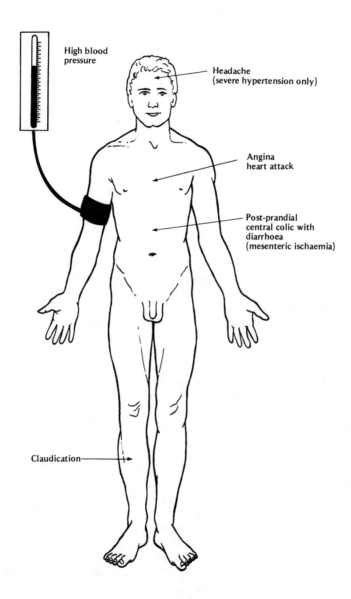

High blood pressure

Headache (severe hypertension only)

Angina heart attack

Post-prandial central colic with diarrhoea (mesenteric ischaemia)

Claudication

Figure 11.8 Symptoms of arteriosclerotic conditions associated with multi-infarct dementia

Parkinson's disease

Dementia occurs ultimately in up to 30% of patients with Parkinson's disease. The typical features of Parkinson's disease are shown in Table 11.29.

Table 11.29   Features of Parkinsonism

• Rigidity	– Expressionless face Immobility of limbs Lack of arm swinging in walking
• Tremor	– Head and limbs
• Slow movement	– Difficulty in talking Difficulty in getting up Short shuffling steps

The patient had no difficulty in standing up or walking and no tremor of the head or limbs, which excludes Parkinson's disease.

Pick's disease

In this degenerative disease the cerebral atrophy is confined predominantly to the frontal lobes, but may sometimes affect the temporal lobes.

It may be difficult to distinguish from the more generalized cerebral atrophy of Alzheimer's disease which will be discussed in more detail subsequently. Some of the features which may help in this differentiation are shown in Table 11.30.

Table 11.30   Differentiation between Pick's disease and Alzheimer's disease

	Pick's disease	*Alzheimer's disease*
Mood	Apathetic Indifferent	Irritable Bad-tempered
Focal neurological deficit	Early	Late
Memory	Fair	Poor
Orientation	Fair	Poor
Speech disorder	Prominent	Minor
Other	Fatuous euphoria Grasp and sucking reflex	

The absence of the typical fatuous euphoria of frontal lobe involvement and the lack of any focal neurological manifestations, especially temporal lobe (Table 11.31), are against the diagnosis of Pick's disease.

Table 11.31 Manifestations of temporal lobe involvement

- Visual and auditory hallucinations
- Partial complex seizures, e.g. *déjà-vu*
- Homonymous quadrantanopia

Huntington's chorea

The features are shown in Table 11.32.

Table 11.32 Features of Huntington's chorea

- Positive family history of condition
- Age 30–45 years
- Jerking involuntary movements arms and legs
- Gradual dementia

Although the patient does have a family history of mental disorder, the late age of onset and the absence of involuntary movements excludes this diagnosis.

Jakob–Creutzfeld disease

This is a rare condition which is thought to be caused by a slow virus. The features are shown in Table 11.33.

Table 11.33 Features of Jakob–Creutzfeld disease

- Progressive dementia
- Cerebellar ataxia
- Spastic paraplegia
- Dysarthria
- Choreo-athetosis
- Cog-wheel rigidity
- Extrapyramidal tremor
- Myoclonic twitches

The lack of difficulty in walking and the absence of involuntary movements excludes this diagnosis in the patient.

Wilson's disease (hepatolenticular degeneration)

This disease is due to an abnormality of copper metabolism which results in deposition of copper in various organs (Figure 11.9).

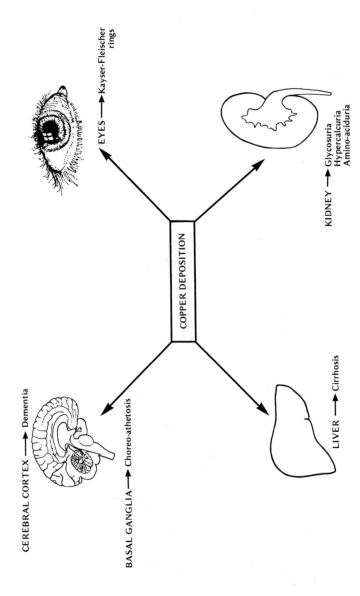

Figure 11.9 Clinical effects of copper deposition in Wilson's disease

The absence of any manifestations of cirrhosis (see Figure 11.6) and the lack of any involuntary movements make this diagnosis very unlikely, but examination of the eyes for Kayser–Fleischer rings and a serum copper estimation are necessary to exclude the diagnosis with certainty.

'Punch-drunk' syndrome

This is due to cerebral atrophy as a result of repeated blows to the brain in boxers. The features are shown in Table 11.34.

Table 11.34   Features of punch-drunk syndrome

• History of professional boxing
• Dementia

• Disorder of movement   – broad-based
                              shuffling
                              unsteady

• Parkinsonism   – slow movement
                              tremor
                              cog-wheel rigidity

As the patient had never been a boxer, this diagnosis is irrelevant.

Multiple sclerosis

Dementia is occasionally an early manifestation of multiple sclerosis.

The diagnosis is made by a history of focal neurological symptoms disseminated in time and space (through the central nervous system), especially optic neuritis. The patient had no previous neurological episodes which might suggest multiple sclerosis.

Chronic epilepsy

The personality change which may develop in chronic epileptics is attributable to several factors:

(1)   Social disadvantages of a disabling restrictive condition.
(2)   Cerebral damage caused by repeated anoxia in tonic phase of grand mal epilepsy.

Table 11.35   Personality change in chronic epilepsy

• Irritability
• Depression
• Slowness of thought and action
• Failure of memory
• Deterioration of intellect

(3)   Effect of chronic anticonvulsant drugs.

The nature of the personality change is shown in Table 11.35 and may simulate dementia.

Since the patient was not an epileptic this diagnosis can be excluded.

Alzheimer's disease

This degenerative condition is the most frequent cause of primary dementia.

The distinction between presenile dementia, designated Alzheimer's disease, and senile dementia is false since Alzheimer's presenile dementia and senile dementia are clinically and pathologically indistinguishable.

The features are shown in Table 11.36.

Table 11.36   Features of Alzhelmer's
disease

- Familial incidence
- Late fifties or early sixties
- Insidious onset
- Loss of short term memory early
- Progressive decline in intellect
- Focal neurological disturbances late
- Death in 5–10 years

The patient's age, family history, insidious onset and memory loss for recent events point to the diagnosis of Alzheimer's disease.

Past history

There was no past history of psychiatric disorder, which makes depression unlikely.

There were no recurrent confusional episodes to suggest hypoglycaemia or porphyria.

There was no past history of liver disease or kidney disease.

Family history

The occurrence of mental disorder associated with loss of memory in his sister and grandfather are likely to be relevant.

A familial incidence has been shown in Alzheimer's disease.

A genetic background also exists for Huntington's chorea and Pick's disease.

CONCLUSIONS FROM THE HISTORY

The patient showed all the symptoms of an organic dementia:

- previous normal intelligence
- loss of memory
- progressive intellectual deterioration
- disorientation in time and place
- change in personality
- blunting of emotional response
- normal level of consciousness.

The likely diagnosis is Alzheimer's disease because:

- he is the right age
- he has a family history of mental disorder
- memory loss was a prominent symptom
- other conditions causing true dementia or pseudo-dementia have been excluded on the basis of the history.

ANALYSIS OF THE EXAMINATION

Physical examination

The analysis of the physical examination in the patient is concerned with excluding organic disease which might be associated with pseudo-dementia or true primary dementia.

General

The absence of arcus senilis and xanthelasma are against premature arteriosclerosis which might cause multi-infarct dementia.

He did not look myxoedematous, which is against the totally reversible 'myxoedema madness'.

He did not have the mask-like face of Parkinson's disease.

The absence of a 'butterfly' rash is against systemic lupus erythematosus.

The absence of anaemia and atrophic glossitis is against vitamin B_{12} deficiency, another reversible cause of pseudo-dementia.

The absence of spider naevi, liver palms, clubbing and white banded nails is against liver failure with encephalopathy.

The lack of any lymph node enlargement is against carcinoma or lymphoma which may be associated with multifocal leukoencephalopathy (MLE), a rare cause of pseudo-dementia.

Cardiovascular system

The normal temporal arteries exclude giant cell (cranial) arteritis.

The regular pulse excludes atrial fibrillation, a cause of multiple cerebral emboli leading to multi-infarct dementia.

There was no thickening of radial or brachial arteries to indicate arteriosclerosis.

The normal blood pressure is another factor against arteriosclerosis.

The absence of valvular heart disease excludes another potential site of cerebral emboli.

The normal peripheral pulses in the feet exclude significant peripheral arterial disease.

Respiratory system

The absence of finger clubbing, neck and/or axillary glands and focal signs in the lungs are against bronchial carcinoma leading to MLE or non-metastatic dementia.

Abdomen

The absence of distended abdominal wall veins, hepatosplenomegaly and ascites excludes cirrhosis with hepatic encephalopathy.

There were no masses to suggest intra-abdominal carcinoma or lymphoma – both causes of MLE.

Nervous system

The normal carotid arteries in the neck and absence of intracranial murmurs are against atherosclerotic intracranial disease which might cause multi-infarct dementia: the absence of focal neurological signs is also against this diagnosis.

There was no papilloedema to suggest an intracranial space-occupying lesion.

The speech disturbance can occur in Alzheimer's disease but also in other conditions such as multi-infarct dementia or Pick's disease. There was no grasp reflex to suggest frontal lobe involvement by Pick's disease.

The normal cerebellar function excludes Jakob–Creutzfeld disease where cerebellar ataxia is a prominent feature.

There was no evidence of peripheral neuritis which might suggest alcoholism.

The intact reflexes, joint sense and vibration sense exclude subacute combined degeneration of the spinal cord due to vitamin B_{12} deficiency.

The normal gait excludes Parkinson's disease.

The absence of involuntary movements such as chorea or myoclonic twitches is against Huntington's chorea, Wilson's disease and Jakob–Creutzfeld disease.

Mental examination

The main findings are summarized in Table 11.37.

The loss of insight, disorientation, loss of recent memory and deterioration in reasoning ability are characteristic of dementia.

Table 11.37 The patient's mental findings

• Loss of insight
• Orientation – Time: lost
Space (driving): lost
• Memory – Immediate: lost
Recent: lost
Remote: retained
• Reasoning – Calculation: lost
Logic: lost
Abstract: lost
• Speech impaired

CONCLUSIONS FROM THE EXAMINATION

- There were no findings to indicate any systemic organic disease which might lead to pseudo-dementia.

- In particular, there was no evidence of any of the conditions associated with reversibility of dementia (Table 11.38).

- The mental examination shows the characteristic features of dementia.

- The lack of any focal neurological signs (apart from a minimal speech disorder) makes the diagnosis of *Alzheimer's disease more likely* than the other primary degenerative conditions of the brain such as Pick's disease, Jakob–Creutzfeld disease and Huntington's chorea.

Table 11.38 Reversible causes of pseudo-dementia

• Systemic disease	• Vitamin B_{12} deficiency
	• Myxoedema
	• Systemic lupus erythematosus
	• Giant cell arteritis
	• Wilson's disease (possibly)
	• Chronic hypoglycaemia
	• Hepatic encephalopathy
	• Malabsorption
	• Renal dialysis
• Cerebral disease	• Hydrocephalus
	• Space-occupying lesion
	• Neurosyphilis (possibly)

INVESTIGATIONS

In a demented patient the main aims of investigation are:

- To diagnose early cases with a treatable cause.

- To avoid excessive investigation in those patients (the majority) for whom little help or treatment is available anyway.

- To confirm the diagnosis of irreversible cerebral atrophy in doubtful cases.

Necessary investigations

The investigations which are required in all patients with suspected dementia are shown in Table 11.39.

Table 11.39   Necessary investigations in all patients with suspected dementia

• Blood count	– Haemoglobin Packed cell volume Mean corpuscular volume
• Erythrocyte sedimentation rate	
• VDRL test	
• Thyroid function tests	
• X-ray	– Chest X-ray Skull X-ray
• Vitamin B_{12} blood level	

Blood count

Haemoglobin
This is to detect anaemia.
   The two conditions relevant to the diagnosis of dementia are: (1) vitamin B_{12} deficiency and (2) occult neoplasm.

Packed cell volume
This is to detect polycythaemia which may encourage multiple cerebral infarction leading to dementia.

Mean corpuscular volume
An increase indicates macrocytosis which may be associated with vitamin B_{12} deficiency.
   The patient's blood count was entirely normal.

Erythrocyte sedimentation rate (ESR)

An increased ESR is found in several conditions which may lead to dementia (Table 11.40).
   The patient's ESR was normal.

Table 11.40 Conditions with a raised ESR which lead to dementia

- Temporal arteritis
- Systemic lupus erythematosis
- Neoplasia   –   carcinoma
                         lymphoreticular
- Sarcoidosis   (multifocal leukoencephalopathy)
- Tuberculosis   (multifocal leukoencephalopathy)

Serological tests for syphilis

Wasserman reaction
This is now outdated.

VDRL test
This is the most widely-used test and is based on finding a non-specific reaginic antibody to syphilitic infection.

Specific treponemal antibody test
This is a more sensitive test for syphilis than the VDRL test.

The patient's blood VDRL and treponemal antibody tests were negative and c.s.f. analysis was therefore not considered necessary.

Thyroid function

This is an important test in all cases of dementia because 'myxoedema madness' is totally reversible.

The most helpful single measurement in diagnosing primary myxoedema is an increased level of thyroid-stimulating hormone (greater than 5 units). This is accompanied by a low serum thyroxine level in myxoedema.

The patient's thyroid function was normal.

Chest X-ray

The purpose of the chest X-ray is to detect carcinoma, either primary (Figure 11.10) or secondary (Figure 11.11). The patient's chest X-ray was normal.

Skull X-ray

The skull X-ray may show evidence of neoplasia (Table 11.41). The patient's skull X-ray was normal.

Table 11.41 Evidence of neoplasia in skull X-ray

- Pineal displacement
- Metastases in bone of skull
- Calcified tumour – meningioma
                        oligodendroglioma
- Erosion of clinoid processes by pituitary tumour

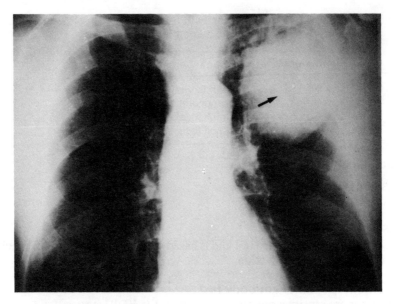

Figure 11.10   Chest X-ray showing primary carcinoma

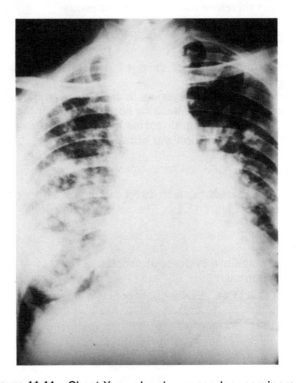

Figure 11.11   Chest X-ray showing secondary carcinoma

Serum B$_{12}$ level

Since the neurological complications of vitamin B$_{12}$ deficiency, including pseudo-dementia, may occur in the absence of anaemia, it is necessary to estimate the serum B$_{12}$ level in all patients.

It was normal in the patient.

Optional investigations

There are other investigations which may be helpful in individual patients but cannot be regarded as necessary in all patients (Table 11.42).

Table 11.42 Optional investigations in dementia

- Lumbar puncture
- Electroencephalogram
- CT scan
- Air encephalography
- Cerebral arteriography
- Isotope scan

Lumbar puncture

The value of this test is in showing neurosyphilis or carcinoma. The changes in neurosyphilis are shown in Table 11.43.

Table 11.43 Cerebrospinal fluid changes in neurosyphilis

- Raised protein
- Increased white cells
- Paretic Lange curve (4443332100)

There was no justification for lumbar puncture in the patient.

Electroencephalogram (e.e.g.)

The e.e.g. may show several possible abnormalities in demented patients (Table 11.44).

Table 11.44 Electroencephalogram changes in dementia

• Focal dysrhythmia	– non-specific
• Flattened waves	– Huntington's chorea
• Generally slow waves	– Alzheimer's disease

The patient's e.e.g. showed a diffuse slowing of both theta and delta waves consistent with Alzheimer's disease.

Computerized tomography (CT) scan

This is a valuable test in dementia in three ways:

- Confirmation of cerebral atrophy.
- It may show a focal lesion, subdural haematoma, brain tumour, or multiple infarcts.
- It may show hydrocephalus.

The presenile dementias are always associated with cortical atrophy.

Hydrocephalus is distinguished from cortical atrophy by the normal or reduced size of the subarachnoid space and the extension of oedema beyond the anterior horns of the lateral ventricles.

The patient's CT scan confirmed cortical atrophy consistent with Alzheimer's disease (Figure 11.12).

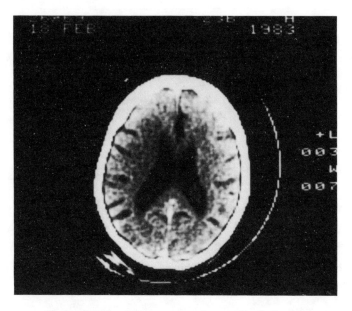

Figure 11.12 CT scan showing cortical atrophy

Air encephalogram

This is a test which can only be carried out if the intracranial pressure is normal as judged by the absence of symptoms (headache, vomiting, visual deterioration) and of papilloedema on examination. The value of the test in dementia is in confirming cerebral atrophy as shown by ventricular dilatation.

It is a painful test and may lead to the exacerbation of the dementia.

It is largely superseded by the CT scan.

Cerebral arteriography

This is a potentially hazardous test which is of little value in the diagnosis of dementia. It may show evidence of brain tumour.

Isotope scan

Intravenous radioactive technetium may show a focal vascular cerebral lesion such as a tumour, but is of very little diagnostic help in dementia.

Intraventricular isotopes may also be used to detect hydrocephalus.

An isotope scan was not considered necessary in the patient because of its limited value.

Other investigations

There are some other tests which may be useful in specific conditions (Table 11.45).

Table 11.45 Special tests in dementia

• Hypocalcaemia	– Serum calcium
• Hypoglycaemia	– Blood sugar
• Porphyria	– Urinary porphyrins
• Hepatic encephalopathy	– Liver function tests
	Blood ammonia level
• Renal failure	– Blood urea
	Serum creatinine
• Malabsorption	– Fat content of stool
	Glucose tolerance test
	Xylose excretion test
	Radiology
	Endoscopy and biopsy

MANAGEMENT OF DEMENTIA

Hospital assessment

It is desirable to admit all patients with suspected dementia to hospital initially for the following reasons.

- To diagnose primary irreversible dementia.

- To detect and initiate treatment of reversible dementia due to systemic or intracranial disease.

- To assess the degree of the patient's incapacity and the measures necessary to support him and his family at home.

Once it has been established that the patient has an untreatable progressive dementia, it is necessary to explain fully, simply and clearly to responsible members of his family the medical facts, prognosis and, most important, the support that can be offered initially at home and later in an institution if this becomes necessary.

General management of dementia

Work environment

In the early stages of dementia it might be possible for the patient to continue work at a reduced level, providing he can be spared unnecessary responsibility and can be protected from any injury which he might sustain as a result of his reduced mental ability.

It would be wise, however, to be prepared for early retirement which will inevitably follow.

Home environment

The important consideration here is to maintain as stable a home environment as possible with a regular unchanging daily structured routine. Some simple measures which may help are shown in Table 11.46.

Table 11.46 Simple measures for demented patients in their home environment

- Daily exercise – walk round house
- Simple tasks   – drying less-breakable crockery
- Regular visits to lavatory to help sphincter control

The relatives need the support of the social services (Table 11.47).

Attendance at a day hospital and holiday admission will reduce the severe stress on the family.

The relentless progressive deterioration will require plans for long term institutional care. It is cruel and wrong to delay these once the family is unable to cope.

Symptomatic treatment

There are a number of conditions associated with dementia which can be offered symptomatic help (Table 11.48).

It is better, if possible, to avoid regular potent sedation which might further dull the patient's declining thought processes. It is acceptable to use such drugs temporarily to tide the patient over a crisis situation.

Table 11.47 Social services help in dementia

• District nurse	– Patient mobilization
	Detect early infection
	lungs
	legs
	urinary tract
	Attention to pressure areas
• Home Help	– To reduce work load of housework
	To allow more attention to patient
• Meals on wheels	– To reduce work of cooking
	To allow more attention to patient
• Social (psychiatric welfare)	
worker	– To mobilize appropriate local facilities
• Voluntary	– MIND and other agencies
• Day Centres	– To occupy
	To relieve pressure on the family
• Hospital	– Holiday relief
	Long-term admission

Table 11.48 Symptomatic treatment in demented patients

Condition	Treatment
Physical	
Seizures	Anticonvulsants
Anaemia	Iron, folic acid
Infection	Antibiotics
Heart failure	Diuretics
Self-neglect	Adequate diet and vitamins
Mental	
Restlessness	⎫ Promazine (Sparine) 25–100 mg 3–4 times/day
Nocturnal wandering	⎬ Chlorpromazine (Largactil) 25–50 mg t.d.s.
	Haloperidol (Serenace) 5–10 mg daily
Insomnia	Nitrazepam (Mogadon) 5–10 mg
	Chloral 0.5–2 g
Depression	Amitriptyline (Tryptizol) 50–100 mg/day
	Imipramine (Tofranil) 75–100 mg/day
	Dothiepin (Prothiaden) 75–100 mg/day

When using these drugs in elderly patients, the dose should be decreased because of reduced renal excretion and impaired hepatic detoxication of the drug.

Specific treatment

There is no specific treatment of proven value in dementia.

Various drugs have been tried but objective evidence of their value is lacking

(Table 11.49). However, treatment of this type may be of psychological value to the family and, provided no harm ensues to the patient, may be justifiable if the frustration of the relatives warrants it.

Table 11.49 Drugs used in
dementia

- Vitamins
- Hormones
- Cerebral vasodilators
- 'Nerve tonics'

New approaches to specific treatment

There are two interesting new developments in the specific treatment of dementia.

Alzheimer's disease

On the basis of the possible role of acetylcholine in sustaining intellectual function in the brain, the use of oral choline bromide has had some encouraging results in this condition.

Vasopressin

This drug has been found to improve memory in patients with memory defects of varying aetiology.

It continues to be investigated in dementia.

NATURAL HISTORY OF DEMENTIA

Prevalence

The prevalence of dementia is shown in Figure 11.13. Five per cent of the population over the age of 65 have dementia due to cerebral degeneration of Alzheimer's type.

It has already been pointed out that the distinction between presenile dementia, hitherto called Alzheimer's disease, and senile dementia is artificial since there are no clinical or pathological differences between the conditions whatever the age group.

This figure of 5% over 65 years of age rises to 20% over the age of 80 years. In the United Kingdom, this produces an overall prevalence of dementia in 10% of the population.

In addition to established dementia it has been estimated that by the age of 65 years, a further 10% of the population are showing some clinical manifestations of dementia (Figure 11.14).

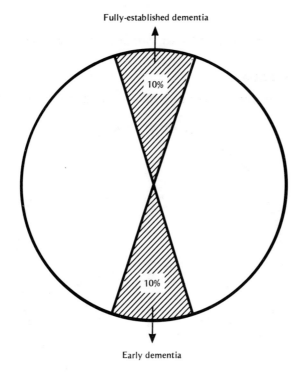

Figure 11.13 Overall prevalence of dementia in the population

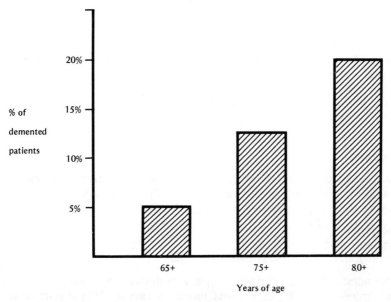

Figure 11.14 Age incidence of dementia in the population

393

Sex incidence

Women are more frequently affected with dementia than men.

Types of dementia

The distribution of the types of dementia is shown in Figure 11.15.

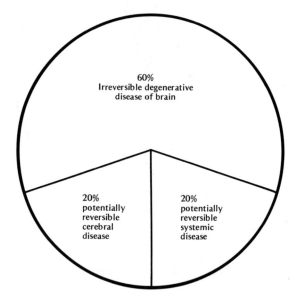

Figure 11.15   Distribution of types of dementia

The incidence of potentially reversible cerebral disease is shown in Figure 11.16 and systemic disease in Figure 11.17.

The incidence of irreversible cerebral degenerative disease is shown in Figure 11.18.

Prognosis

Virtually all patients with dementia due to cerebral degenerative disease will eventually require long term institutional care if they do not die at home first.
If living alone the patient may die of:

- accident
- malnutrition
- infection.

When admitted to hospital 60% of patients die within 6 months. This high overall figure contrasts with a lower mortality rate of 33% if only arteriosclerotic multiple infarct patients are considered.

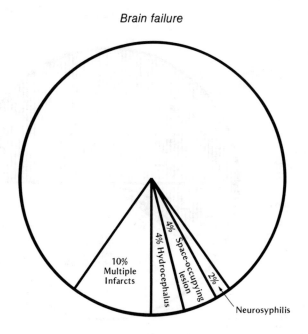

Figure 11.16 Potentially reversible cerebral disease causing dementia

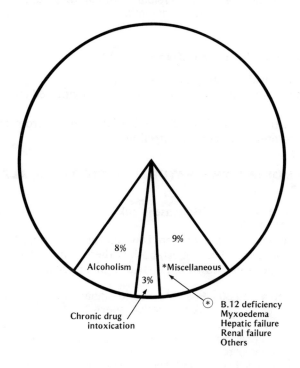

Figure 11.17 Potentially reversible systemic conditions causing dementia

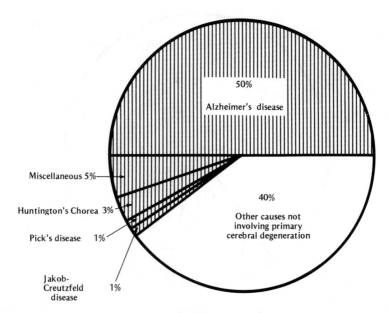

Figure 11.18 Incidence of irreversible cerebral degenerative disease in dementia

Prognosis in Alzheimer'a disease

The normal survival is 5–10 years from diagnosis.

Motor and sensory function and vision remain unaffected until the terminal stages.

Eventually, the patient will become bedfast and die from an aspiration pneumonia or other intercurrent infection.

CAN WE MODIFY THE NATURAL HISTORY OF ALZHEIMER'S DISEASE?

The aetiology of Alzheimer's disease is unknown. The theories suggested are shown in Table 11.50.

As the aetiology is unknown there is no means of primary prevention.

Once the disease has become established there is no known means yet of modifying the inevitable down-hill course ending in death within 5–10 years.

Table 11.50 Possible aetiological factors in Alzheimer's disease

---

- Impairment of cholinergic transmission in brain
- Infectious agent (slow virus)
- Small cerebral vessel pathology (not atheroma)
- Genetic (associated with Down's syndrome)

USEFUL PRACTICAL POINTS

- Mental illness beginning in middle or later life is likely to be due to either organic brain disease or to depression. Neurosis rarely begins at this stage of life.

- There are no clinical or pathological differences between presenile and senile dementia. They are both due most frequently to Alzheimer's disease causing cerebral degeneration and atrophy.

- Demented patients do not get delusions or hallucinations. These features should always suggest schizophrenia.

- Always remember hypothyroidism and vitamin B_{12} deficiency as possible causes of dementia since both conditions are reversible.

- Vitamin B_{12} deficiency can occur in the absence of anaemia so estimate the serum B_{12} level in all cases of dementia.

- When in doubt whether a patient is demented or severely depressed always try a course of antidepressive treatment. Significant improvement will follow only in depressive states.

12

Increase in weight

PRESENT HISTORY

A 34-year-old housewife presented with an increase in weight of $1\frac{1}{2}$ stone (9.5 kg) over the previous year.

Increase in weight

She had been steadily gaining weight over the last 12 months so that now she was having difficulty putting on her skirt. She did not consider that she was eating more than usual – she was in fact trying to reduce her food intake as she was becoming increasingly worried about her gain in weight.

Other relevant facts on direct enquiry

General

She had not noticed any change in her voice. She had not noticed any change in her skin but had been told recently by her hairdresser that her *hair was dry* and tending to come out more than usual when combed. She thought that her face had become *puffy*. She wondered whether her *neck* was a bit *swollen*. She had noticed this for about 6 months. She had no difficulty in swallowing, and no difficulty in breathing when lying down in bed, either on her back or lying on her side.

She had no weather preference.

Alimentary system

She admitted to constipation for many years, opening her bowels usually every 2 or 3 days. She thought, however, that she was becoming more constipated over the last few months.

Respiratory system

She had a 'smoker's cough' for many years, but it had eased a lot since she gave up smoking a year ago.

Menstruation

Her periods had been getting heavy over the last few months and were continuing for up to 10 days at a time, whereas previously they lasted for 5 days only. She denied any hot flushes.

Central nervous system

When asked about paraesthesiae, she had noticed '*pins and needles*' in her left hand for the previous few months. This mainly affected the thumb and index finger. These symptoms were always worse in the morning when she woke up. Occasionally, she had also experienced a severe ache in the left wrist spreading up into her forearm.

She denied any headache.

She thought that her *memory* was not quite as good as it used to be.

She had no deafness.

PAST HISTORY

There were no relevant illnesses.

FAMILY HISTORY

Neither parent was obese and there were no significant illnesses.
One older sister had a goitre and was having tablets for this.

PERSONAL HISTORY

She worked as a part-time office cleaner and was able to cope quite well with this job and looking after her family, comprising her husband and two children, up to a few months ago. She found it much more of an effort now and seemed to *tire more easily* which was unlike her usual energetic self.

She had smoked 15 cigarettes a day for the past 20 years but had stopped 1 year ago.

She drank very little alcohol – on rare social occasions only.

DRUG HISTORY

She was not taking a contraceptive pill.
She was on no regular drug treatment.

EXAMINATION

The abnormal findings are summarized in Figure 12.1.

General

She weighed $11\frac{1}{2}$ stones (73 kg). The distribution of the obesity was general and not confined to the trunk. There was no 'buffalo hump'.

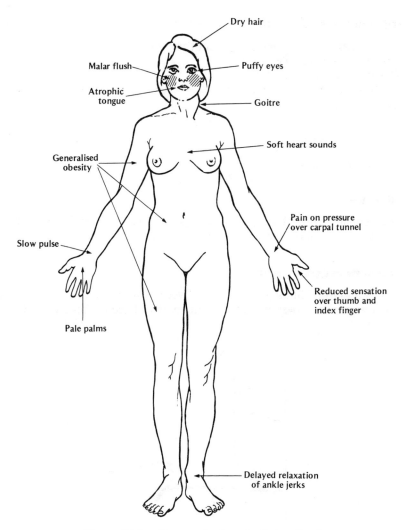

Figure 12.1 Abnormal signs in the patient

The face was *puffy*, especially around the eyes, and there was a *malar flush*.
There was no hirsutes. The tongue showed *atrophic glossitis*. The
conjunctivae were *pale* as were the palms of the hands also. There was no
koilonychia.

Thyroid gland

There was firm diffuse enlargement of the thyroid gland; there were no bruits
audible over the gland. There was no exophthalmos, lid retraction or lid-lag.
There was no finger tremor and the palms were cool and dry.

Cardiovascular system

The pulse was 64/min, regular and poor volume.
The blood pressure was 150/85.
The apex beat was not palpable.
The heart sounds were very soft; there were no gallop rhythm, murmurs or pericardial friction.

Respiratory system

The lungs were normal.

Abdomen

There were no purple abdominal striae. The abdomen was difficult to palpate adequately because of obesity. No abnormality was found.

Central nervous system

The only abnormal finding in the motor system was delayed relaxation of the ankle jerk, which is best elicited with the patient kneeling on a chair (Figure 12.2).

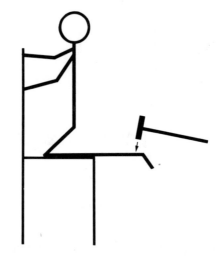

Figure 12.2   Best way of eliciting the ankle jerk

In the sensory system, there was *impairment of cotton wool sensation* and slight *blunting of pinprick* over the left thumb and index finger. Pressure over the left carpal tunnel also produced paraesthesiae in these digits, which was made worse when the pressure was accompanied by forcible wrist flexion.
There was no weakness of the thumb muscles.

Cervical spine

Neck movements were free and painless and no crepitus was felt in the neck with movement.

ANALYSIS OF THE HISTORY

Obesity

This was the main presenting complaint. The causes of obesity are shown in Table 12.1.

By far the most frequent cause of obesity is primary or 'simple' obesity due to excess of calorie intake over expenditure. Factors which predispose to this type of obesity are shown in Table 12.2.

Table 12.1 Causes of obesity

• Primary	– Excess of calorie intake over output
• Secondary	• Hypothyroidism
	• Cushing's disease
	• Insulinoma
	• Hypothalamic disorders

Table 12.2 Factors predisposing to 'simple' obesity

• Genetic	– familial tendency
• Sex	– women more susceptible
• Psychological	– emotional deprivation
	depression
• Lack of physical activity	
• Social class	– more prone in classes IV and V
• Economic	– inability to buy more expensive less-fattening foods
• Stopping smoking	

Simple obesity

This is a possible diagnosis to be considered in the patient.

The excessive weight is generalized, as in the patient.

There was no family history of obesity and there were no symptoms to suggest depression or emotional deprivation.

She was reasonably active in her work as a cleaner.

She was in a lower social class but had no serious financial problems preventing a well-balanced diet.

Hypothyroidism

In addition to obesity, there are a variety of other symptoms which are common in hypothyroidism (Table 12.3).

The patient had increasing constipation, loss of hair, heavy periods and thought that her memory was becoming poor.

Hypothyroidism remains, therefore, a possible diagnosis in this patient.

Table 12.3   Symptoms of hypothyroidism

- Obesity
- Cold intolerance
- Physical and mental slowing
- Increasing constipation
- Hoarse voice
- Dry skin
- Loss of hair
- Menorrhagia
- Deafness

Cushing's syndrome

The symptoms associated with Cushing's syndrome are shown in Table 12.4. None of these symptoms was evident in the patient.

Table 12.4   Symptoms of Cushing's syndrome

- Truncal obesity
- Hirsutes and acne in females
- Muscle weakness
- Amenorrhoea
- Diabetes mellitus   – thirst
                               polyuria
- Spontaneous bruising
- Loss of vision   – pituitary adenoma

Insulinoma

This is a rare condition.

An insulinoma is a functioning adenoma of the β-cells of the islets of

Table 12.5   Symptoms of hypoglycaemia

- Weakness
- Hunger
- Sweating
- Palpitations
- Tremor
- Faintness
- Headache
- Mental confusion
- Fits

Langerhans in the pancreas. It produces an excess of insulin which leads to recurrent attacks of hypoglycaemia. Obesity is another consequency of an insulinoma.

The clinical diagnosis is made on the basis of the symptoms of hypoglycaemia (Table 12.5). Confirmation of the diagnosis is based on finding an excessively high plasma insulin level both in the fasting state and in response to a provocative injection of intravenous tolbutamide.

The patient had no symptoms to suggest recurrent hypoglycaemia.

Hypothalamic disorders

Hypothalamic dysfunction is a very rare cause of obesity, usually in boys. It produces the characteristic picture of the 'Pickwickian Fat Boy' of Fröhlich's syndrome. The features of this type of hypothalamic disorder are shown in Table 12.6.

Obviously, the syndrome is not relevant in the patient.

Table 12.6 Features of Fröhlich's syndrome

• Gross obesity
• Hypogonadism
• Diabetes insipidus
• Visual impairment
• Mental retardation

Swelling of the face

The patient had admitted puffiness of the face. The causes of swelling of the face are shown in Table 12.7.

Table 12.7 Causes of swelling of the face

• Renal	• nephrotic syndrome
	• acute nephritis
• Endocrine	• myxoedema
	• Cushing's syndrome
	• steroid treatment
• Mediastinal obstruction	
• Angioneurotic oedema	
• Skin sensitivity	• drugs
	• cosmetics
	• hair dyes

Renal disease

The lack of swelling of the legs and swelling of the abdomen (ascites) is against the diagnosis of nephrotic syndrome.

The absence of preceding sore throat, haematuria, oliguria and oedema elsewhere excludes acute diffuse glomerulo-tubular nephritis.

Endocrine disease

Myxoedema remains a likely cause of the puffiness of the face.

Cushing's syndrome leads to a round red hirsute face. The absence of symptoms of this disease has already been discussed.

The patient had not been taking any regular steroid treatment.

Mediastinal obstruction

The features of mediastinal obstruction are shown in Table 12.8. The typical appearance is congestion of the head and neck and distended veins in the neck and over the upper part of the chest.

None of these features was present in the patient.

Table 12.8   Features of mediastinal obstruction

- Obstructed superior vena cava
  - oedema and cyanosis of head and neck
  - oedema of upper limbs
  - distended neck veins
  - distended thoracic veins
- Tracheal compression
  - dyspnoea
  - stridor
  - brassy cough
- Oesophageal compression
  - dysphagia
- Recurrent laryngeal nerve involvement
  - hoarse voice

Angioneurotic oedema

The features of this condition are shown in Table 12.9.

The patient's history did not suggest angioneurotic oedema.

Table 12.9   Features of angioneurotic oedema

• Past history of allergy	– hay fever
	asthma
• Recurrent swelling	– face (especially eyes)
	lips
	tongue
• Laryngeal oedema	– severe dyspnoea

Skin sensitivity

The patient had not taken any drugs which might have caused a sensitivity reaction.

She had not used any new or unusual cosmetics or hair dyes which might have led to a contact dermatitis.

Swelling of the neck

The causes of swelling of the neck which ought to be considered and their distinctive features are shown in Table 12.10.

Table 12.10   Causes of swelling of the neck

• Thyroid enlargement	– midline
	base of neck
• Lymph node enlargement	– discrete swelling
	side of neck
• Carotid body tumour	– carotid bifurcation
	pulsatile
	syncope on pressure
• Pharyngeal pouch	– upper side of neck
	fills after meals
• Branchial cysts	– anterior triangle of neck
• Thyroglossal cyst	– midline
	elevates when tongue put out

Apart from thyroid enlargement and swollen lymph glands, all the other conditions are very rare.

A central swelling at the base of the neck, as in this patient, is highly likely to be a goitre due to thyroid enlargement.

If a goitre is present, it is important to exclude pressure on the trachea (stridor in bed) and on the oesophagus (dysphagia): neither was present in the patient.

Constipation

The patient gave a long history of constipation, which had, however, been getting worse recently. The causes of constipation are shown in Table 12.11.

Table 12.11   Causes of constipation

• 'Imaginary'
• Lazy bowel habits
• Inadequate roughage in diet
• Irritable bowel syndrome
• Colonic obstruction
• Painful anal conditions
• Drugs
• Myxoedema

'Imaginary' constipation

'Imaginary' constipation is based on the false assumption that it is necessary and normal to have a bowel action every day.

The patient's longstanding constipation may have been of this type.

'Lazy bowel habits'

These are due to taking inadequate time, for various reasons, to have regular bowel actions. Re-establishment of a daily ritual, together with an increase of bulk and roughage in the diet, may help to overcome this problem.

The patient did admit that she was 'always in a rush' when she was young and this may therefore have been a contributory factor in her constipation.

Inadequate roughage

Her diet appeared to contain sufficient roughage, since she ate a lot of fruit and cabbage. She was also a regular user of wholemeal bread. Roughage did not therefore seem to be her problem.

Irritable bowel syndrome

Although, in the irritable bowel syndrome, diarrhoea is more common, constipation may sometimes occur.

The lack of abdominal pain and 'rumbling' and the absence of flatulence makes this diagnosis very unlikely as a cause of her constipation.

Colonic obstruction

The most important cause to consider in *recent* constipation is carcinoma of the colon leading to obstruction.

This condition is usually associated with loss of weight and often with blood in the stools. Neither was present in the patient.

Painful anal conditions

Conditions such as painful piles, perianal abscess and anal fistula may inhibit defaecation. None was evident in the patient.

Table 12.12   Drugs causing constipation

• Bismuth-containing antacids
• Aluminium-containing antacids
• Anti-cholinergic drugs
• Opiates
• Ganglion-blocking drugs (hypertension)

Drugs

The drugs which may cause some constipation are shown in Table 12.12.
The patient was not taking any drugs regularly.

Myxoedema

Myxoedema remains a likely cause of the patient's constipation, since constipation is a very frequent symptom in this condition.

Menorrhagia

This may be due to local uterine causes (Figure 12.3) or general disease (Table 12.13).
There was no past history of pelvic infection such as salpingitis. Pelvic examination is necessary to exclude fibroids.

Table 12.13   General causes of menorrhagia

• Thyroid disease	• thyrotoxicosis
	• myxoedema
• Bleeding tendency	• liver disease
	• anticoagulant treatment
• Blood dyscrasia	• thrombocytopenic purpura
	• leukaemia

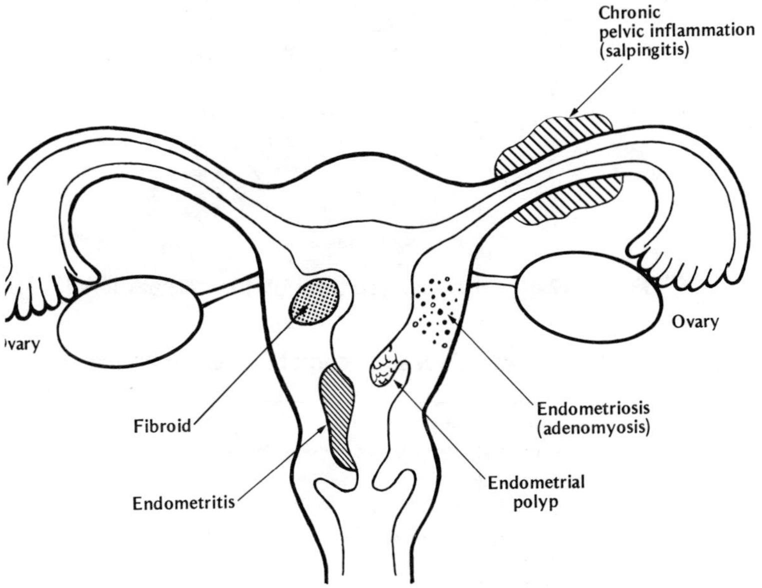

Figure 12.3   Local uterine causes of menorrhagia

A more detailed gynaecological investigation such as dilatation and curettage would be necessary to exclude the other local uterine causes such as endometritis, endometriosis or endometrial polyp.

A generalized bleeding disorder due to liver disease or blood dyscrasia would be expected to produce bleeding elsewhere also, e.g. skin or gastrointestinal tract, and its absence in the patient makes a bleeding disorder very unlikely.

Both thyrotoxicosis and myxoedema can lead to menorrhagia. The other symptoms are very suggestive of *myxoedema* and this is therefore the most likely cause of the menorrhagia in this patient.

Paraesthesiae in the left hand

Paraesthesiae affecting the thumb and index finger indicate median nerve involvement.

The occurrence of these symptoms on waking in the morning is very suggestive of median nerve pressure by the *carpal tunnel syndrome.*

The anatomy of the carpal tunnel is shown in Figure 12.4. It indicates clearly how median nerve compression can occur by involvement of any of the structures forming the carpal tunnel. The causes of the carpal tunnel syndrome are shown in Table 12.14.

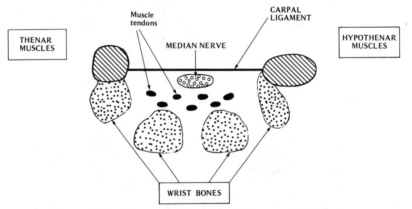

Figure 12.4   Cross-section through the carpal tunnel

Table 12.14   Causes of carpal tunnel syndrome

• Tenosynovitis
• Rheumatoid arthritis
• Myxoedema
• Pregnancy oedema
• Premenstrual oedema
• Amyloidosis
• Acromegaly
• Granulomatous disease e.g. tuberculosis

Localized tenosynovitis of unknown aetiology may occur in middle-aged women. It produces severe and more constant pain along the tendons which inhibits finger movement and may be associated with 'creaking' along the line of the tendon. This picture was not evident in the patient.

There was no history to suggest rheumatoid arthritis of the wrist or fingers.

The symptoms were not related to her periods, and she was not pregnant.

There were no symptoms to suggest amyloidosis (Table 12.15).

There were no other symptoms to suggest acromegaly (Table 12.16).

The patient had no fever, night sweats or constitutional symptoms to suggest tuberculosis.

Myxoedema, therefore, remains the most likely diagnosis of the patient's carpal tunnel syndrome.

Table 12.15   Symptoms of amyloidosis

• Gut	–	diarrhoea
• Kidney	–	generalized oedema
• Liver	–	abdominal swelling (ascites)
• Heart	–	dyspnoea
		palpitations
• Lungs	–	dyspnoea
• Glands	–	localized swellings
• Skin	–	plaques

Table 12.16   Symptoms of acromegaly

- Increasing hand size (gloves)
- Increasing foot size (shoes)
- Joint pains
- Muscle weakness
- Diabetes
    thirst
    polyuria
    loss of weight
- Excessive sweating
- Deepening of the voice
- Headache (expanding pituitary tumour)
- Visual deterioration

Family history

Her sister's thyroid disease might be relevant since there is a familial predisposition in some types of thyroid disease (Table 12.17).

411

This would support the diagnosis of myxoedema due to Hashimoto's thyroiditis in the patient.

Table 12.17   Hereditary types of thyroid disease

- Graves' disease   –   young women
                          exophthalmos
                          diffuse vascular goitre
                          thyrotoxicosis
- Hashimoto's thyroiditis
- Idiopathic myxoedema

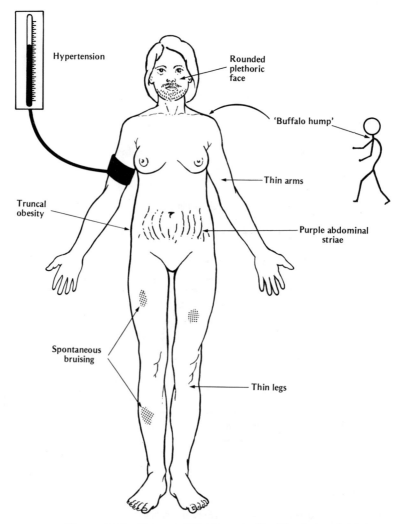

Figure 12.5   Abnormal findings in Cushing's syndrome

CONCLUSIONS FROM THE HISTORY

- The patient has symptoms of hypothyroidism.

- The association of a goitre with the hypothyroidism suggests Hashimoto's disease.

- She has a left carpal tunnel syndrome due to the myxoedema.

- The positive family history of thyroid disease confirms the auto-immune basis of the hypothyroidism.

ANALYSIS OF THE EXAMINATION

Obesity

The generalized obesity excludes Cushing's syndrome.

The other signs of Cushing's syndrome are shown in Figure 12.5. None of these signs was present in the patient.

A typical patient with Cushing's syndrome is shown in Figure 12.6.

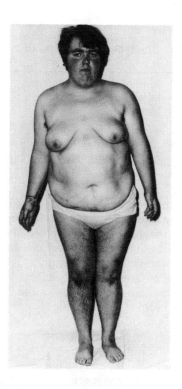

Figure 12.6   Typical patient with Cushing's syndrome

413

Facial appearance

The puffy face with a malar flush suggests the so-called 'strawberries and cream' appearance of myxoedema.

The other causes of a malar flush are shown in Table 12.18.

The dry hair supports the diagnosis of myxoedema.

Table 12.18   Causes of a malar flush

- Myxoedema
- Mitral stenosis
- Systemic lupus erythematosus
- Pernicious anaemia early after treatment with Vitamin B_{12}

Pallor

The pale conjunctivae, pale tongue and pale palms indicate anaemia.

There are three types of anaemia which may be associated with myxoedema (Table 12.19).

Table 12.19   The types of anaemia in myxoedema

- Normocytic normochromic
- Microcytic hypochromic
- Macrocytic

The most frequent type of anaemia with myxoedema is *normocytic* and *normochromic*. It is due to depressed bone marrow function caused by deficiency of thyroxine.

Female patients with myxoedema frequently have menorrhagia. This leads to chronic iron-deficiency anaemia which is *microcytic* and *hypochromic*. The patient does have menorrhagia which is therefore likely to be a contributory factor in her anaemia, though she did not have koilonychia which is frequently associated with chronic iron-deficiency anaemia.

Approximately 10% of myxoedematous patients will also have *pernicious anaemia*. This applies particularly to the auto-immune type of myxoedema due to Hashimoto's thyroiditis. The atrophic tongue is suggestive of an associated pernicious anaemia in this patient.

Goitre

The association of a goitre with hypothyroidism may have several causes (Table 12.20).

Table 12.20   Causes of goitre with hypothyroidism

- Iodine deficiency
- Goitrogenic drugs
- Subacute thyroiditis (De Quervain's thyroiditis)
- Hashimoto's thyroiditis

Iodine deficiency

The metabolic pathway in the formation of thyroxine is shown in Figure 12.7.

Iodide deficiency may cause *endemic goitre* but is rare now in the United Kingdom. It usually begins at puberty or during pregnancy. If the degree of iodide deficiency is very severe, it will also cause hypothyroidism.

The goitre is usually diffuse unless there is an intermittent deficiency of iodide in the diet, when it will become nodular.

The development of the goitre in the fourth decade, and the normal diet, especially the fish content, excludes iodide deficiency in this patient.

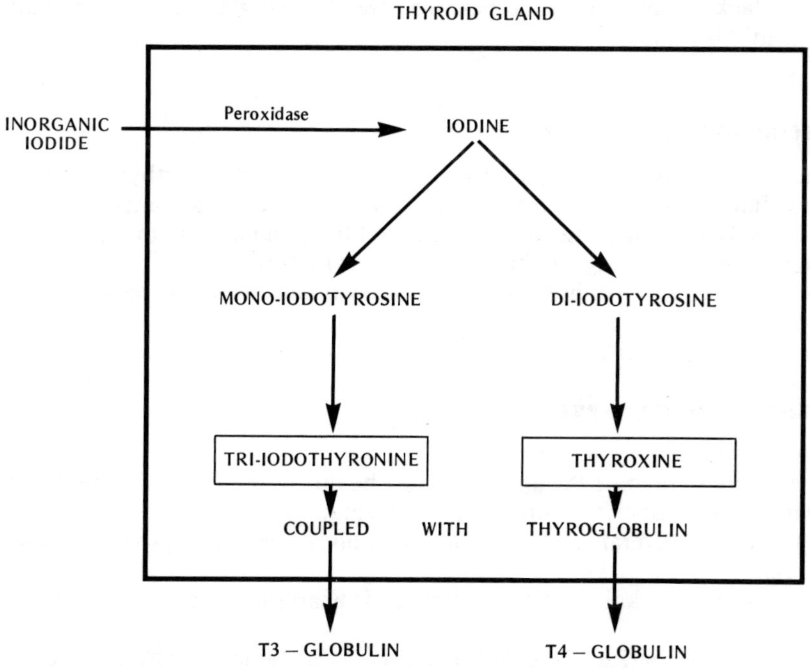

THYROID GLAND

Figure 12.7   Metabolic pathway of thyroid hormones

Goitrogenic drugs

The antithyroid drugs which can cause goitre and hypothyroidism are shown in Table 12.21.

The patient had not taken any of these drugs.

Table 12.21 Goitrogenic drugs

• Para-aminosalicylic acid	(tuberculosis)
• Phenylbutazone	(arthritis)
• Sulphonamides	(infections)
• Sulphonylureas	(diabetes)
• Aminoglutethimide	(breast carcinoma)
• Lithium	(depression)
• Iodides	(asthma)

Subacute thyroiditis (De Quervain's disease)

This is a very painful thyroid disorder associated with a goitre and hypo-thyroidism. Less commonly, hyperthyroidism may occur.

It is thought to be due to a virus infection. It may follow a respiratory tract infection or, sometimes, mumps. The erythrocyte sedimentation rate is usually high. The condition improves spontaneously after weeks or months.

The lack of pain and tenderness over the thyroid gland excludes the diagnosis in this patient.

Hashimoto's thyroiditis

This is the commonest cause of goitre associated with hypothyroidism. It is often familial and occurs most frequently in middle-aged women.

The enlargement of the thyroid gland is diffuse and firm, as in the patient. It rarely gives rise to any significant pressure symptoms.

Hashimoto's thyroiditis is the most likely diagnosis in this patient.

Cardiovascular system

The slow pulse is typical of myxoedema.

Inability to palpate the apex beat may be due to the patient's obesity or to heart disease associated with the myxoedema.

There are several cardiovascular complications of myxoedema (Table 12.22).

There are no manifestations of ischaemic heart disease in the patient (Table 12.23).

The signs of pericardial effusion are shown in Table 12.24. The patient had an impalpable apex beat and the heart sounds were very soft; the other signs were not evident. This could be due to a pericardial effusion but further investigation is required to confirm the diagnosis. This will be discussed later (p. 423).

It was impossible to detect cardiac enlargement since the apex beat was not palpable. Percussion of the heart is rarely practised now, and is unlikely to be accurate enough to detect minor degrees of cardiac enlargement anyway.

The patient had no signs of heart failure (Table 12.25).

Table 12.22   Cardiovascular complications of myxoedema

> • Ischaemic heart disease
> • Pericardial effusion
> • Cardiac enlargement
> • Cardiac failure

Table 12.23   Clinical manifestations of ischaemic heart disease

• History	• Angina
	• Myocardial infarction
	• Heart failure – dyspnoea
	– ankle swelling
	• Arrhythmia – palpitations
• Examination	• Arcus senilis
	• Thickened arteries
	• Cardiac enlargement
	• Gallop rhythm
	• Pulmonary congestion

Table 12.24   Signs of pericardial effusion

> • Poor volume pulse
> • Paradoxical pulse – volume falls in inspiration
> • Distended neck veins on inspiration (Kussmaul's sign)
> • Apex beat not palpable
> • Heart enlarged on percussion
> • Soft heart sounds

Table 12.25   Signs of heart failure

• Left ventricular failure	– dyspnoea
	presystolic triple rhythm
	pulmonary congestion
• Right ventricular failure	– cyanosis
	distended neck veins
	oedema
	enlarged liver
	ascites

Central nervous system

The two abnormalities are:

- delayed relaxation of the ankle jerk
- sensory impairment in the left hand.

Ankle jerk

Prolongation of the relaxation time of the deep reflexes is very suggestive, though not pathognomonic, of hypothyroidism (Table 12.26).

The delayed relaxation is best seen in the ankle jerk and best elicited with the patient kneeling on a chair (see Figure 12.2, p. 402).

The test is of little value in the diagnosis of hyperthyroidism – a reduction in the relaxation time is not clinically evident.

Table 12.26 Causes of delayed
relaxation of the ankle jerk

* Hypothyroidism
* Rheumatic chorea
* Treatment with β-blocking drugs

Sensory changes in the left hand

The sensory changes indicate median nerve involvement.

The likely cause is the carpal tunnel syndrome. The causes of this syndrome have already been shown in Table 12.14 (p. 411) and myxoedema considered to be the diagnosis.

Weakness of the thenar muscles may sometimes occur in the carpal tunnel syndrome but was not evident in the patient.

Other neurological complications which may occur in myxoedema are shown in Table 12.27.

Tables 12.27 Neurological complications
of myxoedema

* Cerebellar degeneration
* Psychosis 'myxoedema madness'
* Polyneuritis
* Myopathy
* Myotonia

CONCLUSIONS FROM THE EXAMINATION

* Examination confirms hypothyroidism because of:
   obesity
   puffy face with malar flush
   dry skin and hair
   slow pulse and soft heart sounds
   slow relaxation of ankle jerks.

* The firm diffuse goitre suggests Hashimoto's disease.

- She has signs of median nerve involvement in the left hand confirming carpal tunnel syndrome.

- The pallor and atrophic glossitis suggest pernicious anaemia associated with the myxoedema.

INVESTIGATIONS

Thyroid function tests

The most important tests in the diagnosis of myxoedema are shown in Table 12.28.

Table 12.28   Diagnostic tests in myxoedema

- Serum thyroxine (T_4) level ↓
- Serum thyroid-stimulating hormone (TSH) level ↑

In myxoedema, the level of serum thyroxine (T_4) will be low. As a result of the feed-back mechanism, pituitary thyroid-stimulating hormone level (TSH) production will be increased in an endeavour to stimulate the thyroid gland to produce more thyroxine (Figure 12.8).

Since circulating T_4 is largely bound to plasma thyroglobulin, this should

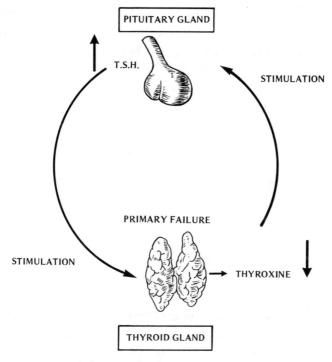

Figure 12.8   Feedback system in myxoedema

419

also be measured to exclude any change which may alter the plasma level of T$_4$.

The conditions which may alter the level of thyroglobulin in the plasma are shown in Table 12.29. Particular attention should be given to the contraceptive pill which is now in widespread use.

Phenytoin and salicylate treatment reduce the serum T$_4$ level by blocking the binding sites for T$_4$ on the globulin molecule.

The differentiation between primary and secondary hypothyroidism is shown in Table 12.30.

The patient's results are shown in Table 12.31. They confirm primary myxoedema.

Table 12.29   Conditions altering level of plasma thyroglobulin

- Increase
  - Pregnancy
  - Oestrogen treatment (includes contraceptive pill)
  - Clofibrate
  - Phenothiazines
- Decrease
  - Hypoproteinaemia – Nephrosis
    - Malnutrition
    - Steroids
    - Androgens
  - Phenytoin
  - Salicylates

Table 12.30   Differentiation between primary and secondary hypothyroidism

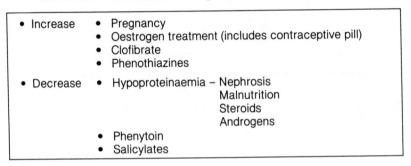

	T$_4$	TSH
Primary	↓	↑
Secondary	↓	↓

Table 12.31   Patient's thyroid function tests

	Results	Normal range
T$_4$	18 nmol/l	(60–170)
TSH	106 u/l	(up to 5.5)
TBG	12.1 mg/l	(8–16)

Thyrotropin-releasing hormone (TRH) test

This is a useful test for both hypothyroidism and thyrotoxicosis when there is doubt about the diagnosis. It is based on the release of thyroid-stimulating hormone from the anterior pituitary gland by an intravenous injection of synthetic thyrotropin-releasing hormone. The responses in primary hypo-thyroidism and thyrotoxicosis are shown in Figure 12.9.

In secondary hypothyroidism due to pituitary disease, the TSH response is either absent or severely impaired.

This test was not considered necessary in the patient, since the very low level of serum thyroxine and very high level of serum TSH have clearly confirmed the diagnosis of primary myxoedema.

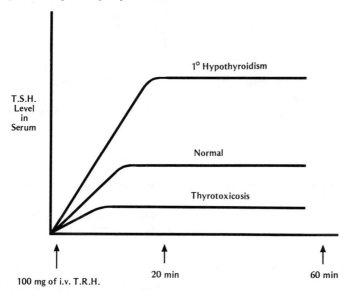

Figure 12.9   TRH test in primary myxoedema and thyrotoxicosis

Thyroid antibody test

This is a necessary test to diagnose auto-immune thyroid disease (Hashimoto's thyroiditis). In this condition, antibodies develop against thyroglobulin and against a microsomal part of the thyroid cells. The patient's antibody results are shown in Table 12.32.

The positive results for both types of autoantibody confirm the diagnosis of Hashimoto's thyroiditis.

Table 12.32   Patient's thyroid-antibody results

• Microsomal	– 6400 (normal <1600)
• Thyroglobulin	– 40 (normal <40)

Blood count

A blood count is required in a myxoedematous patient with clinical evidence

421

Table 12.33 Patient's blood count result

	Result	Normal range
Haemoglobin	8.8 g/dl	(12–16)
Mean corpuscular volume	104 fl	(82–96)
Mean corpuscular haemoglobin	26 pg	(26–32)
Mean corpuscular haemoglobin concentration	32 g/dl	(30–35)
Blood film	macrocytosis anisocytosis poikilocytosis	

of anaemia, to determine which of the three possible types of anaemia is present (see Table 12.19, p. 414).

The patient's blood count is shown in Table 12.33. This confirms macrocytic anaemia, the likely cause being vitamin B_{12} deficiency.

Serum vitamin B_{12} level

This is necessary to decide whether macrocytic anaemia is due to vitamin B_{12} deficiency or folic acid deficiency.

The patient's level was 65 pg/ml, which confirms vitamin B_{12} deficiency as a cause of the macrocytic anaemia (normal B_{12} 200–900 pg/ml).

Bone marrow examination

This is not necessary if the blood film shows clear evidence of macrocytic anaemia, as in this patient.

Blood lipids

Increased serum cholesterol and triglyceride are common findings in myxoedema but of no diagnostic significance.

The patient's cholesterol was increased to 10.5 mmol/l (normal 3.6–7.6) but the triglyceride level was normal.

Electrocardiogram

This may be a helpful test in doubtful cases of myxoedema. The typical findings are shown in Table 12.34.

Table 12.34 Typical e.c.g. findings in myxoedema

- Sinus bradycardia
- Generalized low amplitude complexes
- Flattened or inverted T waves

The patient's e.c.g., in Figure 12.10, shows sinus bradycardia, generally low voltage and flat T waves, consistent with myxoedema.

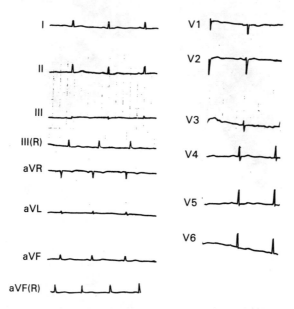

Figure 12.10   Patient's e.c.g. showing changes of myxoedema with sinus bradycardia, low voltage and flat T waves

Chest X-ray

This may be helpful if a pericardial effusion is suspected. If an effusion is present, a 'globular' heart shadow is seen (Figure 12.11).

Cardiac enlargement may also be present in myxoedema, with or without heart failure.

The patient's chest X-ray was normal.

Echocardiography

This test is more accurate than a chest X-ray in detecting pericardial effusion.

The typical changes are shown in Figure 12.12 – the presence of fluid in the pericardial space between the posterior wall of the left ventricle and the posterior wall of the chest, which shows up as a clear space on the record.

Other tests for associated auto-immune disease

There are a number of other auto-immune diseases which may be associated with Hashimoto's thyroiditis. The tests which may be helpful in their diagnosis are shown in Table 12.35.

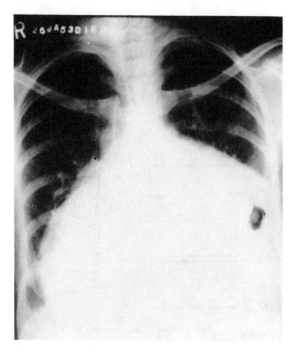

Figure 12.11   Chest X-ray in pericardial effusion showing a 'globular' shadow

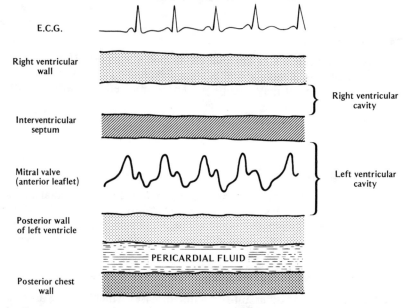

Figure 12.12   Echocardiogram showing the typical changes of pericardial effusion

424

Table 12.35 Diagnosis of auto-immune diseases associated with Hashimoto's thyroiditis

• Chronic active hepatitis	– Liver function tests Hepatitis B antigen Smooth muscle antibodies Liver biopsy
• Rheumatoid arthritis	– Rheumatoid factor X-rays
• Systemic lupus erythematosus	– LE factor (LE cells) Antinuclear factor
• Diabetes	– Blood sugar
• Addison's disease	– Serum cortisol level ACTH stimulation test
• Hypoparathyroidism	– Serum Ca and PO_4 levels

MANAGEMENT OF MYXOEDEMA

The goal of treatment of hypothyroidism is to re-establish a euthyroid state by replacement therapy with thyroxine.

Treatment is lifelong.

Dosage regime

The dosage regime for the uncomplicated adult patient is shown in Table 12.36.

Most patients will remain euthyroid on a maintenance dose of 0.2 mg/day but occasionally 0.3 mg/day is required.

The factors indicating the need for a slower and more cautious build-up of the dose of thyroxine are shown in Table 12.37.

Table 12.36 Dosage regime of thyroxine in the uncomplicated adult patient with myxoedema

Time	Dose
To start	0.05 mg/day
After 2 weeks	0.10 mg/day
After 4 weeks	0.15 mg/day
After 6 weeks	0.20 mg/day
Maintenance	0.20 mg/day

Table 12.37 Factors modifying dose of thyroxine for myxoedema

• Elderly patient	
• Heart disease	• angina • heart failure • arrhythmias

Thyroxine may precipitate heart failure in an elderly patient with subclinical heart disease. It may also exacerbate established angina, heart failure or tachyarrhythmias.

In these patients, therefore, it is best to start with a smaller dose of thyroxine, say 0.025 mg/day and to increase more cautiously and at longer intervals, say monthly, up to a maximum of 0.10–0.15 mg/day. Careful assessment should be made before each increment to exclude cardiac complications.

Dose administration

When thyroxine is taken on an empty stomach, 70% of the dose is absorbed, but when taken with food only 50% of the dose is absorbed. It is important therefore that the patient is consistent in the relationship of dose to food, otherwise fluctuation in blood thyroxine levels may occur.

The long half-life of thyroxine means that the total daily requirement can be given in a single daily dose.

Regular reassessment

Regular clinical and biochemical reassessment should be carried out.

Clinical review

Initially, this should be at fortnightly intervals in the uncomplicated patient but weekly in the elderly patient or if cardiac complications are present. The intervals between assessments are then gradually extended to monthly, 3-monthly or longer according to progress.

At each review, clinical progress is assessed, in relation to symptoms of myxoedema (Table 12.38) but also to heart function. Apart from symptomatic improvement, one of the most useful objective tests of progress is the return of ankle-jerk relaxation time to normal.

Table 12.38   Symptoms of myxoedema

- Mental and physical slowing
- Cold intolerance
- Increasing weight
- Constipation
- Hoarseness of voice
- Loss of hair

Biochemical progress

Periodic measurement of the serum TSH level is the best single index of improvement. This is done initially after 3 months, 6 months, 1 year and then annually. The aim of treatment is to reduce this level to within normal limits.

The level of serum thyroxine (T_4) is also usually measured and should be maintained within the normal range.

SPECIAL CONSIDERATIONS IN THE TREATMENT OF MYXOEDEMA

Myxoedema coma

This is a medical emergency which requires prompt and effective treatment. The clinical features are shown in Table 12.39.

The factors which may precipitate coma are shown in Table 12.40.

The treatment of myxoedema coma is shown in Table 12.41.

Table 12.39 Clinical features of myxoedema coma

- Coma
- Icy-cold skin
- Very low temperature (rectal thermometer)
- Poor respiration
- Bronchopneumonia common
- Cardiac arrhythmia
- Heart failure

Table 12.40 Factors precipitating myxoedema coma

- Infection
- Exposure to cold
- Sedatives and narcotics

Table 12.41 Treatment of myxoedema coma

- Intravenous tri-iodothyronine
- Intravenous hydrocortisone
- Cover to conserve heat but no active warming
- Intravenous glucose–saline
- Effective treatment of infection
- Positive-pressure ventilation if required

Infancy and childhood

Routine screening programmes have shown the prevalence of neonatal hypothyroidism to be 1: 3500–4000 infants.

The clinical recognition of hypothyroidism in a new born baby is very difficult and some symptoms and signs are not manifest until 4–6 weeks of age. The clinical features which may occur are shown in Table 12.42.

Table 12.42 Clinical features of neonatal hypothyroidism

• Symptoms	• Poor feeding
	• Hoarse cry
	• Regurgitation
	• Lethargy
	• Constipation
• Signs	• Coarse facial features
	• Large tongue
	• Dry skin
	• Bradycardia
	• Delayed relaxation of tendon jerks
	• Umbilical hernia

A useful pointer to the possibility of hypothyroidism is the baby who seems too *good* – an inactive, tranquil baby who seldom cries.

Early diagnosis is essential if mental function is to be preserved.

If hypothyroidism is recognized before 3 months of age, 80% of children will develop normally with treatment. After this age, normal development will occur in only 20%.

Infants and children require doses of thyroxine which are disproportionately large in relation to their body size. The dose required will depend on age (Table 12.43).

Table 12.43 Dose of thyroxine in childhood myxoedema

Age	Dose (µg/kg/per day)
<3 months	10–12
3 months–1 year	8–10
1–5 years	6
5–15 years	4–6
>15 years	normal adult dose

Secondary myxoedema

In patients with hypothyroidism secondary to pituitary disease, appropriate dose of steroids should be given to treat the associated adrenal insufficiency, as well as thyroxine for the myxoedema.

Doubtful cases of myxoedema on treatment with thyroxine

If there is a doubt whether longstanding treatment with thyroxine was based on a valid diagnosis of myxoedema, the thyroxine can be discontinued.

Reassessment should be made after 6 weeks and evidence of hypothyroidism sought (Table 12.44). If present, thyroxine can be restarted; if absent, further supervision without treatment is justifiable.

Increase in weight

Table 12.44 Evidence of hypothyroidism after discontinuing
thyroxine

• Clinical symptoms
• Low serum thyroxine level
• Raised serum TSH

MANAGEMENT OF PERNICIOUS ANAEMIA

The patient has pernicious anaemia associated with the myxoedema. The diagnosis was based on the features shown in Table 12.45.

The basis of the association is that both conditions are due to auto-immune disease in which organ damage occurs as a result of antibodies which develop against the patient's own tissues.

It is often the case that when one auto-immune disease is present, others coexist (Table 12.46).

Table 12.45 Diagnosis of pernicious anaemia in the patient

• Clinical – pallor
atrophic tongue
• Tests – anaemia
increased mean corpuscular volume
macrocytosis on blood film
low serum B_{12} level

Table 12.46 Auto-immune diseases
associated with each other

• Hashimoto's thyroiditis
• Pernicious anaemia
• Rheumatoid arthritis
• Other collagen disease
• Ulcerative colitis
• Crohn's disease
• Hypoparathyroidism

Dose of vitamin B_{12}

Treatment is started with intramuscular vitamin B_{12} (hydroxycobalamin) $1000 \, \mu g$ on alternate days, for 1 week. The large initial dose is necessary to replenish the depleted stores of vitamin B_{12} in the liver.

The next stage is weekly injections of $1000 \, \mu g$ of B_{12} until the blood count is normal. Treatment is then continued with monthly injections of B_{12} which can be extended to every 2 or 3 months provided the blood count remains normal. *B_{12} treatment must be continued for the rest of the patient's life.*

Neurological complications

If subacute combined degeneration of the spinal cord is present, it is advisable to maintain high-dose treatment with B_{12} 1000 µg every fortnight for at least 6 months in the hope of neurological improvement, though this is often very limited.

Associated iron deficiency

Iron deficiency may become manifest when improvement in the macrocytic anaemia starts to develop with B_{12}. This would be particularly likely in this patient with menorrhagia.

It would be prudent, therefore, to treat her with an iron preparation from the start until the blood count has been restored to normality.

NATURAL HISTORY OF MYXOEDEMA

Incidence

The incidence of hypothyroidism is shown in Table 12.47. The significance of these figures in an average British general practice is shown in Table 12.48.

Table 12.47 Incidence of hypothyroidism

Type	Sex	Incidence
Adults	Females	1 in 70
	Males	1 in 1000
Congenital		1 in 4000

Table 12.48 Incidence of hypothyroidism in average family practice

• Total no. of patients	2500
• No. of adults	1000
• Hypothyroid women	7
• Hypothyroid men	1
• Congenital hypothyroidism	Unlikely

Causes

The causes of hypothyroidism are shown in Table 12.49.

Table 12.49   Causes of hypothyroidism in the population

• Primary (95%)	• Idiopathic – great majority
	• Chronic thyroiditis
	Hashimoto's disease
	Riedel's thyroiditis
	• Radioactive iodine treatment of thyrotoxicosis
	• Surgical treatment of thyrotoxicosis
• Secondary (5%)	• Pituitary disease

'Latent' hypothyroidism

3% of the population have microsomal antibodies in their blood associated with an increased TSH level, though no overt clinical features of myxoedema. The risk of minor degrees of hypothyroidism in these subjects with thyroid antibodies is 20:1 in men and 13:1 in women.

The incidence rate of overt hypothyroidism developing in subjects with circulating thyroid antibodies is 3% per year, so that half of these subjects will have developed myxoedema in 17 years and all of them in 34 years.

Hashimoto's thyroiditis

This is the most frequent type of auto-immune thyroid disease. The clinical characteristics are shown in Table 12.50.

It is likely that most cases of idiopathic myxoedema are the end-result of Hashimoto's thyroiditis.

Table 12.50   Clinical features of Hashi-moto's disease

• Goitre
• Hypothyroidism
• Circulating thyroid autoantibodies

Riedel's thyroiditis

This is a much rarer type of thyroiditis. It may be clinically indistinguishable from Hashimoto's thyroiditis.

The most important differentiating feature is that the gland is very hard, owing to progressive fibrosis.

CAN WE MODIFY THE NATURAL HISTORY?

Infancy

The most important measure for modifying the natural history of hypothyroidism in infancy and childhood is *screening* of newborn babies.

Screening for neonatal hypothyroidism

The desirability of a screening programme for neonatal hypothyroidism is based on the following considerations.

- Serious physical and mental defects ensue.
- The condition is completely reversible if treated early enough.
- Clinical diagnosis is very difficult before 4–6 weeks.

Screening is a very simple procedure, involving the collection of a small sample of blood onto a filter paper by a heel-prick 5–7 days after birth. The blood is then assayed for level of thyroid-stimulating hormone (TSH) and thyroxine (T_4). The typical change in hypothyroidism is a high TSH and a low T_4.

A sample of this kind is currently widely taken by the hospital or community midwife for phenylketonuria. The same sample can be used for assay of TSH and T_4.

If hypothyroidism is diagnosed at this time by this screening procedure, immediate treatment with an appropriate dose of thyroxine (see Table 12.43, p. 248) will ensure normal physical and mental development.

Adult myxoedema

In relation to adult myxoedema, it is important to detect Hashimoto's thyroiditis which is the commonest cause of hypothyroidism associated with a goitre. In these patients, with a goitre and circulating thyroid autoantibodies, there may be minimal or even no clinical manifestations of hypothyroidism, and very little change in their serum T_4 and TSH levels. However, these patients will almost invariably progress to fully-established hypothyroidism in the course of time. It is advisable therefore to treat them with full replacement thyroxine therapy for life.

With established myxoedema, the prognosis is excellent if permanent full-dose thyroxine replacement therapy is maintained.

Compliance with permanent replacement therapy may be a problem and becomes more evident with increasing age and the passage of time. Possible reasons for thyroxine being discontinued are shown in Table 12.51.

Table 12.51　Reasons for stopping thyroxine treatment

• Patient feels well – considers treatment unnecessary
• Patient forgets to renew prescription
• New doctor doubts original diagnosis

It is desirable for the family doctor to maintain a list of all patients on thyroxine treatment and arrange to see them annually. It would also be helpful if a means is established to *detect whenever such patients fail to renew their prescriptions* for thyroxine. Finally, it is important to impress the patient's relatives with the necessity of continuing *daily thyroxine treatment for life* if normal function is to be maintained.

USEFUL PRACTICAL POINTS

- Always consider hypothyroidism in any middle-aged or elderly patient, especially female, who slows up physically or mentally for no obvious reason.

- Remember the likely development of hypothyroidism in any patient treated for thyrotoxicosis with drugs, surgery or radioactive iodine.

- The commonest cause of hypothyroidism associated with a goitre is Hashimoto's thyroiditis.

- A goitrous patient with circulating thyroid autoantibodies requires life-long thyroxine treatment even in the absence of clinical or biochemical evidence of hypothyroidism.

- Myxoedema coma may result from exposure to cold in elderly patients, with severe hypothyroidism. It is a medical emergency and requires prompt admission to hospital and treatment with intravenous thyroid hormone and steroids.

13

Tiredness

PRESENT HISTORY

A 39-year-old-female social worker presented with increasing weakness, tiredness and lassitude for about 1 year.

Weakness and lassitude

She had not felt well for about a year. Over this period she complained of weakness, undue tiredness and lack of energy.

At first the weakness had only occurred when she had a lot to do and was under stress. More recently, however, she seemed to lack energy all the time, and it had been bad enough on some occasions to keep her off work. As a result she was having difficulty keeping up with her case load and she was losing interest in her work.

Other relevant facts on direct enquiry

Alimentary system

Her *appetite* had become poor over the previous year.

She denied indigestion or abdominal pain but did admit to recurrent bouts of *nausea*. She occasionally vomited clear fluid during these bouts.

There had been no recent change in her bowel habits.

She had *lost weight* over the past year, about half a stone (3 kg). She attributed this to her poor appetite.

Dizziness

She had noticed occasional episodes of dizziness: by this, she meant light-headedness and not vertigo. The dizziness would only last a few minutes and tended to occur in the morning on getting out of bed.

She had also noticed this light-headedness on getting up after kneeling, as when she was gardening. She had never lost consciousness.

Mental symptoms

She admitted to *irritability* and *depression* over the past year. She thought this was due to not being able to cope with her work.

Menstruation

Her periods were becoming irregular and scanty over the past year.

Negative points

She denied chronic respiratory disease.
She was not subject to night sweats.
She had no urinary symptoms, and in particular, no polydipsia or polyuria.

PAST HISTORY

She had a bad attack of '*pneumonia*' when she was 12 years old. This had kept her in hospital for 6 weeks and she had been told afterwards that it had left her with a 'scar on her lung'.

FAMILY HISTORY

Her mother suffered with *diabetes*. Otherwise there was nothing relevant.

PERSONAL HISTORY

She had two children aged 11 and 9 years. There had been no difficulties in either pregnancy, and in particular no bleeding after the births.
She did not smoke.
She drank very little alcohol, on social occasions only.

DRUG HISTORY

She was not on the contraceptive pill or any other type of regular drug treatment.

EXAMINATION

The abnormal physical signs are shown in Figure 13.1.

Skin

Her face and neck appeared sun-tanned. The nipples showed dark areolae. The palmar skin creases were pigmented. An appendicectomy scar was pigmented. There was a patch of brownish discolouration in the epigastric area.

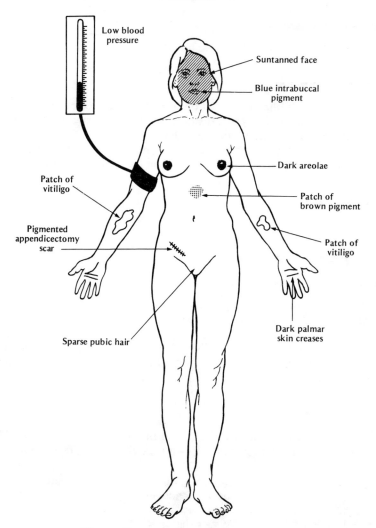

Figure 13.1 Abnormal physical signs

There was an area of depigmented skin (vitiligo) on each forearm.
Pubic and axillary hair were less than expected in a woman of this age.

Cardiovascular system

The pulse was regular but *poor volume*.

The blood pressure was 105/75 (lying) and 90/60 (standing).

The apex beat was difficult to feel and so could not be accurately localized.

The heart sounds were *very soft* but there was no other auscultatory abnormality.

437

Respiratory system

There were no abnormal signs in the lungs.

Alimentary system

There was a patch of bluish pigment on the buccal surface of the right cheek. There was a similar patch in the left side of the mouth between the base of the gum margin and the inside surface of the lower lip.

The only abdominal abnormalities were a small patch of *brown skin in the epigastric area* and a *brownish discolouration* of her *appendicectomy scar*.

Nervous system

No abnormality was found.

ANALYSIS OF THE HISTORY

Tiredness and lack of energy

These were the main presenting symptoms.

Tiredness is often encountered in general practice and is a difficult symptom to evaluate.

The first requirement is to establish whether the patient is complaining of *generalized fatigue* and lack of energy or *actual weakness* associated with loss of power in a particular limb or group of muscles.

Muscle weakness

If this is the real complaint it is helpful to find out whether it is episodic or persistent, since this finding may help with the diagnosis (Table 13.1).

Table 13.1   Some causes of episodic and persistent muscle weakness

• Episodic	• Myasthenia gravis
	• Multiple sclerosis
	• Transient ischaemic attacks
	• Hypokalaemic periodic paralysis
• Persistent	• Cerebrovascular disease
	• Parkinson's disease
	• Polyneuritis
	• Brain tumour
	• Muscle dystrophy

Generalized fatigue

Where the complaint is general tiredness and lack of energy, as in the present patient, it is important to decide whether the cause is likely to be *organic* or *psychogenic*. Table 13.2 shows some helpful pointers.

Table 13.2 Differentiation between organic and psychogenic tiredness

Psychogenic	Organic
'Lifelong'	Recent
Intermittent	Sustained
Only on waking	Later in the day
Exaggerated description	Factual description
May follow emotional trauma	No preceding stress
Other symptoms of anxiety	No anxiety symptoms

The patient's lassitude was recent, initially episodic but later sustained, factually described, not associated with any obvious stress and there were no accompanying symptoms of anxiety. This indicates that the patient's tiredness is likely to be organic.

Organic causes of tiredness

Table 13.3 shows some important causes of organic tiredness.

Table 13.3 Organic causes of tiredness

• Anaemia	
• Infections	• viral
	glandular fever
	hepatitis
	• tuberculosis
	• infective endocarditis
	• brucellosis
• Endocrine	• myxoedema
	• Addison's disease
	• hypopituitarism
• Metabolic disease	• uraemia
	• cirrhosis
• Drugs	• sedatives
	• tranquillizers
• Malignancy	
• Cardiorespiratory disease	

Anaemia

Anaemia is often responsible for tiredness, especially in women. Figure 13.2 shows the most likely causes of anaemia.

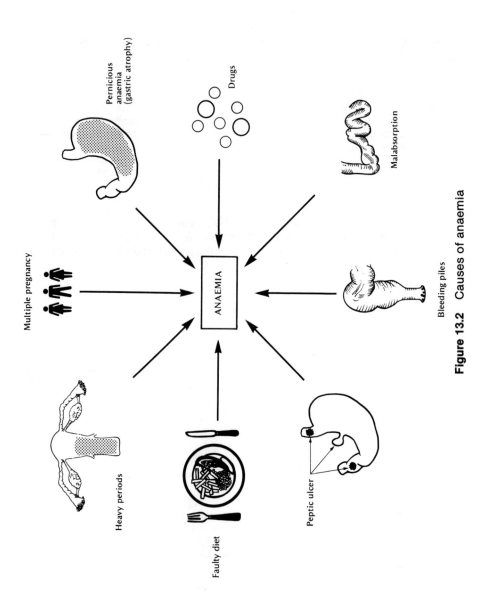

Figure 13.2   Causes of anaemia

If anaemia is present, there are symptoms present other than fatigue (Table 13.4).

Table 13.4 Symptoms of anaemia

> - Fatigue and lassitude
> - Breathlessness on exertion
> - Palpitations
> - Faintness or giddiness
> - Swelling of the legs

The absence of any other symptoms and the lack of any of the likely causes of anaemia excludes this diagnosis.

Infections

Occult infections are frequently overlooked.

Viral infections. Viral infections are accompanied by fever, muscle aching and malaise. Glandular fever will result also in sore throat and enlarged glands, while hepatitis causes upper abdominal discomfort and jaundice. The absence of any of these symptoms makes viral infection very unlikely.

Tuberculosis. Active pulmonary tuberculosis results in profuse night sweats, which were absent in this patient, and there were no respiratory symptoms. Extrapulmonary tuberculosis is also unlikely because of the lack of night sweats.

Infective endocarditis. The absence of a past history of rheumatic fever or chorea, rheumatic heart disease or recent dental treatment makes infective endocarditis unlikely.

Brucellosis. There was no contact with cattle, which would be expected in brucellosis.

Endocrine causes of tiredness

Myxoedema. Excessive tiredness is one of the predominant symptoms of myxoedema. The other symptoms are shown in Table 13.5; none of them was experienced by the patient, thus excluding myxoedema.

Table 13.5 Symptoms of myxoedema

> - Tiredness
> - Cold intolerance
> - Mental and physical slowing
> - Increasing weight
> - Constipation
> - Hoarseness of the voice
> - Loss of hair and dryness of skin

Addison's disease. The symptoms are shown in Table 13.6. The patient does have anorexia, nausea and vomiting, postural dizziness, scanty periods and depression. Addison's disease therefore remains a possible diagnosis based on the history.

Table 13.6   Symptoms of Addison's disease

- Excessive tiredness and fatigue
- Gastrointestinal
    anorexia
    nausea, vomiting
    abdominal pain (in crisis)
    constipation/diarrhoea
- Postural dizziness
- Darkening of the skin
- Depression
- Impotence and amenorrhoea

Hypopituitarism. The symptoms are shown in Table 13.7. The patient does have symptoms consistent with adrenal insufficiency. However, the absence of previous postpartum haemorrhage, and the lack of any symptoms of hypothyroidism, make it unlikely that the adrenal insufficiency is secondary to pituitary failure.

Table 13.7   Symptoms of hypopituitarism

- History of postpartum haemorrhage
- Loss of libido
- Amenorrhoea
- Symptoms of hypothyroidism (see Table 13.5)
- Symptoms of adrenal deficiency (see Table 13.6)

Metabolic disease
Metabolic disorders such as uraemia and cirrhosis may be insidious. The symptoms which might suggest renal disease leading to *uraemia* are shown in Table 13.8. The patient had none of these symptoms.

Table 13.8   Symptoms suggesting uraemia

- History of kidney disease
- Polyuria and polydipsia
- Itching of the skin
- Hiccoughs
- Diarrhoea (may be bloody)
- Muscle twitching
- Drowsiness
- Bleeding tendency
- Paraesthesiae or limb weakness (neuropathy)

The symptoms of *cirrhosis* are shown in Table 13.9. Apart from anorexia and nausea, the patient had no symptoms to suggest cirrhosis.

Table 13.9 Symptoms suggesting cirrhosis

- History of alcoholism
- History of jaundice or liver disease
- Flatulence, anorexia, nausea, vomiting
- Abdominal swelling (ascites)
- Swelling of the legs
- Bleeding tendency – spontaneous bruising
                          gastrointestinal
- Drowsiness, confusion, coma

Drugs
Psychotropic drugs such as tranquillizers often cause excessive tiredness. The patient had not been taking any drug.

Occult neoplasm
Occult cancer is very difficult to exclude on the history alone. Some of the sites often missed are shown in Figure 13.3.

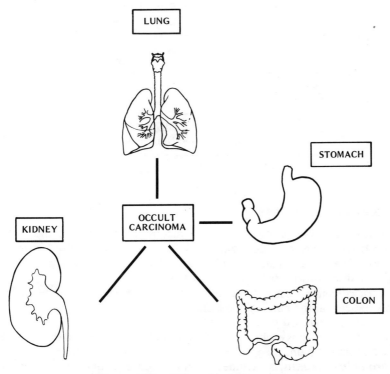

Figure 13.3 Sites of occult carcinoma

Apart from anorexia the patient had no symptoms pointing to any of these sites but further investigation would be necessary to exclude occult carcinoma with any certainty.

Cardiorespiratory disease
Severe heart or lung disease resulting in a grossly impaired oxygen supply to the tissues causes excessive fatigue.

In these circumstances, the fatigue is overshadowed by the other symptoms of the cardiorespiratory disease, especially breathlessness.

The lack of breathlessness excludes severe heart or lung disease.

Anorexia

The patient's appetite had deteriorated during the course of her illness.

Anorexia is often due to organic disease and the main causes are shown in Table 13.10.

Table 13.10   Causes of anorexia

• Gastrointestinal	• Gastritis
	• Carcinoma of stomach
	• Hepatitis
	• Pancreatitis
	• Crohn's disease
• Endocrine	• Addison's disease
	• Hypopituitarism
	• Hyperparathyroidism
• Chronic renal failure	
• Malignancy	
• Cardiorespiratory disease	
• Drugs	• Digitalis
	• Alcohol
	• Narcotics

Gastrointestinal disease

Gastritis is caused by excessive intake of alcohol or of irritant drugs, such as aspirin or the other non-steroidal anti-inflammatory drugs used in treating arthritis. The patient had not taken any drugs of this type and had no epigastric discomfort attributable to gastritis.

Gastric carcinoma is notorious for causing anorexia and cannot be excluded in this patient on the basis of the history alone.

Hepatitis is excluded by the lack of jaundice.

Acute pancreatitis is excluded by the length of the history and the absence of acute abdominal pain.

Chronic pancreatitis is excluded by the absence of diarrhoea with bulky offensive stools resulting from the associated malabsorption.

The absence of abdominal pain (especially in the right iliac fossa), bloody diarrhoea and perianal inflammation and the lack of involvement of skin, eyes, joints and spine excludes *Crohn's* disease.

Endocrine disease

Anorexia is frequent in *Addison's disease.*

It has already been pointed out that the patient has other symptoms consistent with Addison's disease (Table 13.6) and it remains therefore a likely diagnosis.

Hypopituitarism has also been discussed and excluded.

The symptoms of *hyperparathyroidism* are shown in Table 13.11.

Table 13.11   Symptoms of hyperparathyroidism

• Gastrointestinal	– anorexia nausea and vomiting
• Renal	– renal colic dysuria
• Musculoskeletal	– limb weakness bone pain
• Psychiatric	– depression personality change

The patient had no renal or musculoskeletal symptoms, which makes this diagnosis unlikely, though a serum calcium estimation would be required to exclude it with certainty.

Chronic renal failure

This diagnosis has been discussed already and excluded by the absence of the relevant history and other symptoms (Table 13.8, p. 442).

Malignancy

Occult malignancy has also been discussed and the desirability of perspicacious investigation pointed out.

Cardiorespiratory disease

Anorexia is a minor symptom in chronic cardiorespiratory disease and is overshadowed by the features of the heart or lung disease.

There was nothing to suggest chronic heart or lung disease in the patient.

Drugs

Digitalis is the most likely offender, especially in elderly patients and is then often accompanied by other symptoms of toxicity (Table 13.12).

Table 13.12 Symptoms of digitalis toxicity

- Anorexia
- Nausea
- Faintness (bradycardia or heart block)
- 'Missed' beats (ventricular ectopics)
- Palpitations (atrial tachycardia)

The patient was not taking digitalis, was not an alcoholic and had not had any form of narcotic.

Psychiatric causes of anorexia

Apart from organic disease, anorexia may be due to psychiatric disturbance (Table 13.13).

Table 13.13 Psychiatric causes of anorexia

- Anxiety
- Depression
- Anorexia nervosa

Anxiety
Anxiety may cause anorexia. Other symptoms are often present (Table 13.14).

Table 13.14 Symptoms of anxiety

- Palpitations
- Left inframammary pain
- Breathing difficulty
- Sweating
- Shakiness or tremors
- Anorexia
- 'Pins and needles'

Although the patient admitted anxiety about her work, there were none of the other symptoms to suggest an acute anxiety state.

Depression
The symptoms of depression are shown in Table 13.15 but none was present in the patient.

Table 13.15 Symptoms of depression

- Anorexia
- Insomnia
- Early morning waking
- Inability to concentrate
- Forgetfulness
- Fatigue
- Constipation
- Headache
- Weeping spells

Anorexia nervosa

Severe anorexia in a young girl should always suggest the possibility of anorexia nervosa. Amenorrhoea and marked loss of weight are invariable accompaniments.

The patient's age and the lack of marked anorexia or severe loss of weight and the presence of periods, although scanty, are against the diagnosis of anorexia nervosa.

Loss of weight

The patient had a modest loss of weight of half a stone (3 kg) in the previous year. The first fact to establish is whether the patient is taking a normal diet (Table 13.16).

Table 13.16 Abnormal diets causing weight loss

- Old people living alone
- Young girl obsessed with obesity
- Vegetarian diet (especially vegans)

The patient was not taking an abnormal diet.

Organic causes of loss of weight

The organic causes of loss of weight are shown in Table 13.17.

Most of these causes have been discussed already in the previous sections on tiredness and anorexia, and reference will therefore be made here to conditions not already mentioned.

447

Table 13.17   Organic causes of loss of weight

• Endocrine	• Diabetes mellitus
	• Thyrotoxicosis
	• Addison's disease
• Gastrointestinal	• Chronic vomiting
	• Chronic diarrhoea
• Chronic infection	• Tuberculosis
	• Infective endocarditis
	• Brucellosis
	• Fungal infection
• Malignant disease	
• Chronic renal failure	

Endocrine disease

Diabetes is diagnosed on the typical triad of symptoms shown in Table 13.18. In the absence of thirst and polyuria, diabetes is very unlikely.

Table 13.18   Diagnostic triad of symptoms in diabetes

- Thirst
- Polyuria
- Loss of weight

Thyrotoxicosis presents with typical symptoms (Table 13.19). Apart from weight loss, none of these symptoms was present. Additionally, the patient had a poor appetite.

Table 13.19   Symptoms of thyrotoxicosis

- Heat intolerance
- Excessive sweating
- Nervousness and tremors
- Loss of weight
- Good appetite
- Swelling of neck
- Staring eyes

Addison's disease remains a likely diagnosis.

Gastrointestinal disease

The patient did not have chronic vomiting or diarrhoea.

Chronic infection

Fungal infection often involves the respiratory tract: aspergillosis and candidiasis are the likely conditions.

This type of infection tends to occur in debilitated patients such as diabetics or alcoholics. Associated symptoms of pulmonary involvement, such as a productive cough, wheezing and breathlessness are frequent.

The patient was not debilitated and had no respiratory symptoms so fungal infection is very unlikely.

Psychogenic causes of loss of weight

The psychogenic causes of loss of weight are similar to those of anorexia (Table 13.13, p. 446) and have already been discussed.

Postural dizziness

The patient complained of dizziness on getting out of bed and also on standing upright from the stooped position. The causes of postural dizziness are shown in Table 13.20.

Table 13.20   Causes of postural dizziness

> • Vasovagal attack
> • Prolonged standing
> • Prolonged bed-rest
> • Vertebrobasilar insufficiency
> • Autonomic neuropathy – diabetes
> • Drugs
>   peripheral vasodilators in hypertension
>   L-dopa in Parkinsonism
>   phenothiazines

Vasovagal attacks

Vasovagal attacks produce typical symptoms (Table 13.21).

Table 13.21 Symptoms of vasovagal attack

> • Sense of impending passing out
> • Sweating
> • Nausea
> • Dimness of vision

The patient had none of these symptoms.

Standing and bed-rest

The patient had not been standing a long time prior to her attacks of dizziness; nor had she undergone a period of prolonged bed-rest.

Vertebrobasilar insufficiency

The distinctive feature of vertebrobasilar insufficiency is the precipitation of dizziness by sudden movement of the head. Cervical spondylosis is also associated in many cases, leading to pain and creaking in the back of the neck.

The patient did not relate her dizziness to head movement and had no neck pain or creaking.

Autonomic neuropathy

Autonomic neuropathy is most frequently encountered as a complication of diabetes. Nocturnal diarrhoea is often associated.

The patient had no symptoms of diabetes and no diarrhoea, thus excluding this diagnosis.

Drugs

The patient had not taken any of the drugs listed in Table 13.20, p. 449.

Depression

The patient admitted to recent depression.

Most depressed patients have a psychiatric disorder but depression occasionally results from *physical disease* which should always be excluded (Table 13.22).

Table 13.22   Physical causes of depression

• Febrile illness	– influenza pyelonephritis hepatitis
• Head injury	
• Surgical operation	
• Menopause	
• Puerperium	
• Myocardial infarction	
• Multiple sclerosis	
• Cerebrovascular disease	
• Endocrine disease	– myxoedema Addison's disease

Physical causes of depression

The patient had not had a *febrile illness*; nor had she sustained a *head injury*, *surgical operation* or *heart attack*.

She was not menopausal or in the *puerperium*.

There was no neurological history to suggest *multiple sclerosis*.

There were no limb weakness, paraesthesiae or cranial nerve disturbances to suggest *cerebrovascular disease*.

Myxoedema has already been excluded by the lack of symptoms (Table 13.5).

Addison's disease turns up again and is the likely diagnosis.

Psychiatric depression

Psychiatric depression may be triggered off by a traumatic emotional experience, which was not evident in the patient's history.

Failing periods

The causes of oligomenorrhoea are shown in Table 13.23.

Table 13.23 Causes of oligomenorrhoea

• Psychological	– stress
	anorexia nervosa
• Endocrine	
• Pituitary	– acromegaly
	Simmonds's disease
• Addison's disease	
• Ovarian	– polycystic disease
	tumours
	infection
• Systemic disease	– anaemia
	tuberculosis

Psychological disturbance

Stress
The patient was certainly under stress because of her inability to cope with her work.

The change in her periods, however, preceded the difficulties with her work, which makes stress an unlikely cause.

Anorexia nervosa
Anorexia nervosa was thought unlikely, as anorexia and loss of weight were not severe enough and she showed none of the characteristic restlessness often seen in this condition.

Endocrine causes of oligomenorrhoea

There were no symptoms to suggest *acromegaly* (Table 13.24).

Hypopituitarism has been discussed previously and thought unlikely.

Addison's disease seems once again to be the likely cause of the scanty periods.

Table 13.24 Symptoms of acromegaly

- Headache
- Visual deterioration
- Painful joints in hands and feet
- Symptoms of diabetes
- Excessive sweating
- Skin troubles
    acne
    excessive hair in females

Ovarian disease cannot be excluded on history alone.

Systemic disease, such as anaemia and tuberculosis, has been excluded previously.

PAST HISTORY

The past history of a severe 'pneumonia' which left the patient with a 'scarred' lung may be highly relevant.

The pulmonary infection could have been due to *tuberculosis* and this can result in adrenal involvement with the development of Addison's disease.

FAMILY HISTORY

The history of diabetes in the patient's mother may be relevant.

Addison's disease is often caused by auto-immune disease affecting the adrenal glands. Diabetes may also be the result of auto-immune pancreatic disease since auto-immune disease follows a familial pattern. The patient's Addison's disease may be the result of an auto-immune disturbance transmitted through her mother.

CONCLUSIONS FROM THE HISTORY

The patient's symptoms are:

- increasing tiredness
- anorexia and nausea
- loss of weight
- postural dizziness
- scanty periods
- depression.

The combination of severe fatigue, gastrointestinal disturbance and postural dizziness is very suggestive of Addison's disease.

The oligomenorrhoea and depression also fit in with this diagnosis.

The past history is suggestive of tuberculosis and indicates a likely cause of the adrenal damage leading to Addison's disease.

ANALYSIS OF THE EXAMINATION

Pigmentation

The outstanding finding was the brown pigmentation affecting:

- face
- skin creases
- epigastrium
- appendicectomy scar.

She also had bluish intrabuccal pigment.
The causes of pigmentation are shown in Table 13.25.

Table 13.25   Causes of skin pigmentation

• Racial	
• Sunburn	
• Liver disease	• Haemochromatosis
	• Primary biliary cirrhosis
• Chronic renal failure	
• Malignancy	• Adenocarcinoma (acanthosis nigricans)
	• Malignant lymphoma
	• Ectopic ACTH syndrome
• Drugs	• Psoralens (psoriasis)
	• Phenolphthalein (laxative)
	• Barbiturates (epilepsy)
	• Heavy metals
	silver
	arsenic
	mercury
• Endocrine	• Addison's disease
	• Cushing's syndrome
	• Acromegaly
	• Pregnancy (chloasma gravidarum)
	• Contraceptive pill

Racial

This was not relevant.

Sunburn

There was no history of prolonged or excessive exposure to the sun.

Liver disease

Haemochromatosis
The features of haemochromatosis are shown in Figure 13.4.

The patient's sex together with the absence of any features of cirrhosis, diabetes and heart failure excludes this diagnosis.

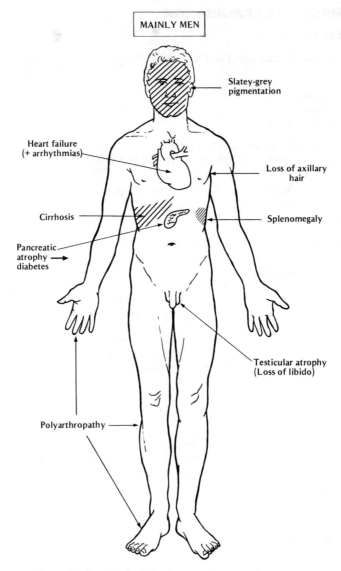

Figure 13.4   Clinical features of haemochromatosis

Primary biliary cirrhosis

The features of primary biliary cirrhosis are shown in Figure 13.5.

The absence of pruritus, jaundice, xanthomata and hepatosplenomegaly excludes this diagnosis.

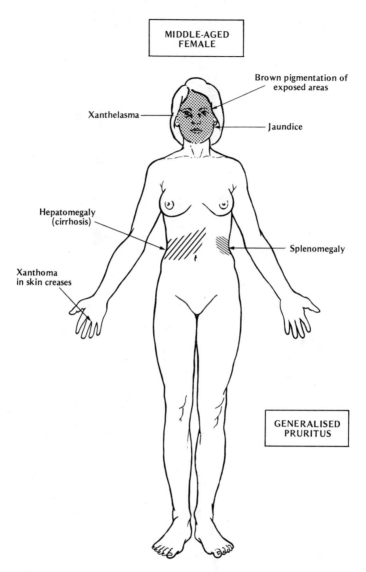

Figure 13.5 Clinical features of primary biliary cirrhosis

Chronic renal failure

This is sometimes associated with hypermelanosis and generalized dusky pigmentation.

Chronic renal failure has been excluded because of the lack of any other relevant evidence (Table 13.8, p. 442).

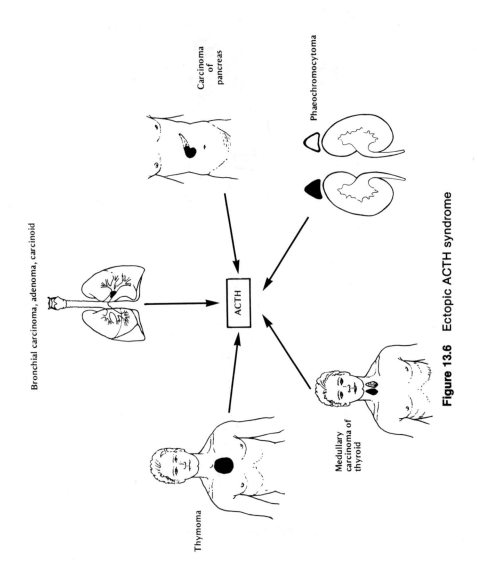

Figure 13.6 Ectopic ACTH syndrome

Malignancy

Acanthosis nigricans
Adenocarcinoma and reticulosis may be associated with acanthosis nigricans, in which there is dark pigmentation especially affecting the neck, axillae and extremities.

There were no focal symptoms or signs to suggest carcinoma of any particular organ.

Lymphoma
The absence of lymph node enlargement is against a diagnosis of malignant lymphoma.

Ectopic ACTH syndrome
The ectopic ACTH syndrome may be associated with various neoplastic conditions (Figure 13.6).

Some features of Cushing's syndrome are frequently present with the pigmentation (Table 13.26). Unlike pituitary or adrenal Cushing's disease, weight gain, truncal obesity and abdominal striae are rare.

Table 13.26   Features of Cushing's syndrome associated with ectopic ACTH syndrome

• Muscle weakness
• Hypertension
• Peripheral oedema
face
feet
• Hirsutes (in women)

The absence of any features of Cushing's syndrome excludes the ectopic ACTH syndrome in this patient.

Drugs

The patient had not taken any of the drugs listed in Table 13.25 (p. 453); nor had she any contact with the heavy metals.

Endocrine disease

Addison's disease
Addison's disease leads to a characteristic distribution of pigmentation (Table 13.27).

The patient's pigmentation closely follows this pattern and therefore Addison's disease is once again suggested as the most likely diagnosis.

Table 13.27 Distribution of pigmentation in Addison's disease

- Exposed areas – face, hands, neck
- Skin creases
- Normally pigmented areas – nipple areola
- Site of skin friction – epigastrium (bending)
- Surgical scars
- Buccal mucosa (bluish patches)

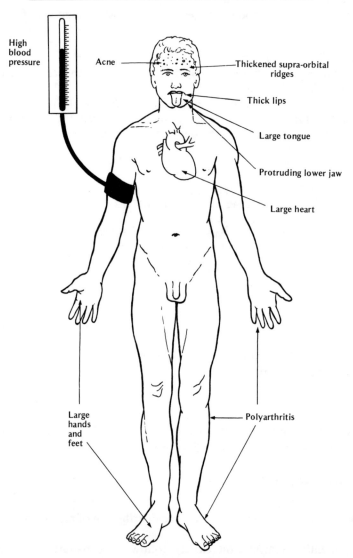

Figure 13.7 Clinical features of acromegaly

Cushing's syndrome
There were no features of Cushing's syndrome, as already mentioned.

Acromegaly
The symptoms of acromegaly have been shown in Table 13.24 and the signs are indicated in Figure 13.7.

There was no overgrowth in the patient's skull or extremities to suggest acromegaly.

Vitiligo

The patient showed patches of vitiligo (depigmented skin) on both forearms. The disorders which may be associated with vitiligo are shown in Figure 13.8.

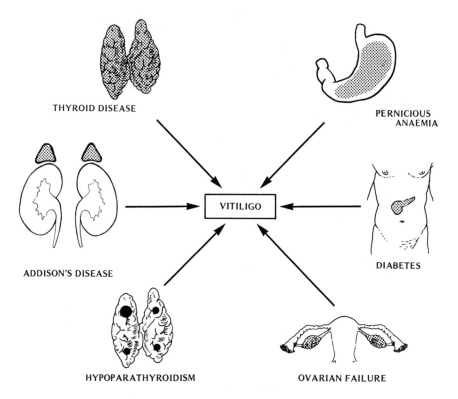

Figure 13.8   Disorders associated with vitiligo

The distinctive feature of all these conditions is the frequent presence of organ-specific autoantibodies to the various organs involved.

Thyroid disease

Hyperthyroidism

Hyperthyroidism may cause vitiligo. Apart from the loss of weight there were no other symptoms to suggest thyrotoxicosis (see Table 13.19, p. 448); nor were there any signs of this condition on examination (Figure 13.9).

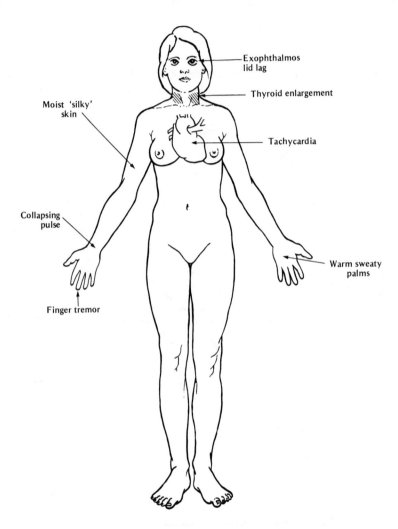

Exophthalmos
lid lag

Thyroid enlargement

Moist 'silky' skin

Tachycardia

Collapsing pulse

Warm sweaty palms

Finger tremor

Figure 13.9   Signs of thyrotoxicosis

Myxoedema
Myxoedema causes vitiligo less frequently than thyrotoxicosis. It is excluded by the absence of symptoms (see Table 13.5, p. 441) and signs (Figure 13.10).

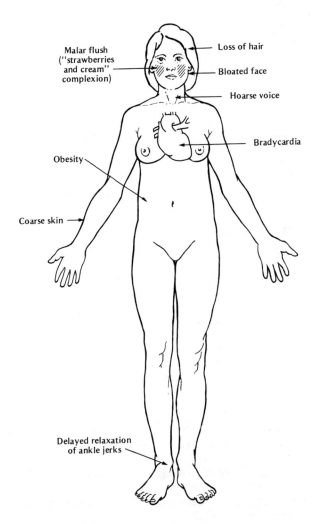

Malar flush ("strawberries and cream" complexion)

Loss of hair

Bloated face

Hoarse voice

Bradycardia

Obesity

Coarse skin

Delayed relaxation of ankle jerks

Figure 13.10 Signs of myxoedema

Pernicious anaemia

The clinical features of pernicious anaemia are shown in Table 13.28; none was present in the patient.

Table 13.28 Clinical features of pernicious anaemia

- Anaemia
- Pale lemon tinge in the skin
- Atrophic glossitis
- Splenomegaly
- Peripheral neuritis
- Subacute combined degeneration of cord
- Prematurely white hair

Diabetes

Diabetes is a rare cause of vitiligo. The unlikelihood of this diagnosis has already been pointed out by the absence of polydipsia and polyuria.

Addison's disease

Addison's disease remains once again the most likely cause of the vitiligo.

Cardiovascular system

The main findings in the patient are summarized in Table 13.29.

Table 13.29 Patient's cardiovascular findings

- Poor volume pulse
- Low blood pressure
- Postural hypotension
- Impalpable apex beat
- Poor heart sounds

The poor volume of the pulse indicates a low cardiac output.

Hypotension is attributable to the depletion of body sodium occurring in Addison's disease with consequent reduction in the circulating blood volume.

The difficulty in feeling the apex beat and the poor quality of the heart sounds indicate impaired cardiac function following the decrease in blood volume produced by sodium depletion.

Other additional factors have been suggested to account for the poor heart function in Addison's disease (Table 13.30).

Table 13.30 Poor heart function in Addison's disease

- Depleted blood volume
- Disturbed myocardial potassium metabolism
- Disuse atrophy in the myocardial cells
- Deposition of haemofucsin in myocardium

CONCLUSIONS FROM THE EXAMINATION

The outstanding findings were:

- pigmentation distributed in the characteristic pattern of Addison's disease
- hypotension and associated poor cardiovascular function typically found in Addison's disease.

In view of these two distinctive features there is little doubt of the diagnosis of Addison's disease.

INVESTIGATION OF ADDISON'S DISEASE

Investigations of adrenal insufficiency involves three aims:

- establishing the diagnosis
- distinguishing primary and secondary disease
- detecting the causal pathology.

Establishing the diagnosis

Serum electrolytes

This is the simplest test available for the diagnosis of Addison's disease.

The typical changes are shown in Table 13.31. They are due to inadequate production of the salt-retaining hormone, aldosterone, by the adrenal cortex.

Table 13.31 Typical electrolyte changes in Addison's disease

- Reduced sodium (Na^+) concentration
- Increased potassium (K^+) concentration
- Increased blood urea level

These alterations in sodium, potassium and urea levels are found only if the adrenal insufficiency is severe, and are particularly marked if the patient is going into an Addisonian crisis.

The patient's electrolyte concentrations and urea levels were all within normal limits.

Plasma cortisol (hydrocortisone) level

The plasma cortisol level is low in Addison's disease.

This is a much better test than serum electrolyte and urea estimation which is non-specific and only abnormal in severe insufficiency.

The patient's fasting cortisol level at 8 a.m. was reduced to $6\,\mu g/dl$ (normal $10-25\,\mu g/dl$).

This confirms adrenal insufficiency.

Urinary steroid excretion

The 24h urinary excretion of 17-oxogenic steroids, which are metabolites of cortisol, is reduced in Addison's disease.

This is not a very reliable test since the same reduction can occur in any chronic debilitating illness. This test was not considered necessary.

Adrenocortical stimulation tests

Because the plasma cortisol level may be within the normal range in a patient with Addison's disease under resting conditions, the definitive way to confirm adrenal insufficiency is to show an impaired response by the adrenal cortex to stimulation with ACTH or with the synthetic bioactive part of the ACTH molecule, tetracosactrin (Synacthen).

Two tests are in use – the *short Synacthen test* and the *depot Synacthen test*.

The short test assesses the response to a single injection after 1 hour and is employed to demonstrate adrenal insufficiency.

The depot test assesses the long term response over 3 days to daily injections of the depot preparations and is used to distinguish between primary adrenal failure and adrenal failure secondary to pituitary disease or long term steroid treatment, when the adrenal gland will respond to prolonged stimulation by Synacthen as it is only partly suppressed by pituitary failure or steroid therapy.

The patient had a short Synacthen test which showed a *persisting low level of plasma cortisol* (below 10 μg/dl). This confirms the diagnosis of adrenal insufficiency.

Differentiation between primary and secondary adrenal insufficiency

The distinction between primary and secondary adrenal insufficiency can be made clinically by the presence of pigmentation in the primary disease and the presence of hypothyroidism, as well as adrenal insufficiency, if the disorder is due to pituitary failure.

A more objective differentiation can be made by tests.

Prolonged ACTH or Synacthen test

The diagnosis of secondary adrenal insufficiency requires a demonstration that the low plasma cortisol level can be induced to rise to normal by ACTH or Synacthen stimulation over several days. In Addison's disease, on the other-hand, no amount of ACTH will restore the cortisol level to normal.

Insulin hypoglycaemia test

This is a test of pituitary function: insulin-induced hypoglycaemia is used to stimulate the pituitary gland to produce ACTH. This will result in cortisol production by the adrenal gland and an increase in plasma cortisol level (Figure 13.11).

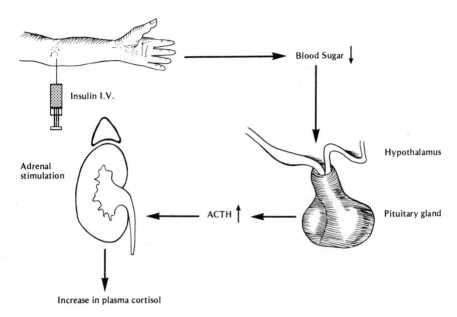

Figure 13.11 Insulin–hypoglycaemia test of pituitary function

If pituitary failure is present, there will be no increase in ACTH secretion by the gland and therefore no increase in plasma cortisol.

Since the adrenal response may be suppressed in longstanding pituitary insufficiency, it may be necessary to give preliminary treatment with Synacthen to restore normal adrenal responsiveness before doing the insulin test.

Estimation of plasma ACTH level

This is a very sophisticated test which can be done in only few centres. It is a very accurate method of distinguishing primary from secondary adrenal insufficiency.

In primary Addison's disease, the ACTH level is high owing to the feedback mechanism between the adrenal and pituitary glands (Figure 13.12).

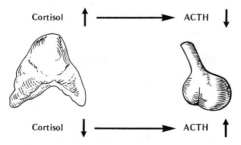

Figure 13.12 Pituitary–adrenal feedback mechanism

465

In adrenal insufficiency secondary to pituitary failure, the plasma ACTH level is low.

In the patient's case it was not considered necessary to carry out any of these tests since it was clear from the marked pigmentation and absence of clinical evidence of hypothyroidism that she had primary Addison's disease.

Detection of causal pathology of the Addison's disease

The causes of Addison's disease are shown in Table 13.32.

Table 13.32   Causes of Addison's disease

- Auto-immune disease
- Tuberculosis
- Secondary carcinoma
- Haemochromatosis
- Amyloidosis
- Sarcoidosis

Auto-immune disease

This is the most frequent cause of Addison's disease.

The diagnosis is based on demonstrating adrenocortical autoantibodies in the circulation which are found more commonly in female patients (80%) than in males (50%) with Addison's disease.

Other autoantibodies may be found also in Addison's disease which may or may not be associated with their corresponding clinical disorders (Table 13.33).

Table 13.33   Auto-immune disease associated with Addison's disease

Antibodies	Clinical disorder
Thyroid	Hypothyroidism
Intrinsic factor	Pernicious anaemia
Gastric parietal cell	
Islets of Langerhans	Diabetes mellitus
Parathyroid	Hypoparathyroidism
Ovarian	Premature menopause

The patient did not have any adrenocortical or other antibodies listed in Table 13.33, thus making auto-immune disorder unlikely as the cause of the Addison's disease.

Tuberculosis

This is the second most frequent cause of Addison's disease.

Chest X-ray
A chest X-ray is useful in showing evidence of previous tuberculosis and this was present in the patient's X-ray (Figure 13.13).

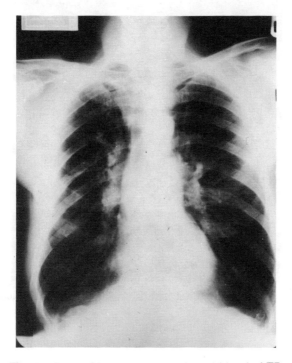

Figure 13.13   Chest X-ray showing old healed TB

The chest X-ray may also show a small and narrow heart in Addison's disease due to the low circulating blood volume consequent on sodium depletion.

Plain X-ray of the abdomen
A plain X-ray of the abdomen should also be done as it may show calcification in the adrenal glands secondary to tuberculosis.

The patient's abdominal X-ray is shown in Figure 13.14, and very clearly demonstrates extensive adrenal calcification. This confirms the diagnosis of tuberculosis as the cause of the patient's Addison's disease.

467

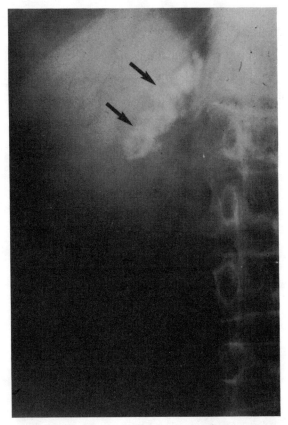

Figure 13.14 Abdominal X-ray showing adrenal calcification

Tuberculin test

A tuberculin test may be of value – if it is negative tuberculosis is unlikely. It was not considered necessary in the patient as the diagnosis of tuberculous adrenal glands had been clearly established.

Secondary carcinoma

Unless there is a demonstrable site of primary carcinoma this diagnosis is very difficult to establish during life. There was no obvious primary carcinoma in the patient.

Haemochromatosis

This diagnosis has already been considered and excluded by the absence of appropriate manifestations (see Figure 13.4, p. 454).

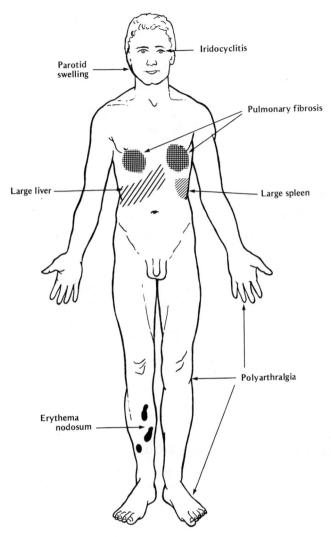

Figure 13.15   Clinical features of sarcoidosis

Amyloidosis

The clinical features of amyloidosis are shown in Table 13.34. None of these features was evident in the patient.

Sarcoidosis

The clinical features are shown in Figure 13.15. There was nothing to suggest sarcoidosis in the patient.

Table 13.34   Clinical features of amyloidosis

• Primary	• Heart failure
	• Peripheral neuritis
	• Large tongue
	• Skin lesions
• Secondary	• Diarrhoea
	• Nephrotic syndrome
	• Hepatosplenomegaly

Other investigations of value in Addison's disease

Electrocardiogram

This is abnormal in Addison's disease but the changes are non-specific (Table 13.35).

Table 13.35   Electrocardiogram changes in Addison's disease

- Sinus bradycardia
- Flat or inverted T wave
- Generally low voltage
- Prolonged Q–T interval
- Conduction defects (20%)

MANAGEMENT OF ADDISON'S DISEASE

If Addison's disease is suspected in general practice, urgent referral to hospital is desirable because of the risk of adrenal crisis. This will be discussed subsequently.

General management

Education

The first requirement is to explain the nature of the disease to the patient and his immediate family fully and simply. The possible hazards should be pointed out and the necessity to seek urgent medical advice if the patient feels at all ill.

Information

The patient should carry a steroid card or wear an appropriate pendant or bracelet to indicate that he suffers from Addison's disease and his current dose of cortisol.

Intercurrent infection

He should be advised to double his dose of cortisol if he develops an intercurrent infection and there is any difficulty or delay in obtaining medical advice.

Exercise

During periods of excessive exercise, especially if associated with marked sweating or in hot weather, the patient should be advised to increase his intake of salt by taking sodium chloride tablets 300 mg.

Specific treatment

The basis of specific treatment in Addison's disease is *cortisol replacement therapy*. The drugs available are shown in Table 13.36.

Table 13.36 Drugs used in treating Addison's disease

- Cortisol (hydrocortisone)
- Cortisone acetate
- Prednisone/prednisolone
- Dexamethasone
- Fludrocortisone

Cortisol (hydrocortisone)

Most patients respond satisfactorily to 10–15 mg of cortisol twice daily.

An alternative dosage regime is 20 mg in the morning and 10 mg in the evening to mimic the normal diurnal variation in adrenal cortisol output.

Cortisone acetate

There is little point in using cortisone acetate instead of cortisol since the cortisone is converted to cortisol anyway in the body.

Prednisone and prednisolone

Both these drugs may be used in a dose of 2.5 mg twice daily, but have the slight disadvantage of not possessing adequate mineralocorticoid effect.

Dexamethasone

This drug is undesirable in the treatment of Addison's disease because it possesses a natriuretic effect.

Fludrocortisone

Although cortisol alone may provide some mineralocorticoid action, it is standard practice to add the more specific mineralocorticoid preparation fludrocortisone (Florinet) in a dose of 0.1 mg daily.

In secondary adrenal insufficiency due to pituitary failure, a mineralocorticoid is not necessary because aldosterone production by the adrenal gland is not under pituitary control. However, additional replacement therapy with thyroxine, and possibly sex hormones, should always be considered.

Follow-up assessment

The patient should be reassessed initially at fortnightly intervals, extending progressively up to 3 monthly or 6 monthly visits if response is satisfactory.

The most important periodic measurements are indicated in Table 13.37. At each visit, evidence of undertreatment or overtreatment should be sought (Table 13.38).

Table 13.37 Important measurements
in following up Addison's disease

• Body weight
• Blood pressure
• Serum potassium

Table 13.38 Detection of under- or over-treatment
with steroids for Addison's disease

• Undertreatment	–	Fatigue
		Low blood pressure
		Raised blood urea
		Raised serum potassium
• Overtreatment	–	High blood pressure
		Oedema
		Heart failure
		Hypokalaemia

Special therapeutic considerations

Addisonian crisis

An Addisonian crisis occurs because of the inability of the patient to increase the adrenal output of cortisol in response to stress.

The features of an Addisonian crisis are shown in Table 13.39. The types of stress which may precipitate a crisis are shown in Table 13.40.

Table 13.39 Clinical features of an Addisonian crisis

- Acute abdominal pain
- Nausea and vomiting
- Severe hypotension→shock
- Lethargy→drowsiness→coma

Table 13.40 Types of stress precipitating an Addisonian crisis

- Intercurrent infection
- Surgery – including dental extraction
- Other trauma – injury
- Vomiting or diarrhoea with dehydration

In a crisis, it is essential immediately to increase the dose of cortisol and give it parenterally, preferably intravenous. Dehydration is treated by intravenous glucose/saline.

If a general practitioner suspects an impending crisis in an Addisonian patient, he should give an intravenous or intramuscular injection of 100 mg of hydrocortisone sodium succinate and arrange urgent admission to hospital.

Pregnancy

It is not necessary to alter the dose of cortisol during an uncomplicated pregnancy.

If vomiting occurs due to toxaemia the dose of cortisol will need to be increased and the patient carefully monitored for clinical and biochemical evidence of adrenal crisis (Table 13.41).

Table 13.41 Signs of Addisonian crisis

• Clinical	–	acute abdominal pain
		nausea and vomiting
		low blood pressure
		drowsiness
• Biochemical	–	low serum sodium
		high serum potassium
		high blood urea

It is advisable to give 50 mg of intramuscular hydrocortisone every 6 hours during labour to minimize the effect of the stress and prevent acute adrenal insufficiency developing.

NATURAL HISTORY OF ADDISON'S DISEASE

Original description

Addison's original description in 1855 of a disorder consisting of 'general languor and debility, remarkable feebleness of the heart's action, irritability of the stomach and a peculiar change in the colour of the skin' has yet to be improved.

Prevalence

The prevalence has been variably assessed as 12–40 per million of the population.

Auto-immune is twice as common as all other causes of the disease added together.

Sex incidence

Women predominate by 2:1 in the auto-immune type of the disease, but the sex incidence is equal in the other types of Addison's disease.

Prognosis

The death rate from Addison's disease is now just over 1 per million of the population.

Before the advent of steroid treatment death occurred within months of diagnosis, or rarely years. Now, the prognosis of successful steroid-treated patients should approximate to that of the general population. The requirements for this favourable prognosis are shown in Table 13.42.

Table 13.42   Requirements for favourable prognosis in Addison's disease

• Blood cortisol and electrolytes kept normal
• Increased steroid given for all forms of stress
• An identity card or bracelet is always available

The prognosis may be more adverse if other disease is present such as diabetes or amyloidosis, and will then depend on the prognosis of the systemic disease itself.

CAN WE MODIFY THE NATURAL HISTORY?

The only measure currently available to produce any significant prevention of the disease is the detection and effective treatment of tuberculosis. Measures which may be helpful are shown in Table 13.43.

Table 13.43   Measures to improve management of tuberculosis

• Raise resistance of population	• Better housing
	• Better jobs
	• Better nutrition
• BCG vaccination	• Young people
	• Health workers
• Detection of tuberculosis by mass mobile X-rays	• Teachers
	• Nurses
	• Bus conductors
	• Mental hospital inmates
	• Prisoners
• Eradicate tuberculosis from cows	

Once Addison's disease has become established the most important measure is to ensure that the dose of steroid is adequate whenever a stressful situation develops.

USEFUL PRACTICAL POINTS

- Brown pigmentation of the exposed areas, scars and skin creases is the single most helpful pointer to the diagnosis of Addison's disease. Additional confirmation is given by bluish pigment in the mouth.

- Addison's disease may be asymptomatic until an infection, operation or gastrointestinal upset occurs.

- The most important differentiating feature between Addison's disease and adrenal insufficiency secondary to pituitary failure is the presence of pigmentation in the primary disease.

- It is essential for all patients with Addison's disease to carry some means of identification of their disorder, with an up-to-date record of their steroid dose.

- Patients with Addison's disease should be advised to double their dose of steroid if they feel ill or develop an infection.

- Any patient with Addison's disease who appears to be developing an acute adrenal crisis should receive an immediate intramuscular or intravenous injection of 100 mg of hydrocortisone and be admitted to hospital as an emergency.

14

Loss of weight and back pain

PRESENT HISTORY

A 60-year-old housewife presented with recent loss of weight and pain in her back.

Weight loss

She had been steadily losing weight over the past few months and her husband was worried because she seemed to be getting very thin. Altogether, she had lost about 1 stone (6.5 kg).

She had not been dieting in any way but did say that her appetite had been getting poor. She wondered whether she was losing weight because she wasn't eating enough food.

Back pain

She had suffered with her back for many years. This usually consisted of pain in the lower lumbar area which sometimes radiated down the back of her right thigh. She had worn a spinal support for this for the last 5 years.

However, she had noticed a different pain in her back recently. It was located higher up in the spine in the middle of the back. This pain had come on about 1 month earlier and was very persistent.

She found that she was having increasing difficulty moving about because of this pain in her back: it was worse if she tried to bend. Her only real relief was when she was in bed lying still.

Although the pain was in the middle of her back, sometimes it would move to below her right shoulder blade.

She thought that the pain was steadily getting worse.

Other relevant facts on direct enquiry

Alimentary system

Her *appetite* had become *poor* over the last few months.

She was beginning to feel *nauseated* with her meals over the same period. She had vomited only once – the fluid was clear and did not contain blood.

There was no previous history of indigestion or heartburn and no current abdominal pain.

She had become *constipated* recently.

Urinary system

Over the last month or two she had noticed *increased frequency* of passing urine, especially at night.

She had also noticed that she seemed to be more *thirsty* and was drinking a lot more fluid.

She denied any dysuria.

She had never had kidney or bladder trouble before.

Nervous system

She had developed a persistent dull *headache* recently over the top and back of her head: it wasn't severe but seemed to interfere with her concentration.

She admitted also that she was getting very *depressed*. She attributed this to the persistent headache and the worry about her loss of weight.

She denied any paraesthesiae, limb weakness or disturbance of bladder control.

She had her menopause when she was 47 years old.

General

She admitted increasing tiredness and lack of energy over recent weeks. Any effort seemed too much and easily provoked *breathlessness* and sometimes *palpitations*.

PAST HISTORY

Although she had not been subject to lung trouble before, over the last few months she had experienced several bad attacks of bronchitis which were very slow to respond to antibiotics.

She had a bad attack of *shingles* (herpes zoster) 3 months earlier. This had affected her right lumbar area. The pain was still troublesome at times.

FAMILY HISTORY

There were no relevant illnesses.

SOCIAL HISTORY

She had been an active woman up to the time of her recent mid-dorsal pain. This had undoubtedly interfered with her looking after her family because it seemed so painful whenever she moved her back.

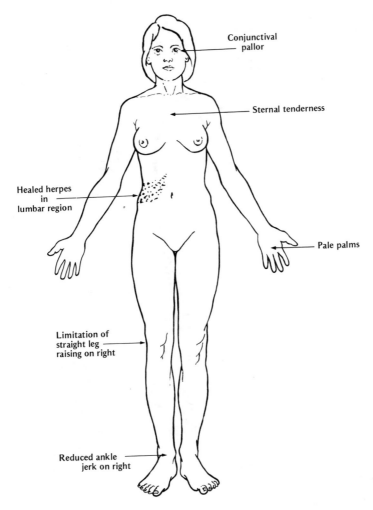

Loss of weight and back pain

Conjunctival pallor

Sternal tenderness

Healed herpes in lumbar region

Pale palms

Limitation of straight leg raising on right

Reduced ankle jerk on right

Figure 14.1 Abnormal physical signs (general)

She did not smoke.
She did not drink alcohol.

DRUG HISTORY

She had used several types of analgesic tablets for her back pain but was now taking frequent paracetamol which only gave limited relief.

EXAMINATION

The abnormal physical signs are shown in Figures 14.1 and 14.2.

479

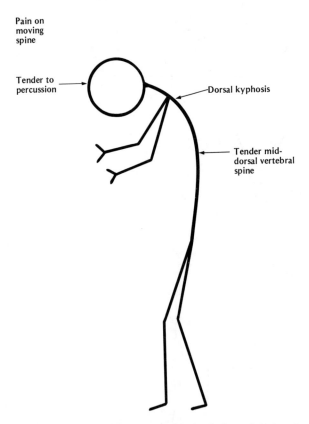

Figure 14.2   Abnormal physical signs (skeletal)

General

The patient looked ill.

She had obviously lost weight.

The conjunctivae and palms were pale. The tongue was normal. There was no koilonychia.

There were no enlarged lymph nodes.

Skeletal findings

Dorsal spine

She had a dorsal kyphosis.

Palpation showed tenderness over the spines of the 5th and 6th dorsal vertebrae. This was even more marked on percussion over the spine.

Forward flexion of the spine was considerably inhibited by pain.

There were no local areas of tenderness over any of the ribs, but there was slight *tenderness over the sternum* both with palpation and percussion.

Lumbar spine

There was no local tenderness over the lumbar vertebrae.

Straight leg raising was limited on the right to 45° because of back pain and pain in the back of the thigh.

Cervical spine

Vertical rotation and lateral flexion were limited and slightly painful. Crepitus was felt on movement.

Skull

Single finger percussion generally over the skull was uncomfortable.

There were several localized areas of more definite tenderness over the vertex.

Cardiovascular system

The blood pressure was 160/90.
There were no abnormal signs.

Respiratory system

There were no abnormal findings.

Abdomen

There was no enlargement of the liver or spleen.
There was no renal tenderness or renal enlargement.

Nervous system

The only abnormal finding was a reduced right ankle jerk.
There were no sensory abnormalities in the right leg.

ANALYSIS OF THE HISTORY

Loss of weight

The main presenting complaint was loss of weight.

The first fact to establish in any patient with loss of weight is whether an

Table 14.1 Deficient diets

• Old people living alone
• Young overweight girls obsessed with weight
• Vegetarians and vegans

abnormal diet is being taken. The groups of people in whom this may be relevant are shown in Table 14.1.

If diet is considered adequate nutritionally, as in this patient, consideration will need to be given to those organic diseases which may be responsible (Table 14.2).

Table 14.2 Organic causes of weight loss

• Endocrine disease	• Diabetes
	• Thyrotoxicosis
	• Addison's disease
• Gastrointestinal disease	• Chronic vomiting
	• Chronic diarrhoea
	• Malabsorption
• Chronic infection	• Tuberculosis
	• Infective endocarditis
	• Brucellosis
	• Fungal infection
• Malignant disease	• Occult carcinoma
	• Reticulosis
	• Myelomatosis
• Chronic renal failure	

Endocrine disease

Diabetes
This is a frequent cause of loss of weight. The typical triad of symptoms is shown in Table 14.3.

Table 14.3 Diagnostic triad of symptoms in diabetes mellitus

• Thirst
• Polyuria
• Loss of weight

Other symptoms relate to the common complications of diabetes (Figure 14.3).

The patient had all three symptoms of the diagnostic triad, but none of those related to diabetic complications.

Diabetes therefore remains a possible diagnosis on the basis of the history.

Thyrotoxicosis
The typical symptoms are shown in Table 14.4.

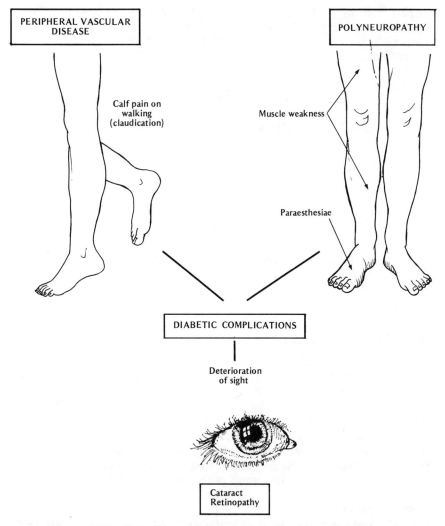

Figure 14.3   Symptoms relating to complications of diabetes

Table 14.4   Symptoms of thyrotoxicosis

- Loss of weight
- Excessive sweating
- Heat intolerance
- Trembling of the hands
- Increase in appetite
- Irritability and short temper

Apart from weight loss, the patient had no symptoms of thyrotoxicosis.

An additional important point against this diagnosis is that the patient's appetite was poor, while in thyrotoxicosis the appetite is often increased or, at the very least, normal.

Addison's disease
The symptoms are shown in Table 14.5.

Table 14.5 Symptoms of Addison's disease

• Excessive fatigue
• Anorexia, nausea
• Postural dizziness
• (Pigmentation)

The patient had anorexia and nausea but no postural dizziness or complaint of skin darkening.

Addison's disease is therefore unlikely but would require further assessment for more certain exclusion.

Gastrointestinal disease

Vomiting and/or diarrhoea
Loss of weight due to gastrointestinal disease may be due to a chronic vomiting and/or diarrhoea, though carcinoma of the stomach may cause profound weight loss in the absence of vomiting. Figure 14.4 shows some causes of chronic vomiting and diarrhoea.

The patient vomited rarely and had no diarrhoea. Her weight loss is not therefore due to any gastrointestinal disease, causing vomiting or diarrhoea. The only proviso is that she could have an occult carcinoma in the alimentary tract which is not causing symptoms other than weight loss.

Malabsorption
Loss of weight occurs with malabsorption. The distinctive feature is the passage of pale, bulky, offensive stools which do not flush away easily.

The patient had no abnormal stools, which excludes this diagnosis.

Chronic infection

Tuberculosis
Extrapulmonary tuberculosis may cause few or no localizing symptoms. The diagnostic clues to tuberculosis are shown in Table 14.6.

Although the patient had some constitutional symptoms, there were no night sweats, which almost invariably occur in all forms of tuberculosis.

This is therefore an unlikely diagnosis though further investigation is necessary to exclude it with certainty.

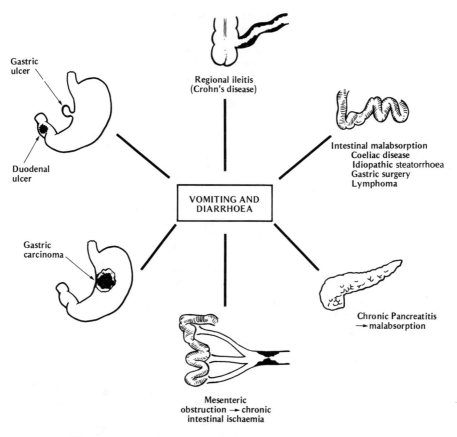

Figure 14.4 Causes of chronic vomiting and diarrhoea

Table 14.6 Diagnostic clues in tuberculosis

- Night sweats
- Constitutional
  - anorexia
  - weakness
  - lack of energy
- Anaemia
  - breathlessness
  - palpitations
  - pallor
  - ankle swelling

Infective endocarditis

The symptoms are shown in Figure 14.5. None was present in the patient.

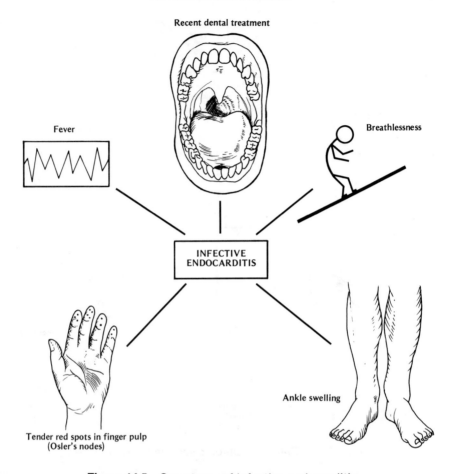

Figure 14.5 Symptoms of infective endocarditis

Brucellosis
This is a rare condition. The symptoms are listed in Table 14.7. The diagnostic clue is contact with cattle.

Table 14.7 Symptoms of brucellosis

- Undulating fever
- Constitutional
  - anorexia
  - sweating
  - weakness
  - headache
- Sore throat
- Pains in joints
- Pain in limb muscles

The patient had no contact with cattle and no fever, sore throat, joint pains or limb pains. Brucellosis is therefore excluded.

Fungal infection
Involvement of the respiratory tract by aspergillosis or candidiasis occurs particularly in debilitated patients such as diabetics, alcoholics and patients with malignant disease. Respiratory symptoms predominate.

The patient was not debilitated by disease and had no respiratory symptoms. Fungal infection is therefore excluded.

Malignant disease

Occult carcinoma
This is very difficult to diagnose unless there are associated localizing symptoms pointing to a particular organ. The commonest sites of occult carcinoma are shown in Figure 14.6.

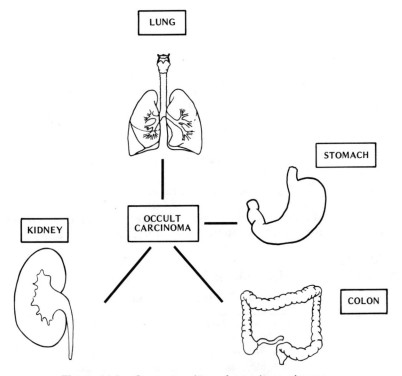

Figure 14.6 Common sites of occult carcinoma

Anorexia and weight loss are almost invariable and the patient had both.

Occult carcinoma remains a possible diagnosis and will need further assessment.

Reticulosis

The symptoms in reticulosis are shown in Figure 14.7.

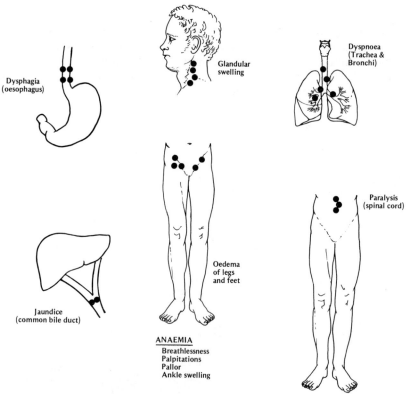

Figure 14.7   Symptoms in reticulosis

There were no symptoms to suggest gland pressure on any organ, and no complaint of enlarged glands. Reticulosis is therefore very unlikely.

Myelomatosis

The symptoms of myelomatosis are shown in Table 14.8.

Table 14.8   Symptoms of myelomatosis

- Loss of weight
- Bone pain
- Susceptibility to infection
- Symptoms of renal failure
- Symptoms of hypercalcaemia

The patient is losing weight, and has back pain and recent respiratory infection and viral infection (shingles). Polydipsia and polyuria can also be attributable to hypercalcaemia.

Myelomatosis remains therefore a *likely diagnosis*.

Chronic renal failure

Chronic renal failure can sometimes present insidiously with loss of weight. Other symptoms which may occur are shown in Table 14.9.

Table 14.9   Symptoms of chronic renal failure

• Past history of kidney disease
• Current urinary symptoms   • polyuria
• dysuria
• haematuria
• Drowsiness
• Hiccoughs
• Pruritus
• Diarrhoea
• Spontaneous bleeding
• Twitching

Apart from polyuria, the patient had no symptoms to suggest chronic renal failure.

Psychogenic disorders

Loss of weight may result from psychiatric disorder.

Depression
This is probably the most frequent psychiatric condition associated with loss of weight. Other symptoms occurring in depression are shown in Table 14.10.

Table 14.10   Symptoms of depression

Insomnia
Early wakening
Loss of interest
Lack of concentration
Loss of libido
Anorexia
Constipation
Loss of weight
Agitation

The patient admitted being depressed and also had anorexia and constipation.

Depression may therefore be a contributory factor in causing loss of weight.

Anxiety

The symptoms of anxiety are shown in Table 14.11. There was nothing to suggest that the patient had an anxiety state.

Table 14.11 Symptoms of anxiety

- Left inframammary pain
- Palpitations
- 'Utter exhaustion'
- Hyperventilation or inability to take a deep breath
- Tension headache

Anorexia nervosa

This occurs predominantly in young women. It is invariably associated with amenorrhoea. Considerable restlessness is often present, described picturesquely as 'bird-like twittering activity'.

The patient's age and lack of other features excludes this diagnosis.

Back pain

The patient had two types of back pain:

- longstanding lower lumbar pain.
- recent mid-dorsal pain

Lower lumbar pain

This longstanding pain radiating down the back of the right thigh indicates a chronic lumbago–sciatica syndrome. The causes are shown in Table 14.12.

Table 14.12 Causes of chronic lumbago–sciatica syndrome

- Prolapsed intervertebral disc
- Osteoarthrosis of the spine
- Ankylosing spondylitis
- Tuberculosis of vertebrae
- Congenital disorders
  - Transitional vertebra
  - Spondylolisthesis
  - Spina bifida
- Psychological backache

Prolapsed intervertebral disc

This is a frequent cause of the lumbago–sciatica syndrome. It presents with recurrent attacks of low back pain and sciatica.

The discs often affected are L4/L5 and L5/S1. Clinical examination will usually show signs of nerve root involvement and will be discussed in more detail later.

The patient's history of recurrent low backache and sciatica for which she has needed to wear a spinal support for 5 years is very suggestive of a chronic prolapsed intervertebral disc.

Lumbar osteoarthrosis
This is also a frequent cause of low backache, especially in elderly patients. It is often associated with some degree of intervertebral disc prolapse. Low backache is the usual symptom and radiation to the buttock or lower limbs may also occur.

This also remains a possible diagnosis in the patient and an X-ray of the spine will be necessary to assess the diagnosis further. Typical X-ray changes of this condition are shown in Figure 14.8.

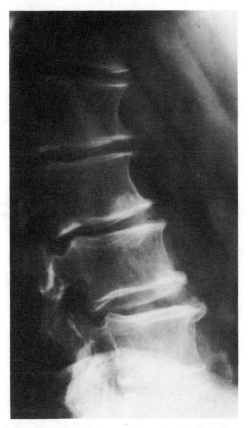

Figure 14.8 Typical X-ray changes in lumbar osteoarthritis

Ankylosing spondylitis
This condition may cause chronic low back pain. The features of this condition are shown in Figure 14.9.

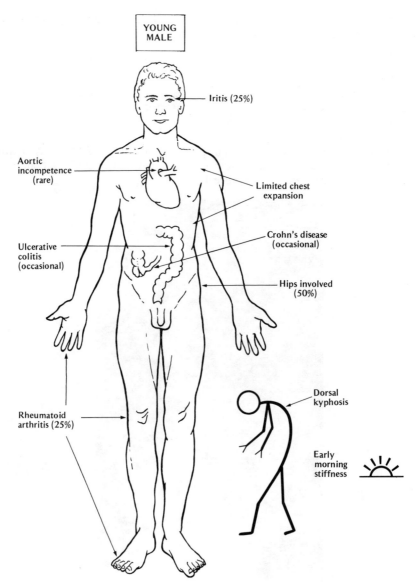

Figure 14.9   Features of ankylosing spondylitis

The patient being an elderly female and the absence of early morning stiffness, respiratory symptoms, eye problems, diarrhoea and polyarthritis exclude this diagnosis.

Tuberculosis of the spine (Pott's disease)
This produces an insidious and prolonged history of backache but may sometimes present acutely with back pain.

492

50% of patients have evidence of tuberculosis elsewhere. There may be constitutional symptoms. Spinal cord compression may occur with weakness or paralysis of the legs.

The patient did have some constitutional symptoms but no night sweats. There were no symptoms to suggest tuberculosis elsewhere, e.g. lungs, and no symptoms of spinal cord compression.

The diagnosis of tuberculosis of the spine cannot be made or excluded accurately on the basis of the history alone. Further investigation will be necessary which includes X-rays, tuberculin test and possibly biopsy of the vertebrae.

Congenital disorders

Spondylolisthesis is an uncommon cause of low back pain and occasionally sciatica also. The diagnosis cannot be made on the history and requires X-ray of the spine.

In the case of *spina bifida* a clue is given by a localized patch of hair in the skin over the site of the lesion.

'Psychogenic' backache

Chronic back pain frequently occurs in depressed or anxious individuals and there is often no evidence of an organic cause even after intensive investigation.

The backache may therefore be due to the psychological state of the patient. Help in arriving at this diagnosis may be given by the gross exaggeration of the symptoms and by the discrepancy between the symptoms and the degree of apparent disability.

There was nothing to suggest psychogenic backache in this patient.

Mid-dorsal pain

The pain in the mid-dorsal region was of recent onset and is likely to be due to *acute organic disease*.

The radiation to the left shoulder blade suggests root pressure involving the 6th–8th thoracic nerves.

The causes of acute pain in the spine are shown in Table 14.13.

Table 14.13 Causes of acute pain in the spine

• Acute prolapsed intervertebral disc	
• Osteoporosis	
• Acute infection	• pyogenic
	• tuberculosis
• Neoplasia	• metastases
	• myeloma
	• lymphoma

Prolapsed intervertebral disc
The occurrence of a prolapsed disc in the midthoracic region is very rare. This diagnosis is therefore highly unlikely.

Osteoporosis
Spinal osteoporosis occurs in postmenopausal women.

The condition often remains symptomless until a crush fracture occurs as a result of trauma. If collapse and compression of several vertebrae occur the patient may become noticeably shorter in height.

Although the patient had no history of severe injury to the spine, even minimal injury may fracture a brittle osteoporotic spine.

This diagnosis remains a possibility until excluded by X-ray of the spine.

Infection

Staphylococcal osteomyelitis
This tends to occur in patients with low resistance, e.g. diabetics or alcoholics. It may follow sepsis elsewhere and may be a complication of surgery, particularly genitourinary surgery.

It produces a painful back with limited movement. Often the back pain is worse on walking when the heel jars the spine with each footstep. Constitutional symptoms are frequent.

The patient was not febrile or debilitated and had no evidence of sepsis elsewhere. There was no complaint of aggravation of the mid-dorsal pain with walking.

Osteomyelitis is therefore very unlikely.

Tuberculosis
Tuberculosis of the spine may present acutely. It may occur with few constitutional symptoms and no obvious tuberculosis elsewhere.

Further investigation is therefore necessary to exclude tuberculosis of the spine.

Neoplasia
Sudden back pain in a patient of this age should always be regarded as neoplastic until proved otherwise.

Metastases
The primary carcinomas which most frequently metastasize to the spine are shown in Figure 14.10.

The patient did not complain of any lumps in her breast.

She had no cough or haemoptysis which might suggest bronchial carcinoma.

There was no loin pain (apart from the recent attack of shingles) and no haematuria which might be due to renal carcinoma.

There had been recent constipation, which raises the possibility of carcinoma of the colon. This will require further assessment and investigation before it can be excluded.

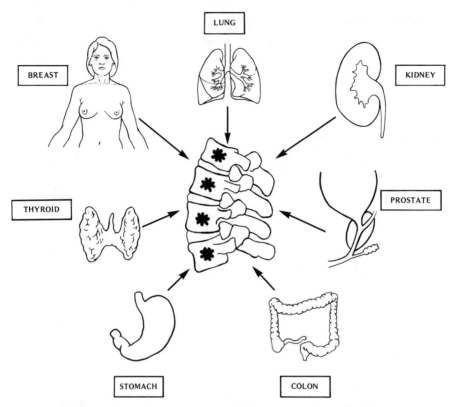

Figure 14.10 Primary carcinomas which frequently metastasize to the spine

Carcinoma of the stomach can be very insidious. She did have a poor appetite and nausea, which with the loss of weight, might well be due to gastric carcinoma. As with colonic carcinoma, further assessment is necessary before this diagnosis can be excluded.

There was no complaint of a swelling in the neck or pressure symptoms, such as dysphagia or stridor, to suggest carcinoma of the thyroid.

Myelomatosis
The possibility of myelomatosis has already been raised on the basis of other symptoms (Table 14.8).

A *myelomatous deposit* in the vertebra possibly with a crush fracture remains therefore, a *likely diagnosis* to account for the acute back pain.

Reticulosis
There was no complaint of lumps in the neck, groin or axilla.

There was no dysphagia, stridor, oedema of the legs, jaundice or paralysis of the legs which might suggest pressure from enlarged lymph nodes (see Figure 14.7, p. 488).

Reticulosis is therefore excluded.

495

Other conditions

There are two other conditions which are worth considering to account for acute back pain:

- dissecting aneurysm of the aorta
- aortic aneurysm.

Dissecting aneurysm of the aorta

This causes acute severe pain in the middle of the back. It is often associated with severe precordial pain which may precede the pain in the back. Typical radiation of the pain may occur (Figure 14.11).

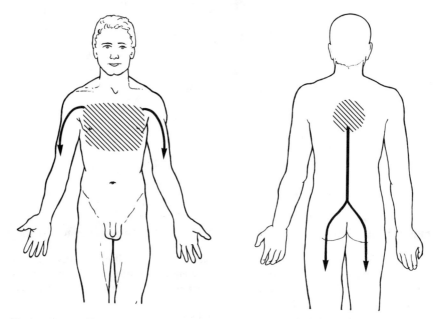

Figure 14.11 Typical radiation of the pain in dissecting aneurysm of the aorta

Dissecting aneurysm is usually a medical emergency and leads frequently to severe circulatory failure.

The site, duration and radiation of the patient's pain was quite unlike that of a dissecting aneurysm.

Aortic aneurysm

An aortic aneurysm produces continuous *boring* back pain due to erosion of the vertebrae and ribs. It may be caused by syphilis or by atherosclerosis.

There may be other symptoms of pressure by the aneurysm such as wheezing, from pressure on the trachea or bronchi, and hoarseness from pressure on the recurrent laryngeal nerve.

There was no past history of syphilis, the patient's pain was not boring and there was no wheezing or hoarseness of the voice. This excludes aortic aneurysm.

Anorexia

The patient had lost her appetite recently.

Anorexia may be caused by involvement of several different systems (Table 14.14).

Table 14.14 System involvement leading to anorexia

- Gastrointestinal disease
- Endocrine disease
- Chronic renal failure
- Malignancy
- Cardiorespiratory disease
- Drugs

Gastrointestinal disease

The causes of anorexia are shown in Figure 14.12.

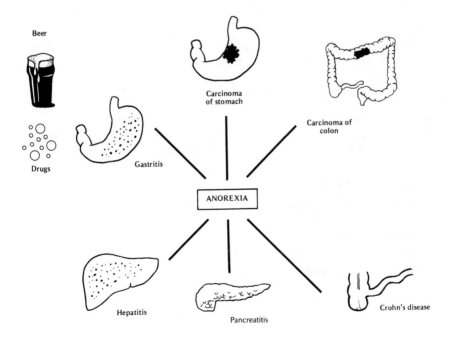

Figure 14.12 Gastrointestinal causes of anorexia

Gastritis

This is caused by excessive intake of alcohol, but may also be induced by drugs (Table 14.15).

Table 14.15 Drugs causing gastritis

- Aspirin
- Non-steroidal anti-inflammatory drugs
- Steroids

The patient did not drink alcohol and was not currently using any other of the listed drugs.

Gastric carcinoma

Occult carcinoma of the stomach obviously remains a diagnostic possibility and requires further assessment.

Carcinoma of the colon

This diagnosis is also possible, especially in view of the recent constipation. Further assessment is necessary.

Hepatitis

This diagnosis is excluded by the absence of jaundice.

Pancreatitis

In acute pancreatitis the anorexia is overshadowed by acute abdominal pain, and in chronic pancreatitis by the malabsorption leading to diarrhoea with pale, bulky, offensive stools.

The patient had neither abdominal pain nor diarrhoea.

Crohn's disease

The anorexia of Crohn's disease is accompanied by abdominal pain and bloody diarrhoea, neither of which the patient had.

Endocrine disease

The three conditions leading to anorexia are shown in Figure 14.13.

Addison's disease

The features are shown in Table 14.16.

Table 14.16 Features of Addison's disease

- Excessive fatigue
- Gastrointestinal   – anorexia
                        nausea
- Postural dizziness
- Pigmentation

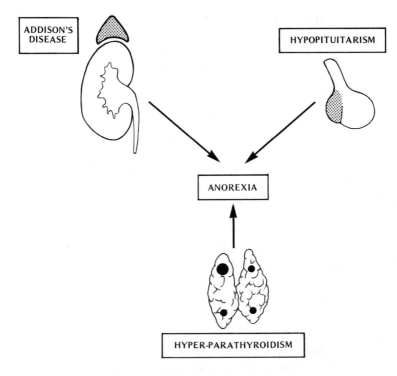

Figure 14.13   Endocrine causes of anorexia

Apart from anorexia, the patient had none of the other symptoms of this condition.

Hypopituitarism
The features are shown in Table 14.17.

Table 14.17   Features of hypopituitarism

- Possible history of postpartum haemorrhage
- Headache and visual disturbance (tumour)
- Symptoms of hypothyroidism
- Symptoms of adrenal insufficiency

The patient had not had a postpartum haemorrhage, and had no deterioration of vision and no symptoms to suggest either thyroid or adrenal insufficiency. This diagnosis is therefore excluded.

Hyperparathyroidism
This condition may be primary, usually due to a parathyroid adenoma, or secondary to chronic renal failure. It has a distinctive clinical picture (Table 14.18).

Table 14.18 Features of hyperparathyroidism

• Gastrointestinal tract	– anorexia
	nausea
	vomiting
• Kidney	– renal colic
	dysuria
• Musculoskeletal system	– muscle weakness
	back pain
• Psychiatric	– depression
	personality changes

The symptoms in the patient relevant to this diagnosis are anorexia, nausea, vomiting and back pain.

This diagnosis will be discussed in more detail later.

Chronic renal failure

This can present with anorexia. The other symptoms have already been indicated and the diagnosis excluded by their absence in the patient.

Malignancy

Anorexia is a common symptom of malignancy.

Carcinoma of the stomach and myelomatosis have already been suggested as possible diagnoses for further consideration but there were no symptoms to suggest reticulosis.

Cardiorespiratory disease

The anorexia of severe cardiorespiratory disease is a minor symptom and is overshadowed by the associated cardiac and respiratory symptoms.

Drugs

Digitalis preparations cause anorexia, especially in old people. The patient had not taken any digitalis preparation.

Constipation

The patient had complained of *recent* constipation which always suggests the possibility of either organic disease or a drug-related problem. The causes which should be considered are shown in Table 14.19.

Inadequate roughage

This is a frequent cause of constipation.

As the patient had been eating less recently this may be a contributory factor in causing her constipation.

Table 14.19   Causes of recent constipation

• Inadequate roughage in the diet	
• Irritable bowel syndrome	
• Colonic obstruction by carcinoma	
• Painful anal conditions	• Piles
	• Fissure
	• Abscess
• Metabolic	• Myxoedema
	• Hypercalcaemia
	• Porphyria
• Drugs	• Bismuth/aluminium antacids
	• Opiates
	• Anticholinergics
	• Ganglion-blockers

Irritable bowel syndrome

This condition may cause either constipation or diarrhoea or both alternating. Associated variable abdominal pain or discomfort is very frequent. Ribbon-like stools or watery diarrhoea often occur also.

The absence of abdominal pain of any sort excludes this diagnosis.

Carcinoma of the colon

Colonic carcinoma causing obstruction is often associated with blood in the stool.

This diagnosis can, however, only be excluded by X-rays or other investigations.

Painful anal conditions

There was no complaint of any of those painful conditions which might inhibit defaecation.

Metabolic disease

Myxoedema

There were no symptoms to suggest myxoedema (Table 14.20).

Table 14.20   Symptoms of myxoedema

• Increasing weight
• Mental and physical slowing
• Cold intolerance
• Loss of hair
• Hoarseness of voice

Hypercalcaemia

The symptoms in this condition are shown in Table 14.21.

Table 14.21   Symptoms of hypercalcaemia

- Nausea and vomiting
- Constipation
- Polydipsia
- Polyuria
- Mental changes • confusion
  - • depression

The patient had nausea and occasional vomiting, constipation, polyuria and polydipsia and depression.

Hypercalcaemia is a likely cause of these symptoms.

Porphyria

The features of acute intermittent porphyria are shown in Table 14.22.

Table 14.22   Features of acute porphyria

- Abdominal colic
- Constipation
- Polyneuritis
- Mental disturbance

The absence of abdominal colic and paraesthesiae or muscle weakness makes this condition very unlikely.

Drugs

The patient had not taken any of the drugs listed in Table 14.19.

Polyuria and polydipsia

The patient had developed recent polyuria and polydipsia. The causes of these conditions are shown in Table 14.23.

Table 14.23   Causes of polyuria and polydipsia

- Diabetes mellitus
- Chronic renal failure
- Hypercalcaemia
- Diabetes insipidus
- Psychogenic

Diabetes mellitus

Diabetes has already been considered a possible diagnosis in the patient because of the presence of the classical triad of symptoms (Table 14.3).

Chronic renal failure

This has been thought unlikely because of the absence of other characteristic symptoms (Table 14.9).

Hypercalcaemia

The likelihood of this diagnosis has been mentioned because of other supportive symptoms (Table 14.21 and p. 482).

Diabetes insipidus

The distinctive features in this condition is the passage of very large amounts of urine – up to 20 litres or more in 24 hours.

The modest amount of urine passed by this patient makes this diagnosis unlikely.

Psychogenic polydipsia

The patient with this condition is psychiatrically grossly disturbed with very bizarre and inconsistent patterns of drinking and passing urine. Withdrawing fluid for 24 hours reduces the urinary output to normal.

The patient did not seem to be a psychiatric problem, and there were no inconsistencies in her patterns of drinking and passing urine.

Headache

The patient complained of recent dull headache with no specific related factors. The causes of headache are shown in Table 14.24.

Table 14.24   Causes of headache

• Migraine
• Tension headache
• Severe hypertension
• Raised intracranial pressure
• Local disease

Migraine

Migraine is excluded by the lack of a throbbing headache, absence of prodromal visual disturbances and terminal vomiting.

Tension headache

Tension headache is often described in exaggerated terms as pressure, heaviness, weights, tight bands in the head. Other symptoms of anxiety are often present. The patient's symptoms did not fit this picture.

Hypertension

Severe hypertension may be symptomless apart from headache. The nature of the headache is typical – occipital, throbbing and early morning. The patient's headache did not have any of these features.

Raised intracranial pressure

Raised intracranial pressure is excluded by lack of a consistent throbbing morning headache with vomiting and visual deterioration.

Local disease

Local disease which may cause headache is shown in Figure 14.14.

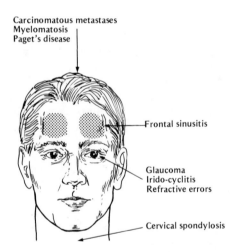

Figure 14.14   Local disease which causes headache

Frontal sinusitis
Frontal sinusitis is excluded by the lack of frontal headache and the absence of associated nasal symptoms, such as purulent discharge and nasal obstruction.

Eye disease
There was no past history of eye disease, no eye pain and no visual deterioration, which excludes the eye conditions listed.

504

Cervical spondylosis

Cervical spondylosis causes pain in the neck or occiput related to head movements, which is quite unlike the patient's symptoms.

Paget's disease

The features of Paget's disease of bone are shown in Figure 14.15. The absence of painful tender deformed long bones makes this an unlikely diagnosis.

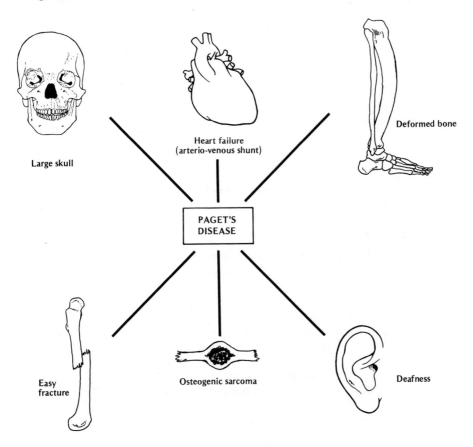

Large skull

Heart failure (arterio-venous shunt)

Deformed bone

PAGET'S DISEASE

Easy fracture

Osteogenic sarcoma

Deafness

Figure 14.15 Clinical features of Paget's disease

Metastatic carcinoma

Metastatic carcinoma from an occult primary source (see Figure 14.6) remains a possibility although there are no symptoms pointing to the primary site.

Myelomatosis

This has already been suggested by other symptoms and therefore remains the most likely diagnosis.

Depression

Depression may be endogenous or reactive.

Endogenous depression

There was no past history of psychological disorder such as mood swings which may precede endogenous depression in later life. Also the patient's personality was not overscrupulous, obsessional or rigid, which may predispose to depression of this type.

Endogenous depression may follow physical disease, such as an operation or severe infection, or cerebral arteriosclerosis.

In the patient's case, another physical cause may be related – *hypercalcaemia*. The features have already been shown in Table 14.21 and include mental disturbance such as depression.

Reactive depression

This occurs as a response to an external happening often involving disappointment, marriage break-up, death of a relative etc.

The patient often has feelings of guilt, unworthiness, self-depreciation.

There were no relevant external events in the patient's history and nothing to suggest feelings of self-abasement.

Past history

She had a past history of repeated respiratory infections and also a recent attack of shingles.

Recurrent respiratory infections

In the absence of a history of chronic lung disease, the repeated infections would suggest a reduced resistance. This could be the result of impaired immunological defence mechanisms which is a distinctive feature of *myelomatosis*. There is a depressed production of normal immunoglobulins required to maintain resistance to infection.

There may also be impairment of cellular immune activity in myelomatosis.

Respiratory infections and urinary infections are particularly prone to occur under these circumstances.

Herpes zoster (shingles)

Herpes zoster also occurs in about 10% of patients with myelomatosis.

This past history therefore lends additional support to the diagnosis of myelomatosis.

Social history

The patient's recent inability to cope with looking after her family may be due to a combination of problems (Table 14.25).

Table 14.25 Problems in the patient coping with her family

- Physical difficulty in moving the painful spine
- Rapid fatigue resulting from anaemia
- Lack of energy caused by malignancy
- Depression

CONCLUSIONS FROM THE HISTORY

- The weight loss is due to malignancy.

- The recent back pain is due to malignant involvement of the spine.

- The headache is also due to malignant involvement of the skull.

- The anorexia, constipation, polyuria, polydipsia and depression are due to hypercalcaemia.

- The symptoms of anaemia could result from marrow replacement by malignancy.

- The increased susceptibility to infections is likely to be due to reduced resistance consequent on suppressed immunological defence mechanisms.

The occurrence of hypercalcaemia with a malignant infiltrative condition of bone would suggest a diagnosis of either *myelomatosis* or *secondary carcinomatosis*.

Hypercalcaemia (serum calcium> 11 mg/dl or 5.44 mmol/l) occurs in 30% of patients with myelomatosis and is less frequent in carcinomatosis.

ANALYSIS OF THE EXAMINATION

Anaemia

The pale conjunctivae and pale palms indicate anaemia.

The absence of koilonychia is against iron deficiency and the normal tongue is against pernicious anaemia.

Anaemia is invariably present in myelomatosis. The causes are shown in Table 14.26.

Table 14.26 Causes of anaemia in myelomatosis

- Bone marrow infiltration by plasma cells
- Low serum iron due to chronic disease
- Haemolysis of abnormal-globulin coated red cells
- Renal failure
- Associated infections
- (Bone marrow suppression by treatment)

Skeletal system

Skull

The causes of localized tenderness are shown in Table 14.27.

Table 14.27 Causes of localized tenderness in the skull

- Osteomyelitis
- Paget's disease
- Malignant infiltration

Osteomyelitis
Osteomyelitis of the skull is a rare condition. The predisposing conditions are shown in Table 14.28.

Table 14.28 Causes of osteomyelitis of the skull

- Chronic sinus infection
- Chronic otitis media and mastoiditis
- Penetrating wounds
- Infected subdural haematoma
- Purulent lung infections

There was no history of sinus disease, ear disease, wound or head injury; there was no infected sputum, or lung signs on examination, to suggest purulent lung infection.

Paget's disease
Paget's disease is excluded by the lack of head enlargement and the absence of painful, tender, deformed, long bones.

Malignancy
Malignant infiltration remains the most likely cause of the local tenderness.

Dorsal spine

The local tenderness and painful limited movement suggest bone destruction,

Table 14.29 Causes of pathological fracture of the vertebrae

- Osteomalacia
- Osteoporosis
- Hyperparathyroidism
- Metastatic carcinoma
- Myeloma

possibly with an associated crush fracture.

The causes of pathological fracture of the vertebrae are shown in Table 14.29.

Osteomalacia

Osteomalacia is due to vitamin D deficiency and the causes are shown in Table 14.30.

Table 14.30 Causes of osteomalacia

* Dietary deficiency
* Malabsorption
* Chronic renal failure
* Chronic anticonvulsant treatment in epilepsy

The patient's diet had been normal though recently reduced. There was no history of diarrhoea with pale, bulky, offensive stools, thus excluding malabsorption. Apart from polyuria there were no features of chronic renal failure (Table 14.9). The patient was not an epileptic.

There was nothing therefore to suggest osteomalacia.

Osteoporosis

Osteoporosis is common in post menopausal women.
This diagnosis can only be excluded by X-rays of the spine.

Hyperparathyroidism

The features of hyperparathyroidism are shown in Table 14.31.

Table 14.31 Features of hyperparathyroidism

• Gastrointestinal	• Anorexia
	• Vomiting
	• Constipation
	• Abdominal pain (acute pancreatitis)
• Renal	• Polyuria
	• Polydipsia
	• Renal colic (stones)
• Skeletal	• Bone pain
	• Pathological fractures
• Mental	• Drowsiness
	• Confusion
	• Depression

The patient has symptoms affecting all the systems listed. Further investigation is therefore necessary before this diagnosis can be excluded.

Carcinomatosis

Secondary carcinomatosis may arise from the primary sources already shown (Figure 14.10).

There were no palpable breast lumps and no axillary glands, thus excluding breast carcinoma.

There was no finger clubbing, no lymphadenopathy in neck or axilla and no localizing lung findings to suggest carcinoma.

There was no renal enlargement or haematuria to suggest renal carcinoma.

There was no lump in the thyroid gland.

There were no abdominal masses, hepatomegaly or lymphadenopathy to suggest gastric or colonic carcinoma.

Secondary carcinoma is therefore unlikely but cannot be excluded with certainty on clinical assessment alone.

Myelomatosis

Sudden pain in the back due to vertebral involvement is one of the commonest presenting symptoms of myelomatosis.

This diagnosis therefore has further support.

The dorsal kyphosis seen in the patient may be a reflection of multiple compression fractures due to a malignant infiltration of the vertebrae.

Sternum

Tenderness on pressure over the sternum suggests involvement by an infiltrative process. This could be due to either metastatic carcinoma or myeloma.

Neurological findings

The patient had impaired straight leg raising on the right, with a reduced ankle jerk but no sensory change.

The impairment of straight leg raising indicates root pressure, most commonly caused by a prolapsed intervertebral disc.

The reduced ankle jerk is also due to root pressure involving the 1st sacral nerve root. The likely cause again is a prolapsed disc.

Prolapsed intervertebral discs most commonly affect the 4th and 5th lumbar and 1st sacral nerve roots. The clinical effects are shown in Figure 14.16.

CONCLUSIONS FROM THE EXAMINATION

The examination findings indicate:

- anaemia, due at least in part to marrow infiltration

- destruction in the mid-dorsal vertebrae

- malignant deposits in the skull

- prolapse of the lumbo-sacral intervertebral disc.

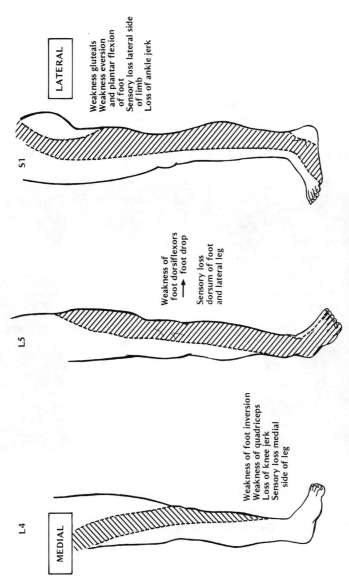

Figure 14.16 Clinical effects of prolapsed intervertebral discs

These findings could be explained by either *carcinomatosis* or *myelomatosis*.

It is not possible on the basis of clinical assessment alone to differentiate the two conditions.

INVESTIGATIONS

X-rays

X-ray of the skull and dorsal spine is mandatory.

Skull

The patient's skull X-ray is shown in Figure 14.17 and indicates extensive osteolytic lesions.

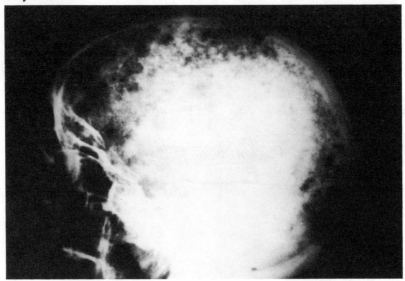

Figure 14.17 Patient's skull X-ray showing myeloma

The most frequent conditions causing this appearance are shown in Table 14.32.

Table 14.32 Causes of osteolytic appearance in the skull X-ray

> - Carcinomatosis
> - Myelomatosis
> - Hyperparathyroidism

Carcinomatosis and *myelomatosis* cannot be differentiated on appearance alone. Further investigation is necessary.

Hyperparathyroidism produces a much finer involvement of the skull with tiny punched-out lesions producing the 'pepper-pot' appearance (Figure 14.18). This is quite unlike the patient's skull X-ray.

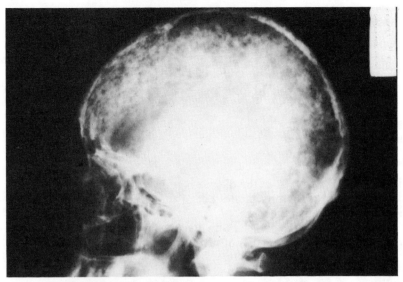

Figure 14.18   'Pepperpot' appearance

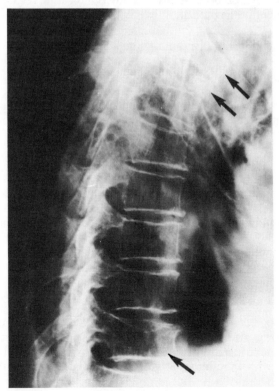

Figure 14.19   Patient's X-ray of the dorsal spine showing myeloma and crush
fractures

Dorsal spine

The patient's X-ray is shown in Figure 14.19. There are destructive lesions in dorsal vertebrae with some compression collapse of the bodies of several dorsal vertebrae.

These appearances could be due either to carcinoma or myeloma.

Urine examination

Bence-Jones protein

This is an important test in the diagnosis of myelomatosis.

Bence-Jones protein precipitates out of the urine on heating to 60 °C then redissolves on boiling the urine.

It is present in 50% of patients with myeloma and was found in the patient's urine, confirming the diagnosis of myelomatosis.

Casts

Protein casts may also occur in myelomatosis indicating renal damage. Casts were not present in the patient.

Blood count

Anaemia

Anaemia is invariable in myelomatosis and will also occur in carcinomatosis. The contributory causes of the anaemia have already been shown in Table 14.26.

Leukopenia and thrombocytopenia

These findings are late developments in myelomatosis and are more common in the closely related condition of macroglobulinaemia.

The patient's blood count showed a moderate normocytic, normochromic anaemia which is a typical finding in myelomatosis; the white count and platelet count were normal.

Erythrocyte sedimentation rate

This is an important but non-specific test in the diagnosis of myelomatosis. The distinctive feature is the very high level, usually above 100 mm/h. The high ESR is due to increased rouleaux formation resulting from the coating of the red cells with the abnormal globulin produced by the plasma cells in myeloma.

The patient's ESR was 122 mm/hr.

Other causes of very high ESR are shown in Table 14.33.

Table 14.33   Causes of very high ESR

- Carcinomatosis
- Myelomatosis
- Giant cell arteritis (temporal arteritis)
- Polymyalgia rheumatica
- Wegener's granulomatosis
- Collagen disease
    e.g. systemic lupus erythematosus
- Left atrial myxoma
- Infections
    - pulmonary
    - urinary tract

Serum electrophoresis

This is probably the most important diagnostic test in myelomatosis.

The typical finding in myeloma is an abnormal M-protein. This is an abnormal homogenous (monoclonal) protein produced by the uncontrolled proliferation of plasma cells which occurs in myeloma. The M-protein, which is an immunoglobulin, can be further refined if necessary into one of the four main types – IgG, IgA, IgM, and IgD.

It is the spillover of this M-protein from the blood into the urine which is detected as Bence-Jones protein.

The patient's electrophoretic pattern showed an abnormal M-protein of IgG type which confirms the diagnosis of myeloma (Figure 14.20).

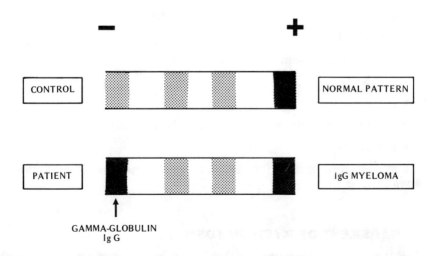

Figure 14.20   Patient's electrophoretic pattern

Bone marrow examination

In myeloma, this shows increased infiltration with abnormal and immature plasma cells.

The cells are large with an eccentric nucleus or sometimes multiple nuclei and intracytoplasmic deposits of protein.

The patient's bone marrow showed infiltration with these abnormal plasma cells.

Serum calcium level

Hypercalcaemia occurs in 30% of patients with myeloma.
The patient's serum calcium was increased to 5.7 mmol/l.
Other causes of hypercalcaemia are shown in Table 14.34.

Table 14.34   Causes of hypercalcaemia

• Immobilization
• Myeloma
• Metastatic carcinoma of bone
• Paget's disease of bone
• Sarcoidosis
• Overdose with vitamin D

CONCLUSIONS FROM THE INVESTIGATIONS

The patient has shown all the distinctive findings of myelomatosis:

- very high ESR

- Bence-Jones proteinuria

- lytic lesions in skull and spine

- abnormal M-protein in serum

- infiltration of marrow with abnormal plasma cells

- hypercalcaemia.

Carcinomatosis is therefore excluded and the *diagnosis confirmed as myelomatosis.*

MANAGEMENT OF MYELOMATOSIS

The treatment of myeloma involves symptomatic measures and specific therapy (Table 14.35).

Table 14.35   Management of myelomatosis

• Symptomatic	–	Hypercalcaemia
		Bone disease and bone pain
		Renal failure
		Infection
		Anaemia
		Hyperuricaemia
		Neurological involvement
		Hyperviscosity
		Amyloidosis
• Specific	–	Radiation
		Chemotherapy

Symptomatic treatment

Hypercalcaemia

The measures which may be helpful are shown in Table 14.36.

Table 14.36   Treatment of hypercalcaemia in myelomatosis

- Encourage physical activity – reduces bone demineralization
- High fluid intake – at least 3 litres a day
- Diuretics – frusemide 40–80 mg/day
- Oral phosphate – 1–3 g/24 h
- Prednisolone – 40–80 mg/day
- Mithramycin – for emergency control
- Calcitonin

Hydration
Adequate hydration is necessary to avoid precipitation of calcium in the kidney. It will also help to prevent renal damage from precipitation of Bence-Jones protein in the kidney.

Diuretics
Diuretic treatment has the same purpose as hydration.

Mithramycin
Mithramycin is a cytotoxic antibiotic which can reduce severe hypercalcaemia within 24 hours. Its main disadvantage is that it can cause marked bone marrow depression leading especially to thrombocytopenic bleeding.

Mild hypercalcaemia
With mild elevation of the serum calcium (11.5–12 mg/dl), intravenous saline and frusemide will suffice until systemic chemotherapy can control the condition more effectively.

Oral phosphate may also help – if renal function is not impaired, with risk of hyperphosphataemia.

Severe hypercalcaemia

Severe hypercalcaemia (serum calcium > 12 mg/dl) is more hazardous because of cardiac toxicity and renal damage. This requires large doses of steroids, mithramycin or calcitonin.

Prednisolone should be given in a dose of 40–100 mg/day until the serum calcium returns to normal, usually within 7–10 days.

The dose of mithramycin is 1.5 g intravenously over 4–6 h.

Bone disease

The measures which are of value are shown in Table 14.37.

Table 14.37   Treatment of bone involvement in myelomatosis

- Radiation
- Surgical fixation
- Spinal support
- Sodium fluoride and calcium carbonate
- Analgesics

Radiation
Severe pain may be quickly and effectively controlled by local radiation in a dose of 2000–3000 rad (20–30 Gy).

Fixation
Painful fractures can be helped by internal fixation.

Spinal support
A spinal support may help a painful back.

Fluoride and carbonate
A combination of sodium fluoride (50 mg b.d.) and calcium carbonate (1 g q.d.s.) may produce increased bone formation.

These drugs should not be given if hypercalcaemia is present.

Analgesics
Analgesics should of course be used as necessary.

Renal failure

This is a major cause of death in myeloma. The two main causes are hypercalcaemia and deposition of Bence-Jones protein in the kidney.

Good hydration and alkalinization of the urine with acetazolamide up to 0.5 g every 12 h may help.

Haemodialysis is a last resort.

Infection

Prophylactic use of antibiotics may be of value in these infection-prone subjects. Prompt investigation and treatment are necessary at the earliest sign of infection.

Penicillin and ampicillin are best.

Nephrotoxic antibiotics (aminoglycosides) should be avoided.

Anaemia

Anaemia can be treated by blood transfusion as necessary.

Occasionally androgens (e.g. testosterone) may help to stimulate erythropoiesis.

Hyperuricaemia

This may be due to renal failure or it may follow specific therapy for myeloma.

Allopurinol, up to 600 mg/day, is the best preventive measure.

Neurological involvement

Spinal cord compression may occur due to vertebral collapse or because of a localized extradural plasmacytoma. The treatment available is shown in Table 14.38.

Table 14.38   Treatment of spinal cord compression in myeloma

- Local irradiation
- Dexamethasone to reduce oedema
- Surgical decompression (laminectomy)

Hyperviscosity

This is due to high concentrations of circulating immunoglobulins such as M-protein of various subtypes. The clinical pointers to this complication are shown in Table 14.39.

Table 14.39   Clinical pointers to hyperviscosity in myeloma

- Mental confusion
- Visual deterioration
- Atypical neurological manifestations
- Bleeding diathesis

Plasmapheresis is of temporary value but must be combined with specific chemotherapy or radiotherapy.

Amyloidosis

This occurs in 10% of patients with myeloma. The diagnostic clues are shown in Table 14.40.

Table 14.40 Diagnostic clues to amyloidosis in myeloma

> - Carpal tunnel syndrome
> - Macroglossia
> - Nephrotic syndrome
> - Refractory heart failure
> - Peripheral neuropathy

The only treatment available is for renal amyloidosis, where short-term haemodialysis may be of value.

SPECIFIC TREATMENT

Chemotherapy

Most patients with myeloma require specific systemic chemotherapy. The most useful cytotoxic drugs are the alkylating agents:

- melphalan
- cyclophosphamide.

Melphalan and cyclophosphamide

The drugs can be given in a continuous low dose, or more usually, in intermittent courses, and are usually combined with prednisolone (Table 14.41). The prednisolone potentiates the effects of the cytotoxic drug.

Table 14.41 Dosage schedules of melphalan and cyclophosphamide in myeloma

Melphalan/prednisolone
    intermittent course for 4 days every 4 weeks
    melphalan 0.25 mg/kg per day
    prednisolone 100 mg/day

Cyclophosphamide/prednisolone
    cyclophosphamide 1 g/m^2 i.v. every 3 weeks
    prednisolone 100 mg/day for 4 days every 3 weeks

If the patient has renal impairment, the doses of the cytotoxic drugs should be reduced by 50% or 75% depending on the degree of renal failure.

Melphalan is tried first; if it is unsuccessful after three courses, *cyclophosphamide* is given.

Patients should be well hydrated and ambulant during treatment with these drugs, to reduce the risk of:

- hypercalcaemia
- hyperuricaemia
- uraemia.

The side-effects of these drugs are shown in Table 14.42.

Table 14.42 Side-effects of melphalan and cyclophosphamide

• Bone marrow depression – anaemia leukopenia – infections thrombocytopenia – bleeding • Nausea and vomiting • Loss of hair

A permanent remission is rarely attained but prolonged remission may occur.

The factors which are helpful in assessing progress and maintenance of remission are shown in Table 14.43. Of these factors, the best indicator of remission is a fall in the level of M-protein in the blood. Treatment should be continued as long as the level continues to fall.

Table 14.43 Evaluation of progress of myeloma in response to treatment

• Clinical assessment	– weight symptoms signs
• Weekly blood count	– neutropenia thrombocytopenia
• M-protein levels in blood and urine every 1–2 weeks initially then every 1–2 months	
• Serum calcium estimation	
• Renal function	– serum creatinine blood urea
• Regular X-rays of lytic lesions in bone	
• Periodic marrow examination	

Newer drugs

Other agents are being investigated especially for use in resistant patients but their place in the treatment of myeloma remains to be established (Table 14.44).

Table 14.44 Newer agents in
the treatment of myeloma

* Nitrosourea
* Carmustine
* Lomustine
* Vinca alkaloids (vincristine)
* *Cis*-platinum
* Interferon
* Levamisole

Radiation treatment

The main use of radiation in myeloma is palliative, to reduce bone pain.

However, there is evidence that high-dose radiation (4000–5000 rad) to regional areas of disease may result in a reduction of the level of circulating M-protein.

Radiation can also induce prolonged remission in solitary myeloma of bone or extramedullary plasmacytoma.

NATURAL HISTORY OF MYELOMATOSIS

Incidence

The annual incidence is 3:100 000 of the population, the same as Hodgkin's disease.

Age and sex

It is predominantly a disease of the middle-aged and elderly.
It is slightly more common in males than females.

Benign monoclonal gammopathy

A Swedish epidemiological study of 7000 individuals over 24 years of age who were quite healthy and asymptomatic showed an abnormal M-protein on serum electrophoresis in as many as 1:100.

This condition has been designated benign monoclonal gammopathy. However, this condition may not be as benign as originally thought, since 10–20% of such individuals have been found to develop a plasma cell or lymphocytic neoplasm within 10 years.

Prognosis

The death rate from myeloma in England and Wales is 4/100 000 a year.

Favourable prognostic features are shown in Table 14.45. The median survival in these patients is 4 years.

Table 14.45 Favourable prognostic features in myeloma

Hb > 10 g/dl
Normal serum calcium
Normal bone (or only solitary plasmacytoma)
Low M-protein level:
   IgG < 5 g/dl
   IgA < 3 g/dl
Normal serum creatinine and blood urea

Adverse prognostic features are shown in Table 14.46. The median survival in these patients is only 2 months.

Table 14.46 Adverse prognostic features in myeloma

Hb <8.5 g/dl
Serum calcium > 12 mg/dl
More than three lytic bone lesions
High M-protein levels:
   IgG > 7 g/dl
   IgA > 5 g/dl
Blood urea> 60 mg/dl

The most useful single prognostic index is the M-protein level doubling time – the shorter the time, the poorer the outlook. Death is usually due to the causes shown in Table 14.47.

Table 14.47 Causes of death in myeloma

- Renal disease
- Infection
- Hyperviscosity
- Haemorrhage
- Acute leukaemia

Development of leukaemia

About 2% of all patients who survive for at least 2 years will develop acute myeloblastic or monocytic leukaemia.

Among patients responding to treatment with alkylating agents, and surviving at least 2 years, the incidence of acute leukaemia increases to 6%. Survival of treated patients for 4 years increases the risk of leukaemia to 15%.

It is thought that the long term treatment with alkylating agents may be the cause of the acute leukaemia in some myeloma patients.

Solitary plasmacytoma

Solitary extraskeletal plasmacytoma, often in the nasopharynx, carries a much better prognosis than patients with skeletal lesions.

Chemotherapy is therefore not needed for these solitary plasmacytomas but local radiation may be of value.

CAN WE MODIFY THE NATURAL HISTORY OF MYELOMA?

The aetiology of myeloma is unknown. The usual factors have been postulated (Table 14.48).

Table 14.48   Postulated aetiological factors in myeloma

• Genetic predispositions
• Oncogenic virus
• Chronic bacterial antigenic stimulation
• Inflammatory stimuli

Since the aetiology is unknown there is no possibility of primary prevention.

The combination of cytotoxic drugs with prednisolone has had a favourable influence in prolonging life.

The median survival for melphalan/prednisolone therapy is about 30 months, and about 15% of patients are alive 5 years after treatment was begun.

USEFUL PRACTICAL POINTS

- Myeloma often presents with sudden back pain due to the involvement of the vertebrae.

- A very high ESR (> 100 mm/h) is a useful, but not specific, pointer to the possibility of myelomatosis, especially in an elderly patient.

- The definitive diagnosis of myeloma requires the demonstration of plasma cell proliferation in the bone marrow, M-protein in the blood and lytic lesions in the skeleton.

- Melphalan and cyclophosphamide are the two most effective specific drugs in treating myeloma. Prednisolone is combined with both.

- The prognosis in myeloma depends on the 'mass' of tumour cells. The clinical guide to this 'mass' is the Hb, serum calcium level and serum level of M-protein.

- The best single indication of disease activity or regression in response to treatment is the rate of change of M-protein level in the serum.

15

Polyarthritis

PRESENT HISTORY

A young lady of 23 years presented with a 9 months' history of pain in her joints.

Joint pains

Over the previous 9 months she was getting recurrent attacks of pain in her joints. The attacks lasted 2–3 weeks at a time.

The joints mainly affected were the metacarpophalangeal and proximal interphalangeal joints of both hands. Other joints affected included wrists, elbows and knees.

During the attack the pains would tend to move from joint to joint and it was rarely the case that all the hand joints were affected at the same time. The joints would become painful, red and swollen during the attack but once it had settled the joints would return to normal.

The attacks were increasing in frequency and duration.

Other relevant facts on direct enquiry

General symptoms

She always felt quite ill during the attacks of joint pains. She felt hot and feverish, would lose her appetite and as a result she thought her weight would tend to go down.

Muscle pains

As well as the joint pains, she would get aching in her muscles during an attack. This would affect her shoulders and sometimes her thigh muscles. The muscle pain would settle with the joint pain.
She had not noticed any residual muscle weakness.

Joints

She denied any morning stiffness in her hands or other joints.
She had never had back pain or stiffness.

Peripheral circulation

Over the past year or so she had noticed that her finger sometimes went 'dead'. This occurred especially in cold weather when the fingers would become white and feel numb. The attack would last about 20 minutes, then the fingers would turn purple and the feeling would come back.

Cardiovascular system

She had no breathlessness or swelling of her feet.

Respiratory system

She had no current cough or sputum.

Alimentary system

She had no abdominal pain or recent alteration in her bowels.
She had lost 10 lb (4.5 kg) in the last 6 months.

Genito-urinary system

Her periods had become irregular over the past year.
She had no urinary symptoms

Nervous system

She had no headache.
   She had experienced a burning discomfort over the soles of the feet recently. She had also noticed tingling in her toes like 'pins and needles'.

Skin rashes

Although she denied any rashes or skin eruptions, she did say that her skin, especially over the face, was getting more sensitive to the sun, so that she would 'burn' much more easily than had always been the case.

Eyes

She denied any eye trouble.

PAST HISTORY

She had never had rheumatic fever or St Vitus' dance.

Two months earlier she had a bad attack of pleurisy affecting her left lung. She could not remember coughing up any sputum, but felt very breathless at the time. Her doctor gave her a course of antibiotics and the pain settled in a few days but she remained breathless for several weeks afterwards. She had no residual cough or sputum.

FAMILY HISTORY

There was no history of arthritis.
There were no other relevant illnesses.

PERSONAL HISTORY

She was not married and had never been pregnant. She was not on the contraceptive pill.
She did not smoke.
She drank very little alcohol – social occasions only.

DRUG HISTORY

Her current treatment was indomethacin 50 mg four times daily.

She would also use paracetamol tablets whenever the pains were especially severe but would get only limited relief.

EXAMINATION

The abnormal signs are shown in Figure 15.1.

General

Fever

The patient was mildly febrile with a temperature of 38.2 °C

Mental state

She was an ill-looking girl with a peculiar, almost euphoric, manner. She kept smiling even when describing the very severe pains in her joints and muscles, and seemed unaffected emotionally by her illness.

Skin

There was a slight erythematous *malar rash* which affected the nose also and was suggestive of a 'butterfly' distribution.

Erythema was also evident at the base of the finger nails (*periungual*

527

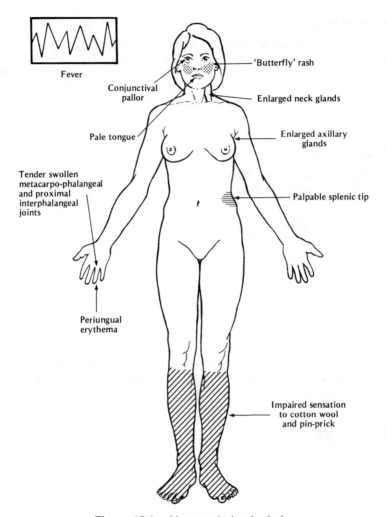

Figure 15.1 Abnormal physical signs

erythema). There were no red tender spots or ulceration in the pulps of the fingers.

There was no abnormal bruising.

There were no gouty tophi in the ears.

Anaemia

The conjunctivae, tongue and palms of the hands were pale. There was no atrophy of the tongue. There was no koilonychia.

528

Joints

There was swelling and redness over several metacarpophalangeal joints and proximal interphalangeal joints in both hands. The joints were tender on palpation and painful to move though there was no restriction of joint movement. There was no joint deformity in the hands.

Wrist flexion was uncomfortable, though not really painful, on both sides. There was no redness, tenderness or swelling of the wrists, and no deformity, especially no ulnar deviation.

All other joints, including cervical spine, seemed normal.

There were no rheumatoid nodules over the bones or tendons.

Glands

There were several firm enlarged glands in the posterior triangle on the left side of the neck: they were not tender.

Slightly enlarged non-tender glands were also present in both axillae.

The groin glands were small and shotty and thought to be normal.

Cardiovascular system

The pulse was 110/min and regular.

The radial arteries were not thickened and the brachial artery was not visible.

The blood pressure was 110/70 and equal in both arms.

The apex was in the normal position and of normal character.

There was a soft, blowing midsystolic murmur over the whole of the precordium, but not conducted to the axilla.

The heart sounds were normal.

There was no pericardial friction.

Respiratory system

There was no residual abnormality following the previous attack of pleurisy, and in particular no evidence of effusion.

No other pulmonary abnormality was found.

Abdomen

The tip of the spleen was palpable. It was not tender.

The liver and kidneys were not felt.

There was no other abnormality.

Nervous system

The fundi were normal.

The cranial nerves were normal.

The motor system (tone, power, reflexes) was normal.

In the sensory system, there was slight but definite blunting of pinprick in both legs in a 'stocking' distribution. Cotton wool sensation was also impaired in this area.

Vibration and joint position sense were intact.

ANALYSIS OF THE HISTORY

Recurrent polyarthritis

The main presenting symptom was recurrent polyarthritis. The common causes of chronic polyarthritis are shown in Table 15.1.

Table 15.1   Causes of chronic polyarthritis

• Rheumatoid arthritis
• Osteoarthrosis
• Gout
• Psoriasis
• Collagen disease   • systemic lupus erythematosus
• polyarteritis nodosa
• scleroderma
• 'mixed' disease
• Reiter's syndrome
• Systemic disease   • ulcerative colitis
• Crohn's disease
• sarcoidosis
• amyloidosis
• malignancy

The diagnostic approach which is helpful in differentiation of these various conditions is shown in Table 15.2.

Table 15.2   Diagnostic approach to polyarthritis

• Onset – rapidity and duration
• Pattern of joint involvement
• Associated systemic involvement
• Associated skin rashes
• Associated eye involvement
• Associated abdominal symptoms

Rheumatoid arthritis

This is the most frequent cause of polyarthritis encountered in clinical practice. The profile of this condition is shown in Figure 15.2.

The young age of the patient, the flitting joint pains, the absence of symmetrical joint involvement, the lack of morning stiffness, the severe con-

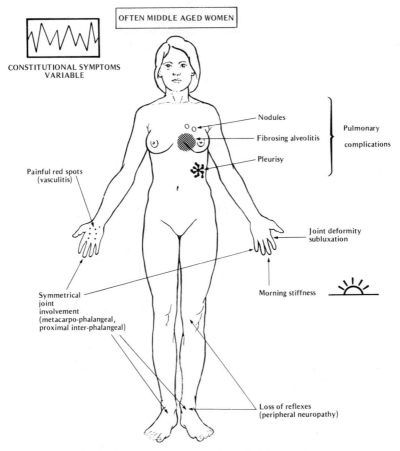

Figure 15.2 Rheumatoid arthritis profile

stitutional symptoms and the absence of any residual joint deformity all make the diagnosis of rheumatoid arthritis unlikely.

Osteoarthrosis

The clinical features are shown in Figure 15.3.

The patient's symptoms do not fit into the pattern of osteoarthrosis in any respect whatsoever.

Although the larger joints, such as the hip and knee, are most often affected by osteoarthrosis, the hands may also be involved. In this case it is always the terminal interphalangeal joints of the fingers which are affected, and Heberden's nodes are very often associated (Figure 15.4).

The spine is also frequently affected by osteoarthrosis.

531

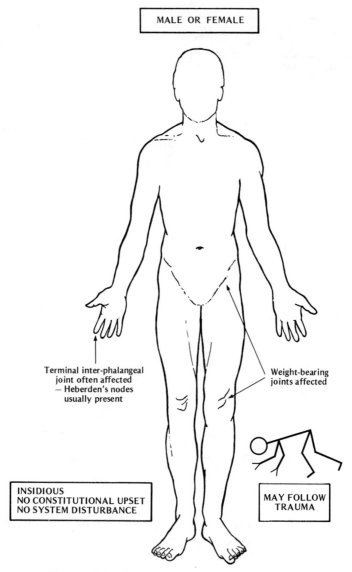

MALE OR FEMALE

Terminal inter-phalangeal
joint often affected
— Heberden's nodes
usually present

Weight-bearing
joints affected

INSIDIOUS
NO CONSTITUTIONAL UPSET
NO SYSTEM DISTURBANCE

MAY FOLLOW
TRAUMA

Figure 15.3   Clinical features of osteoarthrosis

Gout

The clinical features of gout are shown in Table 15.3. Figure 15.5 shows the typical appearance of chronic gout.

The patient's sex, age, lack of involvement of the big toe and absence of residual joint deformity all make gout very unlikely.

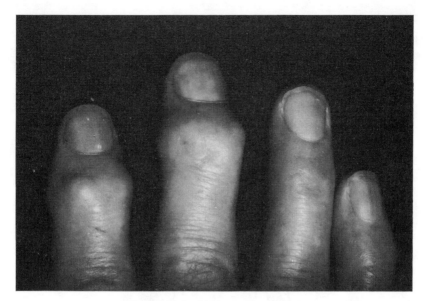

Figure 15.4 Heberden's nodes

Table 15.3 Clinical features of chronic gout

- Positive family history common
- Very rare in women
- Onset usually over 40 years of age
- Acute onset – complete remission in inbetween
- 1st metatarsophalangeal joint frequently affected
- Any joint may be involved
- Joint deformity frequent
- Tophi common – ears
  periarticular tissue

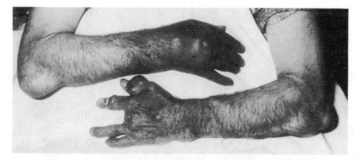

Figure 15.5 Chronic gout

533

Psoriasis

The clinical features of psoriatic arthropathy are shown in Figure 15.6. A typical case is shown in Figure 15.7.

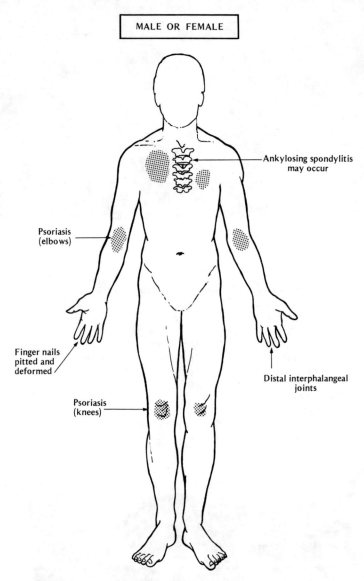

Figure 15.6   Clinical features of psoriatic arthropathy

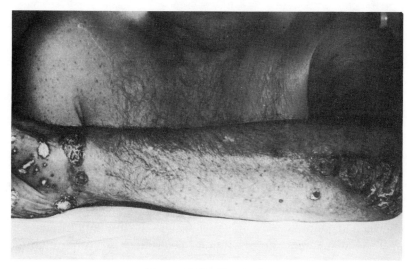

Figure 15.7 Psoriasis

The absence of psoriasis and the lack of involvement of distal phalangeal joints excludes this diagnosis.

Collagen disease

Collagen disease is a much less common cause of chronic polyarthritis than rheumatoid arthritis.

The collagen disorder in which polyarthritis features most prominently is systemic lupus erythematosus. It is a less frequent manifestation in polyarteritis nodosa and systemic sclerosis (scleroderma).

Systemic lupus erythematosus (SLE)

This condition has many manifestations (Figure 15.8).

The patient has experienced a number of symptoms which are typical of SLE. This puts SLE high on the list as the likely diagnosis.

The distinguishing features between SLE and rheumatoid arthritis are shown in Table 15.4.

Polyarteritis nodosa

The clinical features of polyarteritis nodosa are shown in Figure 15.9.

The patient's sex, the involvement of the smaller rather than the larger joints, the absence of asthma and any neurological symptoms to suggest a mononeuritis or focal cerebral arteritis, all serve to exclude this diagnosis on the basis of the history.

Scleroderma

Polyarthritis affecting the small joints is often an early manifestation of

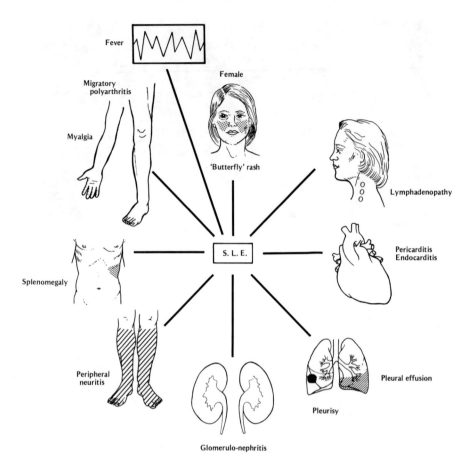

Figure 15.8 Manifestations of SLE

Table 15.4 Differentiation between SLE and rheumatoid arthritis

	SLE	*Rheumatoid arthritis*
Patient	Young woman	Middle-aged woman
Onset	Acute	Gradual
Constitutional	Severe	Variable
Joints	Small – asymmetrical	Small – symmetrical
Pain	Flitting	Constant
Deformity	Very rare	Very common
Morning stiffness	Absent	Common
Other systems	Commonly involved	Occasionally involved
X-rays	Bony disease rare	Destructive bony lesions

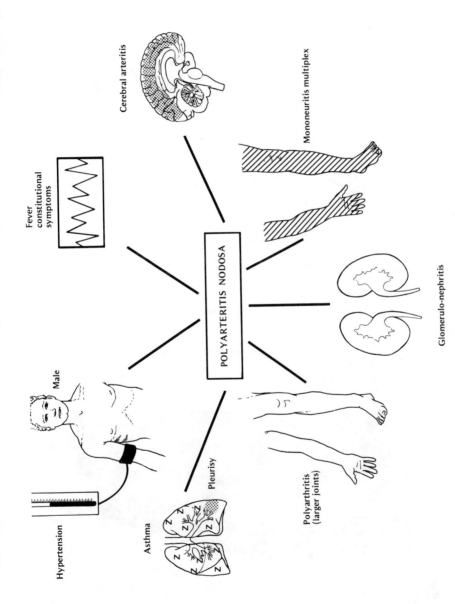

Figure 15.9 Clinical features of polyarteritis nodosa

systemic sclerosis (scleroderma). The other features of the disease are shown in Figure 15.10.

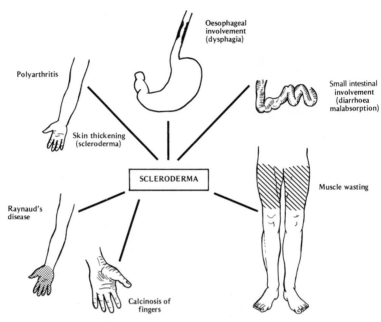

Figure 15.10 Clinical features of scleroderma

Figure 15.11 shows the typical changes of calcinosis in the fingers in a patient with scleroderma.

The absence of dysphagia, bowel disturbance and changes in the skin make this diagnosis very unlikely.

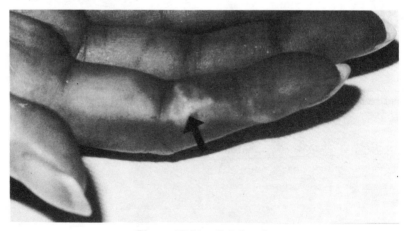

Figure 15.11 Calcinosis

538

'Mixed' disease

This is a mixed connective tissue disease syndrome in which clinical manifestations of systemic lupus erythematosus, scleroderma, and polymyositis overlap.

The diagnosis can be confirmed by serological investigations which will be discussed later.

There is nothing in the patient's history to suggest a diagnosis other than systemic lupus erythematosis.

Reiter's syndrome

Although Reiter's syndrome usually causes an acute episode of polyarthritis it can sometimes continue with recurrent attacks of polyarthritis for years.

The characteristic triad of manifestations in Reiter's syndrome is shown in Figure 15.12. It usually occurs in young males and follows 4–6 weeks after sexual exposure.

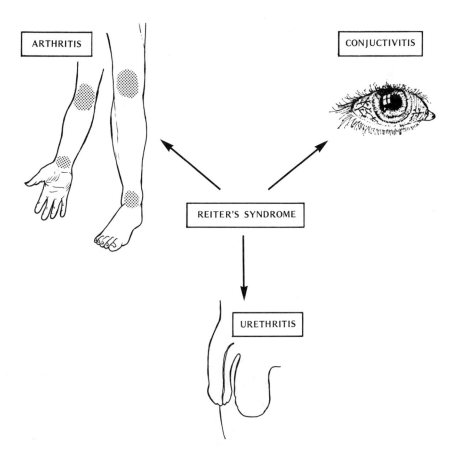

Figure 15.12 Characteristic triad of manifestations in Reiter's syndrome

Apart from polyarthritis there are no features in the patient's clinical picture to suggest Reiter's syndrome.

Systemic disease associated with polyarthritis

There was no abdominal pain or diarrhoea to suggest ulcerative colitis or Crohn's disease.

There were no symptoms to suggest the usual organ involvement of sarcoidosis (Figure 15.13).

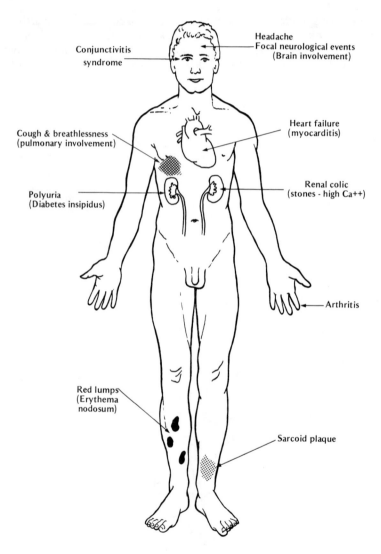

Figure 15.13   Organ involvement in sarcoidosis

Nor were there any symptoms to suggest amyloidosis (Figure 15.14).

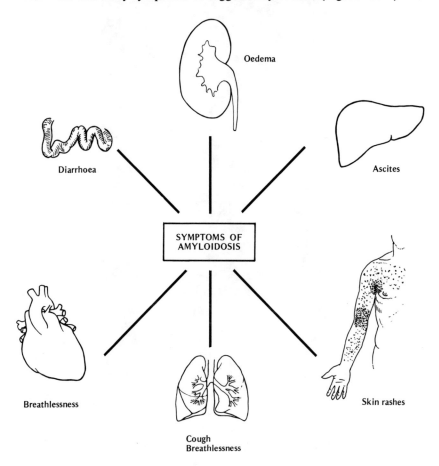

Figure 15.14   Symptoms of amyloidosis

Malignancy

The commonest type of joint involvement in malignancy is hypertrophic pulmonary osteoarthropathy associated with bronchial carcinoma. This leads to finger clubbing and may involve the wrist also (Figure 15.15).

The distal phalanges were not affected in the patient.

There is a rarer type of joint involvement with carcinoma, leading to polyarthritis which may resemble rheumatoid arthritis.

The only way of excluding occult neoplasia is by detailed investigation, since there were no symptoms to suggest carcinoma in the patient.

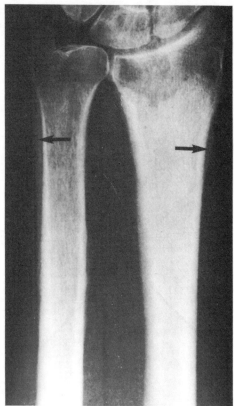

Figure 15.15   X-ray of wrist in hypertrophic pulmonary osteoarthropathy (HPO)

Table 15.5   Causes of acute polyarthritis

• Rheumatic fever	– Previous sore throat
	Migratory polyarthritis
	Erythema marginatum
	Carditis – changing murmurs
	Rheumatic nodules
• Gonococcal arthritis	– Previous urethritis
	Usually large joints
	Tenosynovitis common
	Skin rashes
	papular
	pustular
	haemorrhagic
	necrotic
• Brucellosis	– Contact with cattle
• Rubella	– Rash
• Viral hepatitis	– Jaundice

Acute polyarthritis

There are several other important causes of polyarthritis but as these conditions are more likely to produce an acute episode of polyarthritis and not a recurrent picture, they are not relevant in the patient's diagnosis (Table 15.5).

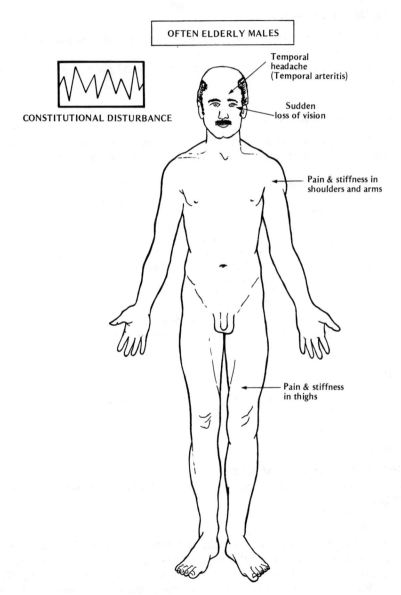

Figure 15.16 Prominent features of polymyalgia rheumatica

Myalgia

Muscle pain associated with polyarthritis is very suggestive of a collagen disorder.

It is very rare in rheumatoid arthritis, though painless muscle wasting associated with diseased joints is not uncommon.

Polymyalgia rheumatica

Muscle pain, affecting the shoulders and thighs, is a prominent feature of this condition (Figure 15.16).

The patient's sex and age, and absence of temporal arteritis excludes this condition.

Raynaud's phenomenon

The 'dead' fingers, first white then blue, in cold weather indicates Raynaud's phenomenon. The causes of this condition are shown in Table 15.6.

Table 15.6   Causes of Raynaud's phenomenon

• Primary
• Secondary   • Collagen disease
• Cervical rib
• Cold agglutinins
• Occupational – pneumatic drill
• Drugs
ergot
methysergide
non-selective β-blockers

Primary

Primary Raynaud's disease usually starts in childhood, which makes it unlikely in this patient.

Secondary

Systemic lupus erythematosus
This had already been suggested by the other symptoms so remains a very likely cause.

Cervical rib
A *cervical rib* compresses the subclavian artery causing the Raynaud's reaction, but often compresses the lowest trunk of the brachial plexus also, causing paraesthesiae along the ulnar border of the forearm (Figure 15.17). The absence of such paraesthesiae is against the diagnosis of a cervical rib but it can only be excluded with certainty by an X-ray of the thoracic inlet.

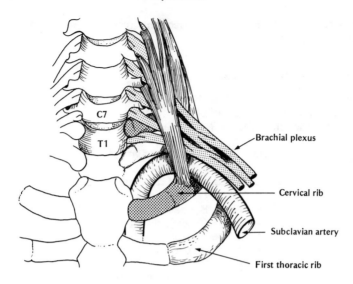

Figure 15.17   Cervical rib causing Raynaud's phenomenon

Cold agglutinins
Cold agglutinins can produce a Raynaud's reaction but the ears, nose and feet are also frequently involved and become purple in cold weather. The most distinctive feature is that there is no preliminary blanching phase to the reaction, and as the patient's fingers always went white this excludes circulatory cold agglutinins as a cause.

Pneumatic drill
This occupational cause is obviously irrelevant.

Drugs
The patient had not taken any of the drugs listed in Table 15.6.

Irregular periods

Dysfunctional uterine bleeding leading to irregular periods in a young woman is very common and has a number of causes (Table 15.7).

Table 15.7   Causes of irregular periods

• Emotional disturbances
• Uterine disease – metropathia haemorrhagica
• Hypothalamic/pituitary disturbance
• Thyroid disease – thyrotoxicosis
myxoedema
• Collagen disease

If the patient has SLE this would account for the menstrual disturbance. Often no cause is found.

Paraesthesiae in the feet

The burning in the soles of both feet and the tingling in her toes indicates a symmetrical peripheral neuritis. The causes of symmetrical peripheral neuritis are shown in Table 15.8.

Table 15.8 Causes of symmetrical polyneuritis

- Diabetes
- Vitamin B_{12} deficiency
- Acute infective polyneuritis
- Collagen disease
- Chronic alcoholism
- Acute porphyria
- Carcinomatous neuropathy

Diabetes

The absence of thirst and polyuria excludes diabetes.

Vitamin B_{12} deficiency

Vitamin B_{12} deficiency causes subacute combined degeneration of the spinal cord with peripheral neuritis. Anaemia is also frequently present, though not invariably. This is a possible diagnosis in the patient since she was anaemic, and needs to be reconsidered in the light of the investigations.

Acute infective polyneuritis

Acute infective polyneuritis (Guillain–Barré syndrome) usually causes acute involvement of all four limbs and may affect chest muscles as well as the facial nerve. Paralysis and sensory loss are produced. This is quite unlike the patient's clinical picture.

Collagen disease

A collagen disease remains a likely cause of the polyneuritis. In SLE the polyneuritis is symmetrical, as in the patient, while polyarteritis nodosa produces a mononeuritis multiplex.

Alcoholism

The patient was not an alcoholic.

Acute porphyria

The features of acute intermittent porphyria are shown in Table 15.9. Some abdominal colic is invariable in acute porphyria; its absence in the patient excludes the diagnosis.

Table 15.9 Features of acute intermittent porphyria

- Polyneuritis
- Acute abdominal colic
- Mental disturbance

Malignancy

Carcinoma is an unlikely diagnosis in a young patient and there were no focal symptoms to suggest a possible site. Occult neoplasia, however, obviously remains a possibility and may not be excluded with certainty even after intensive investigation.

Skin rash

Although the patient denied a skin rash, the recent photosensitivity to sunlight is very relevant since this is a common feature in SLE.

Past history

The past history of pleurisy is likely to be very relevant. The causes that need to be considered in the patient are shown in Table 15.10.

Table 15.10 Possible causes of pleurisy in the patient

- Pulmonary infection
- Pulmonary infarction
- Rheumatoid arthritis
- Systemic lupus erythematosus

The absence of green or yellow sputum with the pleurisy makes an infective cause unlikely.

The absence of haemoptysis and any history of conditions predisposing to venous thrombosis (Table 15.11) is against a diagnosis of pulmonary infarction.

Pleurisy may occur in rheumatoid arthritis but is uncommon, especially in women.

Pleurisy is, however, a *common symptom of SLE* and this condition is once again the likely cause.

Table 15.11 Conditions predisposing to venous thrombosis

- Prolonged immobilization
- Pelvic operation
- Childbirth
- Contraceptive pill
- Heart failure
- Trauma to legs

The persistence of the breathlessness for several weeks after the pleuritic pain has subsided, and the absence of associated cough and sputum, is strongly suggestive of a residual *pleural effusion* which is also a common occurrence in SLE, and less common in rheumatoid arthritis.

Drug history

The importance of an accurate drug history is that a syndrome like SLE can result from the use of several drugs (Table 15.12). The common drugs encountered in practice are hydrallazine and procainamide.

Table 15.12 Drugs causing syndrome like SLE

- Hydrallazine   (hypertension)
- Procainamide   (cardiac arrhythmias)
- Phenytoin   (epilepsy)
- Isoniazid   (tuberculosis)
- Methyldopa   (hypertension)
- L-dopa   (Parkinson's disease)
- Phenothiazines   (tranquillizer)

Renal disease and involvement of the central nervous system are very uncommon in the drug-induced syndrome. Fortunately, the syndrome is reversible on stopping the drug.

The patient had not been taking any of these drugs.

CONCLUSIONS FROM THE HISTORY

The distinctive symptoms in this patient's history are:

- migratory polyarthralgia affecting the small joints

- severe constitutional upset in the attacks

- recent pleuritic pain (followed by dyspnoea probably due to effusion)

- attacks of cold white fingers indicating Raynaud's disease.

In a young woman this combination of symptoms is strongly suggestive of systemic lupus erythematosus.

ANALYSIS OF THE EXAMINATION

Euphoria

Table 15.13 shows some of the causes of euphoria encountered in clinical practice.

Table 15.13   Causes of euphoria

- Manic–depressive psychosis
- Cerebrovascular disease – after a stroke
- Multiple sclerosis
- Steroid treatment
- SLE
- Alcoholism
- Drug addiction

The only likely cause of the patient's euphoria is SLE which produces mental disturbances of various kinds in 15% of the patients.

Facial rash

The typical rash in SLE is a scaly, erythematous rash in a butterfly distribution on the face. The patient's rash is very suggestive of this type of rash, especially when combined with the photosensitivity to sunlight.

The features of chronic cutaneous or discoid lupus erythematosus are shown in Table 15.14.

Table 15.14   Features of discoid lupus

- Focal lesion on head or neck
- Skin atrophy
- Scarring
- Telangiectasis
- Vitiligo
- Hyperpigmentation
- Systemic disease uncommon

Other causes of a malar flush which might be confused with a butterfly rash are shown in Table 15.15.

Table 15.15   Causes of a malar flush

- Mitral stenosis
- Myxoedema ('strawberries and cream')
- Acne rosacea
- Vitamin B_{12} treatment of pernicious anaemia

Anaemia

The pale conjunctivae, pale tongue and pale palms indicated that the patient was anaemic.

Anaemia is a common complication in both rheumatoid arthritis and SLE. There are several kinds of anaemia in rheumatoid arthritis (Table 15.16).

Table 15.16   Types of anaemia in rheumatoid arthritis

• Normocytic normochromic	– Failure of iron release from stores
	Marrow hypoplasia
	Haemodilution
• Hypochromic microcytic	– Blood loss from drugs used
• Haemolytic	– Hypersplenism
• Macrocytic	– Low serum folate

The anaemia in SLE is usually normocytic and normochromic, unless gastrointestinal blood loss from anti-inflammatory drugs causes iron-deficiency anaemia.

The absence of koilonychia makes a chronic hypochromic anaemia unlikely.

Periungual erythema

The erythema at the base of the finger nails is strongly suggestive of the vasculitis which is a common feature of SLE.

Other manifestations of this vasculitis sometimes occur in SLE, such as ulcers in the finger pulps or generalized palmar erythema.

Joint changes

The pattern of joint involvement affecting the metacarpophalangeal and proximal phalangeal joints in the hands, and the wrists, is typical of both rheumatoid arthritis and SLE.

The absence of any persistent spindle-shaped swelling of the joints or other joint deformity is very much against the diagnosis of rheumatoid arthritis. In SLE, however, involvement of bone or articular cartilage is rare so permanent joint changes are very unlikely.

Lymphadenopathy

Lymph node enlargement occurs in almost half the patients with SLE. The glands are not tender in this condition, and this was the case in the patient.

Lymphadenopathy does not occur in rheumatoid arthritis.

Cardiovascular system

Tachycardia

The tachycardia may be due to disease activity or carditis. The absence of cardiac enlargement is against the diagnosis of active carditis.

Systolic murmur

Endocarditis can occur in SLE and affect both the mitral valve and, less commonly, the aortic valve (*Libman–Sachs endocarditis*). Both systolic and diastolic murmurs can result, and may vary with disease activity.

The patient's systolic murmur may be either organic due to endocarditis or functional due to a combination of fever, tachycardia and anaemia.

Further investigation with chest X-ray and electrocardiogram is necessary to decide whether the murmur is organic or functional.

Splenomegaly

Possible causes of mild splenic enlargement are shown in Table 15.17.

Table 15.17   Causes of mild splenic enlargement

• Portal hypertension
• Leukaemia
• Reticulosis
• SLE
• Amyloidosis
• Sarcoidosis
• Infections   • glandular fever
• infective endocarditis

The patient was not an alcoholic and there are no other signs of portal hypertension (Figure 15.18).

There are no features of bone marrow involvement to suggest leukaemia, such as undue susceptibility to infection or spontaneous haemorrhage.

As the patient has lymph node enlargement as well as an enlarged spleen, reticulosis remains a possible diagnosis and needs exclusion by further investigation.

Systemic lupus erythematosus is obviously a likely diagnosis.

Amyloidosis and sarcoidosis have been discussed and excluded on the basis of lack of manifestations of involvement of organs typically affected in these conditions (Figures 15.14, pp. 540–1).

The absence of a sore throat and rash makes glandular fever unlikely.

There were no past history, or present clinical findings, of organic heart disease, no recent dental treatment and no distinctive finger signs of infective endocarditis (Figure 15.19).

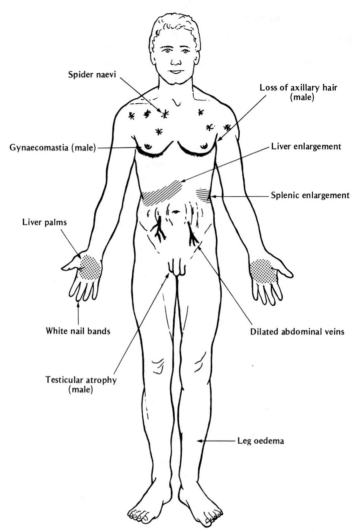

Spider naevi

Loss of axillary hair
(male)

Gynaecomastia (male)

Liver enlargement

Splenic enlargement

Liver palms

White nail bands

Dilated abdominal veins

Testicular atrophy
(male)

Leg oedema

Figure 15.18 Signs of portal hypertension

Peripheral neuritis

The 'stocking' distribution of impaired pinprick and cotton wool sensation indicates a sensory type of peripheral neuritis. The causes have already been discussed (Table 15.8).

The conclusion is that SLE is the most likely cause of the patient's peripheral neuritis.

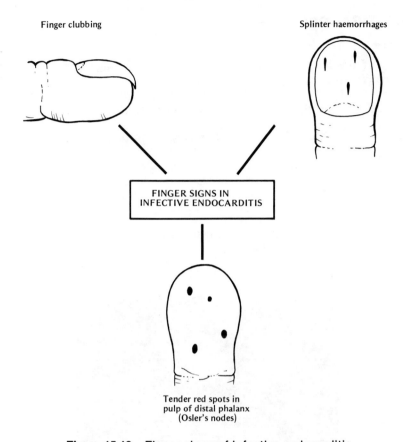

Finger clubbing

Splinter haemorrhages

FINGER SIGNS IN
INFECTIVE ENDOCARDITIS

Tender red spots in
pulp of distal phalanx
(Osler's nodes)

Figure 15.19   Finger signs of infective endocarditis

CLINICAL CONCLUSIONS

There is little doubt that the patient's symptoms and signs point clearly to a diagnosis of systemic lupus erythematosus.

CONCLUSIONS FROM THE EXAMINATION

The distinctive signs are:

- butterfly rash
- periungual erythema
- lymphadenopathy
- splenic enlargement
- peripheral neuritis.

These signs confirm the diagnosis of systemic lupus erythematosus.

INVESTIGATIONS

X-rays

X-rays of the hands are the simplest means of distinguishing SLE from rheumatoid arthritis.

The radiological changes in rheumatoid arthritis are detailed in Table 15.18. A typical X-ray in rheumatoid arthritis is shown in Figure 15.20.

Table 15.18   X-ray changes in the hands in rheumatoid arthritis

> - Juxta-articular osteoporosis
> - Loss of cartilage – narrow joint space
> - Marginal and cystic erosions
>   metacarpal heads
>   proximal phalangeal heads
>   carpal bones
>   head of radius and ulna
> - Dislocations and joint deformity

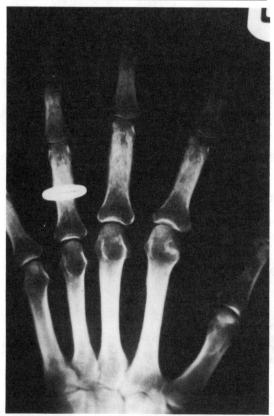

Figure 15.20   X-ray of rheumatoid arthritis

In the great majority of patients with SLE there are no specific radiological changes. A small minority will develop erosive changes resembling rheumatoid arthritis.

The X-rays of the patient's hands showed no bone or joint abnormality.

Radiology of affected joints may also show some distinctive features in other conditions discussed in the differential diagnosis (Table 15.19).

Table 15.19   Distinctive X-ray changes in various arthropathies

Osteo-arthrosis	• Often hip or knee • Osteophytes at joint margins • Subarticular sclerosis • Subluxation of terminal finger joint
Gout	• 1st metatarsophalangeal joint often • Subarticular cysts in bones • 'Punched-out' erosions at joint margin
Psoriatic arthropathy	• Terminal phalanges of fingers/toes • Metacarpal heads may disappear • Spine often affected • Sacro-iliac joints often affected
Reiter's syndrome	• Local periostitis • Sacro-iliitis

Pulmonary osteoarthropathy	• Periostitis
	  metacarpals
	  phalanges
	  radius and ulna

Serological tests

There are several serological tests which help in the diagnosis of SLE (Table 15.20).

Table 15.20   Serological tests in SLE

• Antinuclear antibodies • Antibodies to DNA • LE cell test • Anti-RNP – mixed connective tissue disease

Antinuclear antibodies

The presence of antinuclear antibodies is the most useful screening test for SLE, since they are almost invariably present. It will also help to detect patients on relevant drugs who are in danger of developing a drug-induced syndrome.

Antibodies to DNA

Antibodies to DNA are more specific in the diagnosis of SLE though they may occur occasionally in other conditions (Table 15.21).

Table 15.21 Conditions involving antibodies to DNA

- SLE
- Rheumatoid arthritis
- Polyarteritis nodosa
- Chronic active hepatitis
- Infective endocarditis
- Sarcoidosis

LE cells

The LE cell test is a variation of the antinuclear antibody test and is positive in the great majority of patients with SLE. The test is based on the changes which occur on incubating normal leukocytes with a patient's serum. The test may rarely be positive in rheumatoid arthritis.

When mixed connective tissue disease is present – overlapping features of SLE, scleroderma and dermatomyositis – an antibody to ribonucleoprotein (RNP) may be present.

Rheumatoid factor

The *rheumatoid factor* test is based on an antibody to an immunoglobulin. Table 15.22 shows the conditions in which rheumatoid factor may be present.

Table 15.22 Conditions with rheumatoid factor present

- Rheumatoid arthritis
- Polyarteritis nodosa
- Infective endocarditis
- Sarcoidosis

Arthropathies in which it is very unusual to find rheumatoid factor are shown in Table 15.23.

Table 15.23 Arthropathies where rheumatoid factor is usually absent

- SLE
- Psoriasis
- Ankylosing spondylitis
- Ulcerative colitis and Crohn's disease

The patient's serology is shown in Table 15.24. The results clearly confirm the diagnosis of SLE.

Table 15.24   Patient's serology

Anti-nuclear antibody titre	2000
Anti-DNA titre	> 1280
LE cells	present
Rheumatoid factor	negative

Blood count

This simple test may be useful in the diagnosis of SLE, but is non-specific. The possible changes in SLE are shown in Table 15.25.

Table 15.25   Blood count in SLE

• Anaemia	–	normocytic normochromic haemolytic (auto-immune)
• Leukopenia	–	lymphopenia
• Thrombocytopenia	–	auto-immune

The lymphopenia in SLE, due to circulating antilymphocytic antibodies, distinguishes SLE from polyarteritis nodosa where the leukopenia affects primarily the neutrophils.

The patient's blood count is shown in Table 15.26; it shows changes typical of SLE.

Table 15.26   Patient's blood count

	Results	*Normal range*
Hb	10.3 g/dl	(12–16)
WBC	$3.1 \times 10^9/l$	(4–11)
	neutrophils 80%	(40–75%)
	lymphocytes 12%	(20–50%)
	eosinophils 8%	(1–6%)
Platelets	$120 \times 10^9/1$	(150–400)

ESR and C-reactive protein

These are non-specific tests which are of no diagnostic value in SLE but give a useful guide to its activity and response to treatment.

Urine

The kidney is involved histologically in virtually all patients with SLE, though clinical evidence of disease occurs in only about half (Table 15.27). Clinical renal disease makes the prognosis worse.

Histological changes in the kidney vary from mild to severe (Table 15.28).

Table 15.27 Clinical evidence of renal disease in SLE

- Haematuria
- Proteinuria
- Casts in urine
- Raised serum creatinine or urea

Table 15.28 Histological types of renal disease in SLE

- Mesangial proliferation
- Membranous nephritis
- Focal proliferative glomerulonephritis
- Diffuse proliferative glomerulonephritis
- Glomerular sclerosis
- Necrotizing vasculitis

In view of the frequency of renal involvement in SLE, the urine should be examined in all patients. If urinary abnormality is present, the serum creatinine and blood urea should be checked, and renal biopsy is necessary to help with both treatment and prognosis. The patient's urine showed no significant abnormality.

Chest X-ray

The chest X-ray is of no diagnostic value. It may be helpful if there is any clinical evidence of pulmonary involvement, as in the patient who had pleurisy and effusion.

The patient's chest X-ray showed no residual pleural or pulmonary abnormality.

Electrocardiogram

Like the chest X-ray, this is of no diagnostic value in SLE. It may help to confirm carditis if this is suspected on clinical grounds.

The patient's e.c.g. was normal, thus excluding organic heart disease as a cause of her systolic murmur.

MANAGEMENT OF SYSTEMIC LUPUS ERYTHEMATOSUS

The current views of management of this condition are based on:

- mild disease – symptomatic measures only

- severe disease means systemic involvement
  active treatment required

- guide to progress
  regular clinical assessment
  regular serology.

General measures

Patient education

Since SLE is a chronic relapsing disease, primarily affecting young women, the psychological and social impact may be considerable.

A simple but full explanation of the disease and its treatment to the patient and her family is helpful. Optimistic reassurance is justifiable.

Although the disease is a chronic one, most of the manifestations can be controlled satisfactorily with treatment.

It is also advisable to reassure the patient that any alteration of physical appearance with steroid therapy will improve when the dose is reduced and, hopefully, eventually stopped.

Sun-screening

Since photosensitivity to the sun is a common symptom, the patient should be advised to avoid the sun if acceptable or, if not, to use barrier creams.

Allergy desensitization

Since desensitization for particular allergies, like hay fever, may lead to an exacerbation of the disease, it should be avoided.

Oestrogens

Oestrogen therapy, whether as a contraceptive or for menopausal symptoms, can exacerbate the disease. It should therefore be discouraged.

Infections

Infections also can lead to a flare-up of the disease and should therefore be treated promptly and effectively.

A caution, however, is necessary with the treatment used. Penicillin and sulphonamides may themselves exacerbate the disease, so other antibiotics are preferable.

Rest

Rest is not required unless the disease is very active. The patient should be encouraged to follow normal daily activities as far as possible.

Physiotherapy

This may be of value when muscle weakness occurs following myositis.

Specific treatment of systemic lupus erythematosus

The treatment will depend on disease activity. This can be decided by the clinical features and by laboratory tests, especially blood count and serology.

Clinical indications of severity

The relationship of the clinical features to the severity of the disease is shown in Table 15.29.

Table 15.29   Clinical indications of severity of SLE

• Mild disease	• Fever	
	• Polyarthritis	
	• Polyarthralgia	
	• Myalgia	
• Severe disease	• Heart involvement	– endocarditis
		myocarditis
		pericarditis
	• Lung involvement	– pleurisy
		pneumonia
		pleural effusion
	• Kidney involvement	– clinical evidence
	• CNS involvement	convulsions
		alteration of consciousness
		focal vascular disease
	• Blood involvement	– haemolytic anaemia
		thrombocytopenic purpura
	• Abdominal pain	– vasculitis

Laboratory indications of activity

The tests which are of value in assessing activity of the SLE are shown in Table 15.30.

Table 15.30   Tests of activity of SLE

- Sequential haemoglobin
- ESR
- Lymphocytic count
- Urine examination for protein, red cells and casts
- Serum creatinine and urea
- Anti-DNA antibodies
- Complement

The two most useful tests are the level of complement (C3 and C4) and the titre of anti-DNA antibodies. A falling complement level and an increasing titre of antibodies to DNA indicates a severe exacerbation of the SLE.

The aim of treatment is to normalize C3 and C4 levels in the blood and remove anti-DNA antibodies from the blood.

Mild disease

The drugs of value in mild disease are shown in Table 15.31. They are probably of *symptomatic* value only.

Table 15.31   Drugs used in mild SLE

• Salicylates
• Non-steroidal anti-inflammatory drugs
• Hydroxychloroquine

Salicylates

The drug of choice is aspirin. The dose is up to 0.9 g three times daily.

A common side-effect is gastrointestinal irritation, sometimes with bleeding.

Occasionally aspirin may cause a mild and reversible hepatotoxicity in SLE.

Non-steroidal anti-inflammatory drugs

The drugs in common use are shown in Table 15.32. They share common side-effects (Table 15.33).

Table 15.32   Non-steroidal anti-inflammatory drugs for SLE

Drug	Dose
Phenylbutazone (Butazolidine)	200 mg t.d.s.
Indomethacin (Indocid)	25–50 mg t.d.s.
Naproxen (Naprosyn)	250–500 mg b.d.
Fenbufen (Lederfen)	600 mg once daily
Fenoprofen (Fenopron)	300–600 mg t.d.s.
Ibuprofen (Brufen)	200–400 mg t.d.s.
Ketoprofen (Orudis)	100–200 mg t.d.s.
Diclofenac (Voltarol)	25–50 mg t.d.s.

Table 15.33 Side-effects of non-steroidal anti-inflammatory drugs

- Gastrointestinal discomfort
- Gastrointestinal bleeding
- Fluid retention – oedema
                        hypertension
- Hypersensitivity – angioneurotic oedema
                        asthma
                        rashes
- Headache
- Vertigo and tinnitus
- Blood dyscrasia – rare

As well as controlling the joint symptoms, these drugs may be of value in controlling the pain of pericarditis and pleurisy in the more severe forms of the disease.

Hydroxychloroquine (Plaquenil)

This antimalarial drug is of particular value in the milder form of the disease to control skin and joint involvement. The optimal dose is 6 mg/kg per day.

The most important toxic effect is retinal damage which usually occurs with high doses of the drug and may be irreversible. If the patient is on long term hydroxychloroquine, an ophthalmic check-up is advisable every 6 or 12 months.

Severe disease

The specific treatment used for severe SLE is shown in Table 15.34.

Table 15.34 Specific treatment for severe SLE

- Steroids
- Immunosuppressive drugs
- Plasmapheresis

Steroids

These are the mainstay of treatment in aggressive multi-system involvement. Most patients will require steroids at some stage of their disease. The dose will depend on the system involved but should be kept as low as possible compatible with control of disease activity (Table 15.35).

Table 15.35 Dose of prednisolone in SLE based on system involvement

System	Dose per day
Cardiac involvement	0.5 mg/kg
Renal	
focal glomerulonephritis	0.5–1.0 mg/kg
diffuse glomerulonephritis	1–3 mg/kg
membranous nephritis	1–3 mg/kg
CNS involvement	2–3 mg/kg

As soon as a satisfactory response occurs, the dose of prednisolone should be progressively reduced by 5 mg every 3–4 days to the lowest level compatible with absence of clinical and laboratory activity of the disease. The dose is continued to maintain disease suppression. Any relapses are treated by increasing the dose.

The side-effects of long term steroid therapy should always be kept in mind (Table 15.36).

Table 15.36 Side-effects of long term steroids

- Cushingoid appearance
- Fluid retention – moon face
  -         oedema
  -         hypertension
- Peptic ulcer
- Diabetes
- Spontaneous bruising
- Osteoporosis – pathological fractures
- Psychosis
- Susceptibility to infection

Immunosuppressive drugs

When full-dose steroid therapy fails to control disease activity, *cyclophosphamide* or *azathioprine* can be added. This is often necessary in the more severe forms of renal involvement or when extensive vasculitis is present. The dose and side-effects of the drugs are shown in Table 15.37.

Table 15.37 Dose and side effects of immunosuppressive drugs

Azathioprine	–	1–2 mg/kg per day
Cyclophosphamide	–	100–150 mg/day
Side-effects	–	marrow suppression
		haemorrhagic cystitis
		alopecia
		sterility

Cyclophosphamide combined with prednisolone is more effective than azathioprine with prednisolone.

Skin rashes

Both the acute erythematous rash and the more chronic discoid lesion respond well to local application of steroid cream or hydroxychloroquine.

Plasmapharesis

This may be of value as an adjunct to steroids during the acute phase of the disease. The aim is to remove circulating immune complexes which may exacerbate the inflammatory process.

Sometimes a severe rebound effect may occur; this is best suppressed with cyclophosphamide.

Pregnancy

SLE is not an absolute bar to pregnancy provided the disease is not in an active phase.

Exacerbations tend to occur in the last trimester of pregnancy and in the immediate postpartum period. There is also an increased tendency to deep vein thrombosis and spontaneous abortion.

If there is a relapse of the SLE during pregnancy, high-dose steroids should be used. In addition, it is advisable to use intravenous hydrocortisone routinely during labour to avoid activation of the disease which sometimes occurs when the uterus is emptied.

NATURAL HISTORY OF SYSTEMIC LUPUS ERYTHEMATOSUS

Prevalence

The prevalence of SLE is 50 patients per 100 000 of the population.

Incidence

The annual incidence of new cases is at a rate of 5–7 patients per 100 000 of the population per year.

SLE is predominantly a disease of young women of child-bearing age. The female:male ratio is 9:1. The maximum incidence is in the third and fourth decades. It may, however, occur at any age.

Race

It is twice as frequent in black women as in white women.

Prognosis

Before the advent of steroids, the prognosis was bad. There has been a steady improvement in survival over the last 25 years (Figure 15.21).

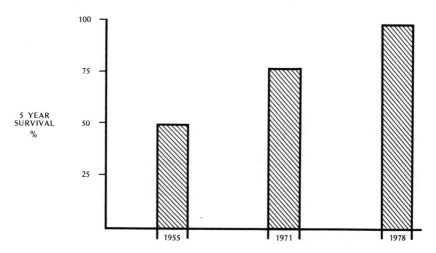

Figure 15.21   5 year survival of SLE

The causes of death are shown in Table 15.38.

The most adverse prognostic features are shown in Table 15.39. The most serious complication is involvement of the central nervous system, which may be particularly intractable to treatment.

Table 15.38   Causes of death in SLE

- Uraemia
- Heart failure
- Haemorrhage
- CNS disease
- Intercurrent infection

Table 15.39   Adverse prognostic features in SLE

- CNS involvement
- Renal disease
- Pulmonary involvement

CAN WE MODIFY THE NATURAL HISTORY?

The aetiology of SLE is unknown. Primary prevention is therefore not possible.

The aetiological factors which have been suggested are shown in Table 15.40. The current view is that the disease is due to an amalgam of these factors – an altered immune response to chronic viral infection in a genetically predisposed individual.

Table 15.40   Possible aetiological factors in SLE

- Basic defect in immune regulation
- Viral infection
- Genetic predisposition
- Endocrine factors

Since the nature of any presumed viral infection is completely unknown, no prophylactic measures can be taken.

However, once the disease has become established there is no doubt that the natural history can be modified by steroid treatment, especially in relation to renal involvement which was a major cause of death prior to the introduction of this treatment.

USEFUL PRACTICAL POINTS

- Flitting polyarthralgia affecting the hands and other small joints in a young woman should suggest the possibility of SLE.

- The recurrent polyarthritis of SLE, unlike rheumatoid arthritis, leaves very little residual joint swelling or joint deformity.

- Renal involvement is very common in SLE but rare in rheumatoid arthritis.

- A scaly erythematous rash in a butterfly distribution in the face is diagnostic of SLE.

- The milder manifestations of SLE (fever, arthralgia, arthritis, myalgia) can be treated by aspirin and other non-steroidal anti-inflammatory drugs. Multisystem involvement requires steroids ± immunosuppressive drugs.

- With modern treatment the prognosis in SLE is good unless there is diffuse renal involvement, and even more advise if the CNS is affected.

Index